"*Process-Based CBT* represents an important adva... behavioral therapy (CBT). It admirably describes how to target relevant and largely transdiagnostic processes to promote healthy growth and development. Treatment manuals, developed for research trials for specific DSM disorders, are often quite limiting, in a way that can impede their effectiveness, especially when there are comorbidities. Learning about the core processes presented in this book will enrich students, practitioners, educators, and researchers."

> —**Judith S. Beck, PhD**, president of the Beck Institute for Cognitive Behavior Therapy, and clinical professor of psychology in psychiatry at the University of Pennsylvania

"Governments and healthcare policy makers, and tens of thousands of psychotherapists around the world, strongly endorse CBT because it works, but it doesn't always work, and even when it does, it is often not as effective as we would all like. In this remarkable book, two of the leading theorists and clinical scientists in the world, Steven Hayes and Stefan Hofmann, make a strong case that going forward CBT must focus on fundamental transdiagnostic psychopathological processes and core behavioral interventions in what they call the process model of CBT. This is clearly the future of our science and profession."

> —**David H. Barlow PhD, ABPP**, professor of psychology and psychiatry emeritus, and founder and director emeritus of the Center for Anxiety and Related Disorders at Boston University

"As an educator, researcher, and clinician, I found *Process-Based CBT* to be a much-needed and stimulating resource. Science has helped us determine what treatments work. We now need to enhance our understanding of the complexities in precisely *how* those treatments work, and *why*. This book, edited by leaders in clinical psychology—Steven Hayes and Stefan Hofmann—brings a new vision for CBT. It superbly ties together undergirding processes through our in-session work and procedures, with an impetus for new diagnostic, formulation, assessment, design, and analytic methodologies. In the short term, these important ideas will inform our training curricula and research studies. In the longer term, these ideas will influence a generation of practitioners. I strongly recommend this book to all those learning, practicing, or researching CBT."

> —**Nikolaos Kazantzis, PhD**, program director for clinical psychology, and director of the Cognitive Behaviour Therapy Research Unit at Monash University in Melbourne, Australia

"This is a cutting-edge book that eloquently makes the case for increasing our focus on core therapeutic processes. It is impressive in its breadth and depth of topics, yet it remains sensitive to historical and philosophical implications. Combined with the expertise from leading international experts, *Process-Based CBT* promises to influence the development of psychotherapy practice and training for years to come."

—**Andrew Gloster**, chair of the division of clinical psychology and intervention science at the University of Basel, Switzerland

"Imagine a roomful of experts in all the essential skills of CBT standing at the ready to help you take the best possible care of your clients. Buy this book and that's what you'll get. An outstanding toolbox for the cognitive behavior therapist who is striving to integrate standard CBT with mindfulness- and acceptance-based approaches."

—**Jacqueline B. Persons, PhD**, Cognitive Behavior Therapy and Science Center, Oakland, CA; University of California, Berkeley

"Paving the way to the future of psychotherapy! This book goes beyond current CBT readers, puts these approaches into a broader, even philosophical context, and hereby opens new perspectives for improving current treatment approaches. It integrates different strands of psychotherapy (traditional CBT, ACT, and MBCT). This book is not only a must-have for anyone who wants to improve treatment skills by improving and personalizing the selection of specific interventions for specific patient problems, but also for psychotherapy researchers who really want to bring the field forward to a new level of developing and systemizing psychological interventions."

—**Winfried Rief, PhD**, board member of the European Association of Clinical Psychology and Psychological Therapy (EACLIPT)

"This is a remarkable and timely book. As the first, to my knowledge, to address in one place the training standards and clinical competencies outlined by the *Inter-Organizational Task Force on Cognitive and Behavioral Psychology Doctoral Education*, it is likely to become a core text in doctoral-level CBT training programs. Moreover, its explication of the epistemologies, theories, basic principles, and core processes that comprise CBT as a field will facilitate the evolution of CBT and the empirically based treatment movement from simply matching interventions and syndromes to one that selects and customizes clinical interventions based on empirically supported theory and contextual analysis."

—**Michael J. Dougher, PhD**, University of New Mexico

"The most challenging task for today's practicing psychotherapists, as well as psychotherapy researchers, is to personalize the process of evidence-based psychotherapy using the available selection of treatment strategies and assessment tools. I cannot imagine a better resource for this task than this outstanding book by the two leading experts: Steven Hayes and Stefan Hofmann. This rich collection of topics integrates the behavioral, cognitive, emotional, motivational, and interpersonal as well as acceptance and mindfulness traditions within psychological treatments. It is a major step forward and provides a new standard for the future of evidence-based psychotherapy. Anyone interested in psychological treatments will find it comprehensive as well as fun to read. It provides an exceptional resource for practicing clinicians as well as clinical training."

—**Wolfgang Lutz, PhD**, department of psychology at the University of Trier, Germany

"Clients are at risk for receiving less-than-optimal services when clinicians fail to follow a science-based approach to clinical intervention. This book by Hayes and Hofmann is the first to present a comprehensive overview of evidence-based core principles, practices, and processes that integrate intervention competencies and strategies across multiple treatment models and multiple syndromes."

—**Stephen N. Haynes**, emeritus professor of psychology at the University of Hawai'i at Mānoa, and editor of the American Psychological Association journal *Psychological Assessment*

"Too many books on this topic have emphasized either the 'C' *or* the 'B' in CBT, the differences between acceptance-based *versus* change-based interventions, or the distinction between branded CBT manuals compared to common, non-specific elements across psychotherapy. Hayes, Hofmann, and colleagues have taken an entirely different approach. They move the field forward by eschewing false dichotomies and unnecessarily simplistic caricatures of CBT, and by embracing the many empirically supported processes of change underlying cognitive and behavioral therapies. What emerges is clear and practical for clinicians: yesterday's CBT has been replaced by today's growing and diverse family of *contemporary* CBTs."

—**M. Zachary Rosenthal, PhD**, associate professor, vice chair, and clinical director at the Cognitive-Behavioral Research and Treatment Program; director of the Clinical Psychology Fellowship Program; and director of the Misophonia and Emotion Regulation Program in the department of psychiatry and behavioral sciences, and the department of psychology and neuroscience at Duke University

# PROCESS-BASED CBT

The Science *and* Core Clinical
Competencies *of* Cognitive
Behavioral Therapy

*Edited by*
STEVEN C. HAYES, PhD
STEFAN G. HOFMANN, PhD

CONTEXT PRESS
An Imprint of New Harbinger Publications, Inc.

## Publisher's Note

*This publication is designed to provide accurate and authoritative information in regard to the subject matter covered. It is sold with the understanding that the publisher is not engaged in rendering psychological, financial, legal, or other professional services. If expert assistance or counseling is needed, the services of a competent professional should be sought.*

Distributed in Canada by Raincoast Books

Copyright © 2018 by Steven C. Hayes and Stefan G. Hofmann
     Context Press
     An imprint of New Harbinger Publications, Inc.
     5674 Shattuck Avenue
     Oakland, CA 94609
     www.newharbinger.com

Figure 1 in chapter 11 is reprinted from Cahill, K., Hartmann-Boyce, J., & Perera, R. (2015). Incentives for smoking cessation. *Cochrane Database of Systematic Reviews, 5*(CD004307). Copyright © 2015 Wiley. Used by permission of Wiley.

Cover design by Amy Shoup

Acquired by Catharine Meyers

Edited by James Lainsbury

Indexed by James Minkin

All Rights Reserved

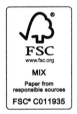
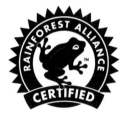

FSC
www.fsc.org
MIX
Paper from responsible sources
FSC® C011935

Library of Congress Cataloging-in-Publication Data on file

20  19  18

10  9  8  7  6  5  4  3  2  1    First Printing

# Contents

## Part 3

# Introduction

Steven C. Hayes, PhD

*Department of Psychology, University of Nevada, Reno*

Stefan G. Hofmann, PhD

*Department of Psychological and Brain Sciences, Boston University*

The goal of this book is to present the core processes of cognitive behavioral therapy (CBT) in a way that honors the behavioral, cognitive, and acceptance and mindfulness wings of this family of approaches. The book is unique not just in its breadth, but in its attempt to lay the foundation for real understanding and common purpose among these wings and traditions.

So far as we are aware, this textbook is the first to be broadly based on the new training standards for teaching the clinical competencies developed by the Inter-Organizational Task Force on Cognitive and Behavioral Psychology Doctoral Education (Klepac et al., 2012). What we will refer to here as the "training task force," organized under the auspices of the Association for Behavioral and Cognitive Therapies (ABCT), brought together representatives from fourteen organizations for four days of face-to-face meetings and several phone conferences spread out over ten months in 2011 and 2012. The organizations ranged across the wings and generations of thought in cognitive and behavioral practice, from the Academy of Cognitive Therapy to the Association for Contextual Behavioral Science, and from the International Society for the Improvement and Teaching of Dialectical Behavior Therapy to the Association for Behavior Analysis International.

This training task force was charged with developing guidelines for integrating doctoral education and training in cognitive and behavioral psychology in the United States. The result was a thoughtful review of the contemporary literature and concrete recommendations that serve as the basis for this book.

No one book could cover all of the areas that the training standards do. We decided to set aside training issues in research methods and assessment, since they are so well covered in existing volumes, and instead focus on areas that seem to us to involve new ideas and new sensitivities that are not well represented in existing volumes.

In the area of scientific attitude, the task force training standards take two strong stands: "The first proposition is that doctoral study in CBP [cognitive and behavioral psychology] includes foundational work in the philosophy of science" (Klepac et al. p. 691), and the "second proposition is that ethical decision making is fundamental to CBP, and should permeate all aspects of research and practice" (p. 692). Both of these stands are woven into section 1 of this book, which addresses the nature of behavioral and cognitive therapies, and are carried forward in other chapters.

To our knowledge, the present volume is the first CBT text to fully explore the implications of what the training standards call "overarching scientific 'world views'" (p. 691). The training task force argues, we believe correctly, that training in the various philosophical worldviews underlying different cognitive and behavioral methods is key to having the ability to communicate across its various wings, waves, and traditions:

> Many psychologists may not be aware of the implicit assumptions that underlie their work, which can lead to considerable confusion and controversy of a sort that impedes progress in the science itself. Different philosophies of science (and especially the epistemologies represented by those philosophical systems) lead not only to different methods of inquiry, but also to different interpretations of data, including at times different interpretations of the very same data. Failure to appreciate differences in preanalytic assumptions can lead to frustration among scholars and practitioners alike, who become puzzled when their colleagues fail to be convinced of the implications of certain clinical observations or research findings. Lack of awareness of one's philosophical assumptions also precludes critical examination and comparison of alternative philosophies of science. (p. 691)

The task force listed seventeen core clinical competencies of known importance and suggested that the focus of education should be on "training in the basic principles behind [these] interventions" (p. 696). These principles were said to emerge from an understanding of several key domains, such as understanding learning theory, cognition, emotion, the therapeutic relationship, and neuroscience.

These guidelines are a key focus in this volume. This book includes chapters for all of the core clinical competencies mentioned in the standards and all of the key process domains, as well as a chapter on evolution science. For each clinical competency, the authors also attempted to focus on core processes and principles that account for the impact of these methods.

We believe that examining evidence-based intervention in light of the ideas in the new training standards allows the field to redefine evidence-based therapy to mean the targeting of evidence-based process with evidence-based procedures that alleviate the problems and promote the prosperity of people. We believe that a focus on process-based therapy will guide the field far into the future. Identifying core processes will enable us to avoid the constraints of using protocol for syndromes as the primary empirical approach to treatment and instead allow us to directly link treatment to theory.

We hope this text serves as one important step in this direction. We intend for it to serve as a reference and graduate text in clinical intervention for behavioral and cognitive therapies, broadly defined. We believe it provides practitioners, researchers, interns, and students with a thorough review of the core processes involved in contemporary behavioral and cognitive therapies and, to some degree, in evidence-based therapy more generally. The focus on evidence-based competencies in this book is designed to make readers step back from the more specific protocols and skills that are often highlighted in different treatments and to *embrace core processes that are common* to many empirically supported approaches. We explicitly mean for it to span the various traditions and generations of different behavioral and cognitive therapies, while at the same time respect what is unique about their different processes of research and development.

This book is divided into three sections. Section 1 addresses the nature of behavioral and cognitive therapies and includes chapters on the history of CBT development—from its inception as a discredited new treatment model to its position today at the forefront of evidence-based therapies, philosophy of science, ethics, and the changing role of practice. Section 2 focuses on the principles, domains, and areas that serve as the theoretical foundations of CBT as a collection of empirically supported treatments; these principles, domains, and areas include behavioral principles, cognition, emotion, neuroscience, and evolution science. Section 3 discusses the core clinical competencies that make up the bulk of CBT interventions, including contingency management, stimulus control, shaping, self-management, arousal reduction, coping and emotion regulation, problem solving, exposure strategies, behavioral activation, interpersonal skills, cognitive reappraisal, modifying core beliefs, defusion/distancing, enhancing psychological acceptance, values, mindfulness and integrative approaches, motivational strategies, and crisis management. Each of these chapters about competencies focuses on the known mediator and moderators that link these methods to the process domains and principles described earlier in the book. The book ends with a summary of what we've learned and future directions for this field.

We, the two editors of this textbook, might seem like an odd couple. In fact, we *are* an odd couple. Although both of us served as president of ABCT, our philosophical backgrounds are quite different. We are both considered prominent figures in the communities representing the two seemingly opposing camps in contemporary CBT: the acceptance and commitment therapy/new generation CBT (Hayes) and the Beckian/more traditional CBT (Hofmann). After a stormy beginning with countless heated debates during panel discussions (often resembling the academic version of boxing matches or wrestling events) and in writing, we became close friends and collaborators. We have been continuously working to identify common ground while respecting our differences and points of view. Our mutual goal has always been the same: moving the science and practice of clinical intervention forward.

Because of our status in different wings of the field, we were able to assemble a diverse and stellar group of contributing authors. They have been able to combine their expertise to produce this groundbreaking, contemporary text that brings together the best of behavior therapy, behavior analysis, cognitive therapy, and acceptance- and mindfulness-based therapies, emphasizing the core processes of change in intervention that every clinician should know. We hope it helps set the stage for a new era of process-based therapy that will move the field beyond its era of silos toward an era of scientific progress that will positively impact the lives of those we serve.

# References

Klepac, R. K., Ronan, G. F., Andrasik, F., Arnold, K. D., Belar, C. D., Berry, S. L., et al. (2012). Guidelines for cognitive behavioral training within doctoral psychology programs in the United States: Report of the Inter-Organizational Task Force on Cognitive and Behavioral Psychology Doctoral Education. *Behavior Therapy, 43*(4), 687–697.

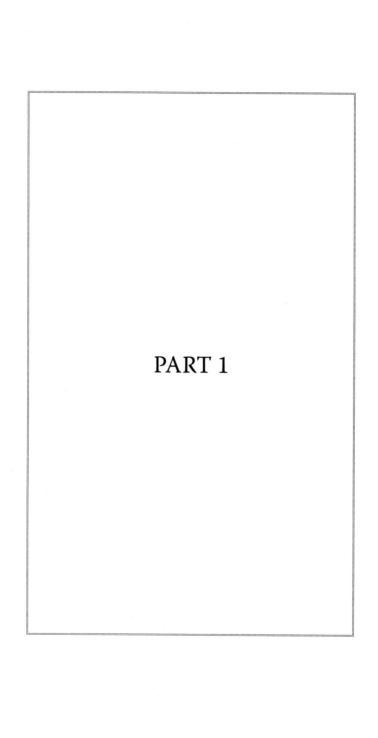

PART 1

# CHAPTER 1

# The History and Current Status of CBT as an Evidence-Based Therapy

Stefan G. Hofmann, PhD

*Department of Psychological and Brain Sciences,
Boston University*

Steven C. Hayes, PhD

*Department of Psychology, University of Nevada, Reno*

The Inter-Organizational Task Force on Cognitive and Behavioral Psychology Doctoral Education, organized by the Association for Behavioral and Cognitive Therapies (Klepac et al., 2012), marks an important step in the arduous journey of clinical psychology toward a mature applied science. The task force developed guidelines for integrated education and training in cognitive and behavioral psychology at the doctoral level in the United States, which seem to us to open up important avenues of training.

A series of important consensus processes has marked the development of evidence-based intervention approaches. A milestone on this journey was the 1949 Boulder conference, which officially recognized that clinical psychology training should emphasize both the practice and the science of the profession (Raimy, 1950). Soon after, in 1952, Hans-Jürgen Eysenck delivered a somber challenge to the nascent field of clinical psychological science in his review of the effectiveness of adult psychotherapies, concluding that psychotherapy was not more effective in treating clients than the simple passage of time:

> In general, certain conclusions are possible from these data. They fail to prove that psychotherapy, Freudian or otherwise, facilitates the recovery of neurotic patients. They show that roughly two-thirds of a group of neurotic patients will recover or improve to a marked extent within about

two years of the onset of their illness, whether they are treated by means of psychotherapy or not. This figure appears to be remarkably stable from one investigation to another, regardless of type of patient treated, standard of recovery employed, or method of therapy used. From the point of view of the neurotic, these figures are encouraging; from the point of view of the psychotherapist, they can hardly be called very favorable to his claims. (pp. 322–323)

Eysenck was known for his strong bias against psychoanalysis, and the development of behavior therapy was, at least in part, an attempt to rise to his challenge. The first behavior therapy journal, *Behaviour Research and Therapy*, appeared in 1965, and within a few years Eysenck's original question—Does psychotherapy work?—changed to a much more specific and difficult question (Paul, 1969, p. 44): "What treatment, by whom, is most effective for this individual with that specific problem, and under which set of circumstances, and how does it come about?" Behavior therapists, and later, cognitive behavioral therapists, pursued at least part of that question by studying protocols of various specific disorders and problems.

By the time Smith and Glass (1977) performed the first meta-analysis of psychotherapy outcomes, they were able to examine 375 studies, representing approximately 25,000 subjects, and to calculate an effect-size analysis based on 833 effect-size measures. The results of this impressive analysis show clear evidence of the efficacy of psychotherapy beyond merely waiting. On average, a typical patient receiving any form of psychotherapy was better off than 75 percent of untreated people, and overall the various forms of psychotherapy (systematic desensitization, behavior modification, Rogerian, psychodynamic, rational emotive, transactional analysis, and so on) were equally effective.

Since then, psychotherapy research has evolved considerably. Enhancements have been made in clinical methodologies and research design, our understanding of diverse psychopathologies, psychiatric nosology, and assessment and treatment techniques. Government agencies, insurance companies, and patient advocate groups have begun to demand that psychological interventions be based on evidence. In line with the more general move toward evidence-based medicine (Sackett, Strauss, Richardson, Rosenberg, & Haynes, 2000), in psychotherapy the term *evidence-based practice* considers the best available research evidence for the effectiveness of a treatment, the specific patient characteristics of those receiving the treatment, and the clinical expertise of the therapist delivering the treatment (American Psychological Association Presidential Task Force on Evidence-Based Practice, 2006). Various agencies and associations worldwide have begun compiling lists of evidence-based psychotherapy methods, such as the National Registry of Evidence-based Programs and Practices (NREPP) of the US Substance Abuse and Mental Health Services Administration.

In a highly influential step in 1995, the Society of Clinical Psychology (Division 12 of the American Psychological Association) created a Task Force on Promotion and Dissemination of Psychological Procedures with the goal of developing a list of research-supported psychological treatments (RSPTs; earlier names for this list were evidence-supported treatments and evidence-based treatments). It should be noted that the Division 12 task force deliberately recruited clinicians and researchers from a number of different theoretical orientations, including psychodynamic, interpersonal, cognitive behavioral, and systemic points of view, in order to avoid allegiance biases (Ollendick, Muris, & Essau, in press).

The Division 12 task force published its first report in 1995, in which it included three categories of RSPTs: (1) well-established treatments, (2) probably efficacious treatments, and (3) experimental treatments. Well-established treatments had to be superior to a psychological placebo, drug, or other treatment, whereas the probably efficacious treatments had to be superior only to a wait-list or no-treatment control condition. Well-established treatments were also required to have evidence from at least two different investigatory teams, whereas probably efficacious treatments were required to have evidence from only one investigatory team. Moreover, the task force required that all treatments specify patient characteristics (such as age, sex, ethnicity, diagnosis, etc.) and that treatment manuals explain the specific treatment strategies. Although not strictly required, the list of RSPTs was largely based on treatments for specific disorders defined by the *Diagnostic and Statistical Manual of Mental Disorders* (DSM; American Psychiatric Association, 2000, 2013).

Finally, it was necessary for treatments to demonstrate clinical outcomes in well-controlled clinical trials or in a series of well-controlled single-case designs. The quality of the designs had to be such that the benefits observed were not due to chance or confounding factors, such as the passage of time, the effects of psychological assessment, or the presence of different types of clients in the various treatment conditions (Chambless & Hollon, 1998). This system of treatment categorization was intended to be a work in progress. Consistent with this goal, the list of RSPTs was placed online and is now maintained and updated at http://www.div12.org/psychological-treatments/treatments.

Most recently, the criteria for RSPTs were revised to include evidence from meta-analytic reviews of multiple trials across multiple domains of functioning (Tolin, McKay, Forman, Klonsky, & Thombs, 2015). Of all treatments, cognitive behavioral therapy (CBT) has by far the largest evidence base. A review of the efficacy of CBT for mental disorders easily filled a large three-volume textbook series (Hofmann, 2014b). It should be noted, however, that some disorders are more responsive to existing CBT methods than others. In the case of anxiety disorders, for example, a meta-analysis of methodologically rigorous, randomized, placebo-controlled studies reported that CBT yields the largest effect sizes for obsessive-compulsive disorder and acute stress disorder but only small effect sizes for panic disorder (Hofmann & Smits, 2008). Moreover, some CBT protocols show disorder specificity; for example, depression changes to a significantly lesser degree than anxiety with a protocol targeting anxiety disorders, and the reverse is true for depressive disorders. This clearly speaks against the argument that CBT lacks treatment specificity. At the same time, this and many other meta-analyses show that there is clearly a lot of room for improvement with contemporary CBT (Hofmann, Asnaani, Vonk, Sawyer, & Fang, 2012).

Despite the well-planned and executed mission, the Division 12 task force report and its list-supported treatments generated heated debates and arguments. Some of the counterarguments focused on fears that the use of treatment manuals would lead to mechanical, inflexible interventions and a loss of creativity and innovation in the therapy process. Another frequently made argument was that treatments that were effective in clinical research settings might not be transportable to "real-life" clinical practice settings with more difficult or comorbid clients (for a review, see Chambless & Ollendick, 2001). The strong representation of CBT protocols (in contrast to psychodynamically or humanistically oriented therapies) among the treatments meeting the RSPT criteria also fueled the intensity of the debates. A final major concern for some psychotherapists was the alignment of empirically supported treatments with specific diagnostic categories.

For example, consider the difference between CBT and psychodynamically oriented therapies. Instead of trying to identify and resolve hidden conflicts, CBT practitioners could encourage clients to utilize more-adaptive strategies to deal with their present psychological problems. As a result of this relative concordance, CBT protocols were developed for virtually every category of the DSM and the tenth revision of the *International Statistical Classification of Diseases and Related Health Problems* (ICD-10; World Health Organization, 1992–1994).

A recent review of the literature identified no fewer than 269 meta-analytic studies examining CBT for nearly every DSM category (Hofmann, Asnaani et al., 2012). In general, the evidence base of CBT is very strong, especially for anxiety disorders, somatoform disorders, bulimia, anger control problems, and general stress, because CBT protocols closely align with the different psychiatric categories. Although generally efficacious, there are clear differences in the degree of CBT's efficacy across disorders. For example, major depressive disorder and panic disorder manifest a relatively high placebo-response rate. Such disorders run a fluctuating and recurring course so that the important question is not so much what are the short-term outcomes, since many treatments may work initially, but rather how effective are treatments in preventing relapse and recurrence in the longer term (Hollon, Stewart, & Strunk, 2006).

The focus on DSM-defined psychiatric disorders has sometimes limited the vision of CBT in its measures and application. For example, with CBT, measures of flourishing, quality of life, prosociality, relationship quality, or other issues that are more focused on growth and prosperity are often less in focus despite client interest in such issues. This limited vision is especially true of behavioral measures, which is unfortunate, because we know that some of the methods used in evidence-based therapy are applicable to health and prosperity issues.

The focus on disorders has led to a proliferation of specific protocols that can make training difficult and can limit the integration of research and clinical literature. Practitioners can get lost in a sea of supposedly distinctive but often overlapping methods.

These issues of breadth of focus, long-term effects, and protocol proliferation touch upon some fundamental ideas about the nature of psychological functioning and of treatment goals. It is the claim of this volume that the field needs a course correction to rise to the challenges of the present moment.

# Problems with the Biomedical Model

The development and refinement of CBT models for the various DSM and ICD-10 diagnoses has permitted therapists and researchers to apply specific treatment techniques across a diverse range of psychopathologies. However, the general alignment of CBT protocols with the medical classification system of mental disorders has had downsides (e.g., Deacon, 2013). For example, classifying people using criteria-based psychiatric diagnostic categories based on presenting symptoms minimizes or ignores contextual and situational factors contributing to the problem (e.g., Hofmann, 2014a). Modern CBT often overemphasizes techniques for specific symptoms at the expense of theory and case conceptualization, limiting the further development of CBT. Health promotion and the whole person can become less of a focus as syndromal thinking dominates. CBT is not at an end state; rather, it needs to continue to evolve with time, generating testable models (Hofmann, Asmundson, & Beck, 2013) and novel treatment strategies (e.g., Hayes, Follette, & Linehan, 2004).

Some authors argue that clinical researchers developing research-based interventions largely ignore common factors (as opposed to specific treatment strategies), and that these factors are primarily responsible for therapeutic change (Laska, Gurman, & Wampold, 2014). Approaching this issue as a dichotomy appears to be an error. It is actually relatively common for clinical researchers developing empirically supported treatments to consider these factors by examining the effects of, for example, the therapeutic alliance in outcomes. The impact of common factors varies from disorder to disorder, and although they can be important, they alone are not sufficient to produce the maximum effects on treatment outcomes. Furthermore, relationship factors can be responsive to the same psychological processes that evidence-based methods target. This suggests that the theoretically coherent processes addressed by CBT may in part account for some common factors. For example, the mediating relationship of the working alliance is no longer significant to outcome if a client's psychological flexibility is added as an additional mediator (e.g., Gifford et al., 2011), suggesting that the therapeutic alliance works in part by modeling acceptance, nonjudgment, and similar processes that may be targeted in modern CBT methods.

Much of the data on the therapeutic alliance is correlational and points to relatively immutable features, such as therapist variables. Common factors become central to practitioners, however, when specific methods to change them are developed and tested against other evidence-based methods. That kind of work is just beginning, and to conduct that work better, therapists need to develop theories about the therapeutic alliance and how, concretely, to change it—precisely the kinds of areas where CBT and evidence-based therapy can be helpful.

It is time for clinical psychology and psychiatry to move beyond picking either common factors or evidence-based psychological treatments in an all-or-none analysis (Hofmann & Barlow, 2014). Instead, we need to isolate and understand the effective processes of change and how best to target them, with relationship factors treated as one such process. This approach will allow the field to focus on any issue that will help our clients improve their lives and will help advance our scientific discipline.

# Defining the Targets of Psychotherapy and Psychological Intervention

In the early days of behavior therapy, specific problems or specific positive growth targets were often the aim of the intervention, but with the rise of the DSM, syndrome and mental disorders became more of a focus. Clinical scientists have engaged in a long and heated debate over how to best define and classify mental disorders (e.g., Varga, 2011). The structure of the DSM-5 and ICD-10 is firmly rooted in the biomedical model, assuming that signs and symptoms reflect underlying and latent disease entities. Earlier versions of these manuals were grounded in psychoanalytic theory, assuming that mental disorders are rooted in deep-seated conflicts. In contrast, the modern versions implicate dysfunctions in genetic, biological, psychological, and developmental processes as the primary causes of a mental disorder.

A prominent sociobiological definition of the term *mental disorder* is "harmful dysfunction" (Wakefield, 1992). The problem is considered a "dysfunction" because having it means that the person cannot perform a natural function as designed by evolution; the problem is considered "harmful" because it has negative consequences for the person, and society views the dysfunction negatively.

Not surprisingly, this definition is not without criticism because it is unclear how to define and determine the function or dysfunction of a behavior (e.g., McNally, 2011). Early critics (e.g., Szasz, 1961) argued that psychiatric disorders are simply labels that society attaches to normal human experiences and represent essentially arbitrary social constructions without any functional value. The same phenomenon that is considered abnormal in one culture or at one point in history may be considered normal or even desirable in another culture or at another point in history.

The official definition of a *mental disorder* in the DSM is "a syndrome characterized by clinically significant disturbance in an individual's cognition, emotion regulation, or behavior that reflects a dysfunction in the psychological, biological, or developmental processes underlying mental functioning" (American Psychiatric Association, 2013, p. 20). Although this definition specifically mentions psychological and developmental processes as possible primary causes in addition to biological ones, psychiatry has long operated primarily within a biomedical framework.

The cognitive behavioral approach is most commonly based on a diathesis-stress model, which assumes that an individual's vulnerability factors in conjunction with particular environmental factors or stressors can lead to the development of the disorder. This perspective makes a critical distinction between *initiating* factors (i.e., the factors that contribute to the development of a problem) and *maintaining* factors (i.e., the factors that are responsible for the maintenance of a problem) (Hofmann, 2011). These two sets of factors are typically not the same. Unlike other theoretical models of mental disorders, CBT is generally more concerned about the maintenance factors because they are the targets of effective treatments for present impairments. Therefore, from a CBT perspective, classifying individuals based on maintenance factors is likely to be of far greater importance than classifying individuals based on vulnerabilities alone, such as genetic factors or brain circuits.

This emphasis is broadly in line with the developmental approach of the behavioral tradition, which may not emphasize vulnerabilities and stressors but recognizes that the historical factors that led to a problem may differ from the environmental factors that maintain it. Functional analysis is focused on maintaining factors for current behaviors precisely because it is these that need to change in order to improve an individual's mental health.

## Why Classify Mental Disorders?

Proponents of the DSM often point out that a psychiatric classification system, no matter how imprecise, is a necessity for the following reasons: First, it provides the field with a common language to describe individuals with psychological problems. This is of great practical value because it simplifies communication among practitioners and provides a coding system for insurance companies. Second, it advances clinical science by grouping together people with similar problems in order to identify common patterns and isolate features that distinguish them from other groups. Third, this information may be used to improve existing treatments or to develop new interventions. This latter purpose is acknowledged by the DSM-5, which states, "The diagnosis of a mental disorder should have clinical utility: it should help clinicians to determine prognosis, treatment plans, and potential treatment outcomes for their patients" (American Psychiatric Association, 2013, p. 20). Despite these lofty goals, however, the DSM-5 offered little new or different material from its predecessors, sparking a great degree of dissatisfaction in the medical and research community.

Aside from political and financial issues (the DSM is a major source of income for the American Psychiatric Association), there are many theoretical and conceptual problems with the DSM. For example, it pathologizes normality using arbitrary cut points; a diagnosis made using the DSM is merely based on subjective judgment by a clinician rather than objective measures; it is overly focused on symptoms; its categories describe a heterogeneous group of individuals and a large number of different symptom combinations that define the same diagnosis, and most clinicians continue to use the residual diagnosis ("not otherwise specified") because most clients do not fall neatly into any of the diagnostic categories, which are derived by consensus agreement of experts (for a review, see Gornall, 2013).

Perhaps one of the biggest conceptual problems is comorbidity (i.e., the co-occurrence of two or more different diagnoses). Comorbidity is inconsistent with the basic notion that symptoms of a disorder reflect the existence of a latent disease entity. If disorders were in fact distinct disease entities, comorbidity should be an exception in nosology. However, disorders are commonly comorbid. For example, among mood and anxiety disorders, the DSM-5 posits that virtually all of the considerable covariance among latent variables corresponding to its constructs of unipolar depression, generalized anxiety disorder, social anxiety disorder, obsessive-compulsive disorder, panic disorder, and agoraphobia can be explained by the higher-order dimensions of negative and positive affect; this suggests that mood and anxiety disorders emerge from shared psychosocial and biological/genetic diatheses (Brown & Barlow, 2009).

Observations like these served as the basis for recent efforts to develop so-called transdiagnostic (Norton, 2012) or unified (Barlow et al., 2010) treatment protocols that cut across diagnostic categories to address the core features of disorders, the goal being to develop more parsimonious and, perhaps, powerful treatments (Barlow, Allen, & Choate, 2004). In addition, this approach might counter the drawback of training clinicians in disorder-specific CBT protocols, which often leads to an oversimplification of human suffering, inflexibility on the part of the clinician, and low adherence to evidence-based practices (McHugh, Murray, & Barlow, 2009).

# Research Domain Criteria

In an attempt to offer a solution to the nosology problems associated with the DSM (and the ICD-10), the National Institute of Mental Health (NIMH) developed the Research Domain Criteria (RDoC) Initiative, a new framework for classifying mental disorders based on dimensions of observable behavior and neurobiological measures (Insel et al., 2010). This initiative is an attempt to move the field of psychiatry forward by creating a classification system that conceptualizes mental illnesses as brain disorders. In contrast to neurological disorders with identifiable lesions, mental disorders are considered disorders with abnormal brain circuits (Insel et al., 2010). Instead of relying on clinical impressions, resulting in arbitrarily defined categories that comprise heterogeneous and overlapping diagnostic groups, the NIMH suggests integrating the findings of modern brain sciences in order to define and diagnose mental disorders (Insel et al., 2010).

The stated goal of this project is to develop a classification system for mental disorders based on biobehavioral dimensions that cut across current heterogeneous DSM categories. The RDoC framework assumes that dysfunctions in neural circuits can be identified with the tools of clinical neuroscience, including electrophysiology, functional neuroimaging, and new methods for quantifying connections in vivo. The framework further assumes that data from genetics and clinical neuroscience will yield biosignatures that can augment the clinical symptoms and signs used for clinical management. For example, in the case of anxiety disorders, the practitioner of the future would utilize data from functional or structural imaging, genomic sequencing, and laboratory-based evaluations of fear conditioning and extinction to determine a prognosis and appropriate treatment (Insel et al., 2010). The concrete product of the RDoC initiative is a matrix that lists different levels (molecular, brain circuit, behavioral, and symptom) of analysis in order to define constructs that are assumed to be the core symptoms of mental disorders.

Whereas neuroscientists generally applauded the RDoC initiative (Casey et al., 2013), others criticized it for various reasons. For example, the project overemphasizes certain kinds of biological processes, reducing mental health problems to simple brain disorders (Deacon, 2013; Miller, 2010). So far the RDoC has had limited clinical utility because it is primarily intended to advance future research, not to guide clinical decision making (Cuthbert & Kozak, 2013). Moreover, the RDoC initiative shares with the DSM the strong theoretical assumption that psychological problems ("symptoms") are caused by a latent disease. In the case of the DSM, these latent disease entities are measured through symptom reports and clinical impressions, whereas in the case of the RDoC they are measured through sophisticated behavioral tests (e.g., genetic tests) and biological instruments (e.g., neuroimaging).

# Moving Toward Core Dimensions in Psychopathology

In the last few decades, considerable progress has been made to identify core dimensions of psychopathology. The RDoC initiative proposes such a dimensional classification system. Similarly, psychologists have been reconsidering dimensions of psychopathology. For example, in the case of emotional disorders, numerous authors have identified emotion dysregulation as one of the core transdiagnostic problems (Barlow et al., 2004; Hayes, Luoma, Bond, Masuda, & Lillis, 2006; Hayes, Strosahl, & Wilson, 1999; Hofmann, Asnaani et al., 2012; Hofmann, Sawyer, Fang, & Asnaani, 2012). This is fully consistent with contemporary emotion research, such as the process model described by Gross (1998). Gross's emotion-generative process model of emotions posits that emotion-relevant cues are processed to activate physiological, behavioral, and experiential responses, and that these responses are modulated by emotion regulation tendencies. Depending on the time point at which a person engages in emotion regulation, the techniques are either antecedent-focused or response-focused strategies. Antecedent-focused emotion regulation strategies include cognitive reappraisal, situation modification, and attention deployment and occur before the emotional response has been fully activated. In contrast, response-focused emotion regulation strategies, such as strategies to suppress or tolerate the response, are attempts to alter the expression or experience of an emotion after the response has been initiated.

There are many more pathology dimensions that cut across DSM-defined disorders, such as negative affect, impulse control, attentional control, rumination and worrying, cognitive flexibility, self-awareness, or approach-based motivation to name only a few. As these dimensions have become more central to the understanding of psychopathology, it has become clearer that employing in a flexible manner the strategies that are most appropriate for a given context and goal pursuit is the most adaptive method for long-term adjustment (Bonanno, Papa, Lalande, Westphal, & Coifman, 2004). Many forms of psychopathology are associated with the negatively valenced responses, such as fear, sadness, anger, or distress, but all of these play a positive role in life. No psychological reaction, and no strategy for addressing a psychological reaction, is consistently adaptive or maladaptive (Haines et al., 2016). The goal of modern CBT is not to eliminate or suppress feelings, thoughts, sensations, or memories—it is to promote more positive life trajectories. Learning how best to target relevant processes that foster positive growth and development is the challenge of modern intervention science and the focus of this volume.

# Moving Toward Core Processes in CBT

It appears that the fundamental question of psychotherapy research formulated by Hans-Jürgen Eysenck (1952), and then revised by Gordon Paul (1969), needs to be revised yet again. The core question is no longer whether intervention works in a global way, nor is it how to make effective technological decisions in a contextually specific manner. The first question has been answered, and the technological emphasis of the second has led to a proliferation of methods that are difficult to systematize in a progressive fashion. Because of their failure to identify functionally distinct entities, both the purely syndromal focus and the largely technological approach need to be de-emphasized.

The movement toward the RDoC contains a key aspect that seems to fit this moment of evolution in the field of psychotherapy. The complex network approach also offers another potentially promising new perspective on psychopathology and treatment (Hofmann, Curtiss, & McNally, 2016). Instead of assuming that mental disorders arise from underlying disease entities, the complex network approach holds that these disorders exist due to a network of interrelated elements. An effective therapy may change the structure of the network from a pathological to a nonpathological state by targeting core processes. Similar to traditional functional analysis, we need to understand the causal relationship between stimuli and responses in order to identify and target these core processes of pathology and change in a contextually specific way. Longitudinal designs are allowing clinicians to develop targeted and specific measures that predict the development of psychopathology over time (e.g., Westin, Hayes, & Andersson, 2008). Clinicians can target these measures for change using evidence-based methods and determine the mediating role of change in these processes (e.g., Hesser, Westin, Hayes, & Andersson, 2009; Zettle, Rains, & Hayes, 2011).

By combining strategies, such as RDoC, functional analysis, the complex network approach, and longitudinal design, researchers are making progress in identifying the core processes of change in psychotherapy and psychological intervention (Hayes et al., 2006). With increasing knowledge of the components that move targeted processes (e.g., Levin, Hildebrandt, Lillis, & Hayes, 2012), researchers are building on that foundation. The goal is to learn which core biopsychosocial processes should be targeted with a given client who has a given goal in a given situation, and to then identify the component methods most likely to change those processes.

The identification of core processes in psychotherapy will guide psychotherapists into the future. These processes will allow us to avoid the constraints of treatment protocols based on a rigid and arbitrary diagnostic system and will directly link treatment to theory. This vision is what animates the present volume—that is, creating a more process-based form of CBT and evidence-based therapy. This vision pulls together many trends that already exist in the field and builds on the strengths of the many traditions and generations of work that make up the cognitive and behavioral approaches to therapy.

# References

American Psychiatric Association (2000). *Diagnostic and statistical manual of mental disorders: DSM-IV-TR* (4th ed., text revision). Washington, DC: American Psychiatric Association.

American Psychiatric Association (2013). *Diagnostic and statistical manual of mental disorders: DSM-5* (5th ed.). Washington, DC: American Psychiatric Association.

American Psychological Association Presidential Task Force on Evidence-Based Practice (2006). Evidence-based practice in psychology. *American Psychologist, 61*(4), 271–285.

Barlow, D. H., Allen, L. B., Choate, M. L. (2004). Toward a unified treatment for emotional disorders. *Behavior Therapy, 35*(2), 205–230.

Barlow, D. H., Ellard, K. K., Fairholm, C., Farchione, T. J., Boisseau, C. L., Ehrenreich-May, J. T., et al. (2010). *Unified protocol for transdiagnostic treatment of emotional disorders (treatments that work series).* New York: Oxford University Press.

Bonanno, G. A., Papa, A., Lalande, K., Westphal, M., & Coifman, K. (2004). The importance of being flexible: The ability to both enhance and suppress emotional expression predicts long-term adjustment. *Psychological Science, 15*(7), 482–487.

Brown, T. A., & Barlow, D. H. (2009). A proposal for a dimensional classification system based on the shared features of the DSM-IV anxiety and mood disorders: Implications for assessment and treatment. *Psychological Assessment, 21*(3), 256–271.

Casey, B. J., Craddock, N., Cuthbert, B. N., Hyman, S. E., Lee, F. S., & Ressler, K. J. (2013). DSM-5 and RDoC: Progress in psychiatry research? *Nature Reviews: Neuroscience, 14*(11), 810–814.

Chambless, D. L., & Hollon, S. D. (1998). Defining empirically supported therapies. *Journal of Consulting and Clinical Psychology, 66*(1), 7–18.

Chambless, D. L., & Ollendick, T. H. (2001). Empirically supported psychological interventions: Controversies and evidence. *Annual Review of Psychology, 52*, 685–716.

Cuthbert, B. N., & Kozak, M. J. (2013). Constructing constructs for psychopathology: The NIMH research domain criteria. *Journal of Abnormal Psychology, 122*(3), 928–937.

Deacon, B. J. (2013). The biomedical model of mental disorder: A critical analysis of its validity, utility, and effects on psychotherapy research. *Clinical Psychology Review, 33*(7), 846–861.

Eysenck, H. J. (1952). The effects of psychotherapy: An evaluation. *Journal of Consulting Psychology, 16*(5), 319–324.

Gifford, E. V., Kohlenberg, B. S., Hayes, S. C., Pierson, H. M., Piasecki, M. P., Antonuccio, D. O., et al. (2011). Does acceptance and relationship focused behavior therapy contribute to bupropion outcomes? A randomized controlled trial of functional analytic psychotherapy and acceptance and commitment therapy for smoking cessation. *Behavior Therapy, 42*(4), 700–715.

Gornall, J. (2013). DSM-5: A fatal diagnosis? *BMJ, 346*: f3256.

Gross, J. J. (1998). Antecedent- and response-focused emotion regulation: Divergent consequences for experience, expression, and physiology. *Journal of Personality and Social Psychology, 74*(1), 224–237.

Haines, S. J., Gleeson, J., Kuppens, P., Hollenstein, T., Ciarrochi, J., Labuschagne, I., et al. (2016). The wisdom to know the difference: Strategy-situation fit in emotion regulation in daily life is associated with well-being. *Psychological Science, 27*(12), 1651–1659.

Hayes, S. C., Follette, V. M., & Linehan, M. M. (Eds.). (2004). *Mindfulness and acceptance: Expanding the cognitive-behavioral tradition.* New York: Guilford Press.

Hayes, S. C., Luoma, J. B., Bond, F. W., Masuda, A., & Lillis, J. (2006). Acceptance and commitment therapy: Model, processes, and outcomes. *Behaviour Research and Therapy, 44*(1), 1–25.

Hayes, S. C., Strosahl, K. D., & Wilson, K. G. (1999). *Acceptance and commitment therapy: An experiential approach to behavior change.* New York: Guilford Press.

Hesser, H., Westin, V., Hayes, S. C., & Andersson, G. (2009). Clients' in-session acceptance and cognitive defusion behaviors in acceptance-based treatment of tinnitus distress. *Behaviour Research and Therapy, 47*(6), 523–528.

Hofmann, S. G. (2011). *An introduction to modern CBT: Psychological solutions to mental health problems.* Oxford, UK: Wiley.

Hofmann, S. G. (2014a). Toward a cognitive-behavioral classification system for mental disorders. *Behavior Therapy, 45*(4), 576–587.

Hofmann, S. G. (Ed.). (2014b). *The Wiley handbook of cognitive behavioral therapy* (Vols. I–III). Chichester, UK: John Wiley & Sons.

Hofmann, S. G., Asmundson, G. J., & Beck, A. T. (2013). The science of cognitive therapy. *Behavior Therapy, 44*(2), 199–212.

Hofmann, S. G., Asnaani, A., Vonk, I. J., Sawyer, A. T., & Fang, A. (2012). The efficacy of cognitive behavioral therapy: A review of meta-analyses. *Cognitive Therapy and Research, 36*(5), 427–440.

Hofmann, S. G., & Barlow, D. H. (2014). Evidence-based psychological interventions and the common factors approach: the beginnings of a rapprochement? *Psychotherapy, 51*(4), 510–513.

Hofmann, S. G., Curtiss, J., & McNally, R. J. (2016). A complex network perspective on clinical science. *Perspectives on Psychological Science, 11*(5), 597–605.

Hofmann, S. G., Sawyer, A. T., Fang, A., & Asnaani, A. (2012). Emotion dysregulation model of mood and anxiety disorders. *Depression and Anxiety, 29*(5), 409–416.

Hofmann, S. G., & Smits, J. A. J. (2008). Cognitive-behavioral therapy for adult anxiety disorders: A meta-analysis of randomized placebo-controlled trials. *Journal of Clinical Psychiatry, 69*(4), 621–632.

Hollon, S. D., Stewart, M. O., & Strunk, D. (2006). Enduring effects for cognitive behavior therapy in the treatment of depression and anxiety. *Annual Review of Psychology, 57,* 285–315.

Insel, T., Cuthbert, B., Garvey, M., Heinssen, R., Pine, D. S., Quinn, K., et al. (2010). Research domain criteria (RDoC): Toward a new classification framework for research on mental disorders. *American Journal of Psychiatry, 167*(7), 748–751.

Klepac, R. K., Ronan, G. F., Andrasik, F., Arnold, K. D., Belar, C. D., Berry, S. L., et al. (2012). Guidelines for cognitive behavioral training within doctoral psychology programs in the United States: Report of the Inter-Organizational Task Force on Cognitive and Behavioral Psychology Doctoral Education. *Behavior Therapy, 43*(4), 687–697.

Laska, K. M., Gurman, A. S., & Wampold, B. E. (2014). Expanding the lens of evidence-based practice in psychotherapy: A common factors perspective. *Psychotherapy, 51*(4), 467–481.

Levin, M. E., Hildebrandt, M. J., Lillis, J., & Hayes, S. C. (2012). The impact of treatment components suggested by the psychological flexibility model: A meta-analysis of laboratory-based component studies. *Behavior Therapy, 43*(4), 741–756.

McHugh, R. K., Murray, H. W., & Barlow, D. H. (2009). Balancing fidelity and adaptation in the dissemination of empirically-supported treatments: the promise of transdiagnostic interventions. *Behaviour Research and Therapy, 47*(11), 946–995.

McNally, R. J. (2011). *What is mental illness?* Cambridge, MA: Belknap Press of Harvard University Press.

Miller, G. A. (2010). Mistreating psychology in the decades of the brain. *Perspectives on Psychological Science, 5*(6), 716–743.

Norton, P. J. (2012). *Group cognitive-behavioral therapy of anxiety: A transdiagnostic treatment manual.* New York: Guilford Press.

Ollendick, T. H., Muris, P., Essau, C. A. (in press). Evidence-based treatments: The debate. In S. G. Hofmann (Ed.), *Clinical psychology: A global perspective.* Chichester, UK: Wiley-Blackwell.

Paul, G. L. (1969). Behavior modification research: Design and tactics. In C. M. Franks (Ed.), *Behavior therapy: Appraisal and status* (pp. 29–62). New York: McGraw-Hill.

Raimy, V. C. (Ed.). (1950). *Training in clinical psychology.* New York: Prentice Hall.

Sackett, D. L., Strauss, S. E., Richardson, W. S., Rosenberg, W., & Haynes, R. B. (2000). *Evidence-based medicine: How to practice and teach EBM* (2nd ed.). London: Churchill Livingstone.

Smith, M. L., & Glass, G. V. (1977). Meta-analysis of psychotherapy outcome studies. *American Psychologist, 32*(9), 752–760.

Szasz, T. (1961). *The myth of mental illness: Foundations of a theory of personal conduct.* New York: Hoeber-Harper.

Tolin, D. F., McKay, D., Forman, E. M., Klonsky, E. D., & Thombs, B. D. (2015). Empirically supported treatment: Recommendations for a new model. *Clinical Psychology: Science and Practice, 22*(4), 317–338.

Varga, S. (2011). Defining mental disorder: Exploring the "natural function" approach. *Philosophy, Ethics, and Humanities in Medicine, 6*(1), 1.

Wakefield, J. C. (1992). The concept of mental disorder: On the boundary between biological facts and social values. *American Psychologist, 47*(3), 373–388.

Westin, V., Hayes, S. C., & Andersson, G. (2008). Is it the sound or your relationship to it? The role of acceptance in predicting tinnitus impact. *Behaviour Research and Therapy, 46*(12), 1259–1265.

World Health Organization (1992–1994). *International statistical classification of diseases and related health problems: ICD-10* (10th rev., 3 vols.). Geneva: World Health Organization.

Zettle, R. D., Rains, J. C., & Hayes, S. C. (2011). Processes of change in acceptance and commitment therapy and cognitive therapy for depression: A mediational reanalysis of Zettle and Rains. *Behavior Modification, 35*(3), 265–283.

CHAPTER 2

# The Philosophy of Science As It Applies to Clinical Psychology

Sean Hughes, PhD

*Department of Experimental Clinical and Health Psychology,*
*Ghent University*

## Introduction

Imagine three scientists out to expand the limits of human understanding. The first is an astronaut busy analyzing soil samples on the cold, dark surface of the moon. The second is a marine biologist trying to find ways to get penguins more active and engaged at a large public aquarium. The third is a primatologist deeply interested in the courting behavior of silverback gorillas, who finds herself wading through a tropical forest in Central Africa. Although all three use the scientific method to understand a specific phenomenon, they approach their goals in very different ways. The fundamental questions they are interested in (e.g., What is the lunar soil composed of? How can the behavior of captive penguins be changed? How do primates behave socially in the wild?) will guide the procedures they use, the theories they generate, the types of data they collect, and the answers they ultimately find satisfactory.

In many ways, clinical psychological science faces a similar situation. Although clinicians and researchers are united by a shared goal (to understand how human suffering can be alleviated and well-being promoted), they often tackle that goal in fundamentally different ways. Some argue that this goal can be best achieved by detecting and correcting the dysfunctional beliefs, pathological cognitive schemas, or faulty information-processing styles that underpin psychological

The Ghent University Methusalem Grant BOF16/MET_V/002, presented to Jan De Houwer, supported the preparation of this chapter. Correspondence concerning this chapter should be addressed to sean.hughes@ugent.be.

suffering (e.g., Beck, 1993; Ellis & Dryden, 2007). Others counter that the best solution requires that we contact and alter the functions of internal events rather than their particular form or frequency (e.g., Hayes, Strosahl, & Wilson, 1999; Linehan, 1993; Segal, Williams, & Teasdale, 2001). In this rich, dense jungle of clinical research and theorizing, different traditions often find themselves in fierce competition, with proponents of one perspective arguing for the logical suprem- acy of their own procedures, findings, theories, and therapies, while others respond with equally and strongly held convictions (see Reyna, 1995, for an example). In such an environment, you might ask yourself, *Is there really a "best" solution to the problem of psychological suffering?* How do clinicians and researchers define what qualifies as "best," and is this a subjective or objective choice? How do they actu- ally determine whether a given procedure, finding, theory, or therapy is satisfac- tory or even better than others?

Even if clinical researchers do not typically operate in the cold vacuum of outer space, the water tanks of an aquarium, or the humid interiors of tropical forests, their activities are nevertheless carried out within a larger context that guides their scientific values and goals. One of the more important aspects of this context is their philosophical worldview. Worldviews specify the nature and purpose of science, causality, data, and explanation. They define what we con- sider the proper subject matter of our field, what our units of analysis will be, the types of theories and therapies we build and evaluate, the methodologies we con- struct, and how findings should be generated and interpreted.

Questions about ontology, epistemology, and axiology can seem highly abstract and far removed from the daily trials and tribulations that make up clini- cal research or therapeutic practice. In what follows I aim to demonstrate how philosophical assumptions are similar to the air we breathe: typically invisible, integral to our daily functioning, and yet often taken for granted. There is no privileged place that allows you to avoid these issues: your worldview silently shapes how you think and act, influencing the theories, therapies, techniques, and data you consider convincing or valid (e.g., Babbage & Ronan, 2000; Forsyth, 2016). It dictates some of your moment-to-moment behavior when interacting with a client. By properly articulating and organizing these assumptions, you gain access to a powerful method of determining the internal consistency of your own scientific views and ensure that your efforts at knowledge development are progressive—when measured against your (clinical) scientific goals.

Scientific endeavors must have criteria to evaluate competing theoretical and methodological accounts if progress is to be achieved. Yet scholars often engage in debates of a different kind: ones that center on the legitimacy, primacy, and value of one intellectual tradition relative to another. Such debates have been labeled "pseudoconflicts," given that they involve applying the philosophical assumptions (and thus scientific goals and values) of one's own approach to the assumptions, goals, and values of others (Pepper, 1942; Hayes, Hayes, & Reese, 1988). For instance, behaviorally oriented therapists may dismiss the value of mental-mediating representations and processes, such as cognitive schemas or biases, given that such explanatory constructs are counter (or even irrelevant) to their own focus on manipulable, contextual variables that can facilitate the prediction and influence of psychological events. Similarly, cognitively oriented researchers might view any analysis that omits reference to the mental machinery of the mind as merely descriptive and nonexplanatory. As Dougher (1995) notes, these respective scholars might wonder why their counterparts "persist in taking such outdated or plainly wrong-headed positions, why they persist in misrepresenting my position, and why they can't see that both logic and data render their position clearly inferior" (p. 215). The failure to recognize the philosophical origins of these debates often leads to "frustration, sarcasm, and even *ad hominem* attacks on the intellectual or academic competence of those holding alternative positions" (p. 215).

Psychological scientists who are capable of articulating their philosophical assumptions are better able to identify genuine and productive conflicts within traditions that drive theory and research forward, and they can avoid wasting time on pseudoconflicts that tend to be degenerative in nature. In other words, appreciating the philosophical underpinnings of your work also allows you to communicate without dogmatism or arrogance to those who hold different assumptions. Such flexibility is central to the theme of this book: helping different wings of evidence-based therapy learn to communicate across philosophical divides. For these reasons and others, a consortium of cognitive and behavioral organizations recently added training in philosophy of science to the training standards for empirical clinicians (Klepac et al., 2012).

Finally, the clinical literature is home to an overwhelming number of perspectives that may tempt students to adopt a vapid form of eclecticism, hoping that by mixing together all plausible theories and concepts, even better therapeutic outcomes will be likely. Disciplined combinations of approaches are possible and helpful, but confusion results if theories and therapies are mixed in ways that are inconsistent (because underlying philosophical assumptions were misunderstood or ignored).

This chapter is divided into three sections. Part 1 provides a brief introduction to the core topics of philosophy of science as they apply to those undergoing clinical training (examples of more extensive treatments are Gawronski & Bodenhausen, 2015; Morris, 1988; Guba & Lincoln, 1994; among many others). In part 2, I introduce a number of worldviews that were originally forwarded by Stephen Pepper in the 1940s, with a focus on mechanism and contextualism in particular. I will demonstrate how these latter worldviews have arguably shaped and continue to drive clinical psychology. Finally, in part 3 I consider the topics of worldview selection, evaluation, communication, and collaboration. If readers then decide to adopt a particular philosophical perspective, they will do so with awareness of the alternatives, how this decision shapes their own thinking and actions, and how they can interact with colleagues who see (or construct) the world in ways that differ from their own.

# Part 1: A Brief Introduction to Philosophy of Science

*Science* is broadly concerned with the development of a systematic body of knowledge that is tied to empirically derived evidence (e.g., Lakatos, 1978; Laudan, 1978). This system of knowledge is built with the intention of understanding and influencing "patterns of relations among phenomena and processes of the experienced world" (Lerner & Damon, 2006, p. 70). *Philosophy of science* refers to the conceptual foundation upon which this systematic body of knowledge is built. Rather than focusing on the particular theories, methods, and observations that define a scientific domain, philosophy of science is concerned with the scientific enterprise itself. The goal is to uncover the assumptions that are often implicit (or taken for granted) in scientific practice and that dictate its course (e.g., how science should proceed, what methods of inquiry should be used, how much confidence should be placed in the findings generated, and what are the limits of the knowledge obtained). In this way, philosophy of science provides a perspective from which to examine and potentially evaluate clinical psychological science.

## *Philosophical Worldviews*

A *philosophical worldview* can be defined as the coherent set of interrelated assumptions that provides the preanalytic framework that sets the stage for scientific or therapeutic activity (see Hayes et al., 1988; closely related terms are "paradigm," Kuhn, 1962; and "research programme," Lakatos, 1978). One's worldview is a belief system that both describes and prescribes what data, tools, theories, therapies, participants, and findings are acceptable or unacceptable. The basic beliefs that make up a worldview typically revolve around the following set of interrelated questions, with the answers to one question constraining responses to the others.

**The ontological question.** *Ontology* is broadly concerned with the nature, origin, and structure of reality and "being." In other words, what does it mean to say that something is "real," and is it possible to study reality in an objective manner?

Many ontological stances can and have been taken. For illustrative purposes, I'll briefly discuss positivism, postpositivism, and constructivism, given their prominence within psychological science, although perspectives other than these are possible.

*Positivism* is a reductionistic and deterministic perspective that often involves a belief in "naïve realism," the idea that a discoverable reality exists that is governed by a system of natural laws and mechanisms. Scientific models and theories are considered useful or valid insofar as they increase our ability to make claims that refer to entities or relations in a mind-independent reality (i.e., truth as correspondence). This type of "knowledge is conventionally summarized in the form of time- and context-free generalizations, some of which take the form of cause-effect laws" (Guba & Lincoln, 1994, p. 109). Scientific progress itself involves the development of theories in which representational nature gradually converges upon a single reality.

*Postpositivism* also assumes that mind-independent reality exists, but it can only be imperfectly and probabilistically understood by humans due to their biased intellectual abilities and the fundamentally intractable nature of phenomena. Postpositivists believe that there is a reality independent of perception and theories about it but also argue that humans cannot know that reality with absolute certainty (e.g., see Lincoln, Lynham, & Guba, 2011). Thus, all scientific claims about reality must be submitted to close scrutiny if we are to converge on an understanding of reality that is acceptable (if never perfect).

*Constructivism*, unlike positivism and postpositivism, takes a relativistic ontological stance. A mind-independent reality is substituted for a constructed one: reality does not exist independently from our perception or theories about it. Instead we interpret and construct it based on our experiences and interactions with the social, experiential, historical, and cultural environments in which we are embedded. Constructed realities are malleable, differ in their content and sophistication, and are not "true" in any absolute sense of the word. Although constructivists tend to acknowledge that phenomena exist, they challenge the extent to which we can rationally know reality outside of our personal perspectives (e.g., see Blaikie, 2007; Lincoln et al., 2011; Von Glasersfeld, 2001). In some forms of this approach, constructivists simply refuse, on pragmatic grounds, to view ontological questions as answerable, useful, or necessary (Hayes, 1997).

**The epistemological question.** *Epistemology*, the theory of knowledge, is concerned with the acquisition and justification of knowledge (i.e., whether we do or can know anything, as well as the validity of that knowledge and how we come to know it). It involves asking questions such as "How certain are we that we have accumulated knowledge?" and "How can we distinguish this knowledge from belief?" When applied to science, "knowledge" refers to scientific theories, explanations, and laws, and "epistemology" involves answering questions such as "In what way does evidence support a theory?" or "What does it mean to say that a theory is true or false?" or "Is the revision and change of theory a rational or irrational process?" Once again, different stances can be taken in the pursuit of scientific knowledge.

Positivism adopts a dualistic and objectivist position: provided that she has access to the proper methodologies, the knower (scientist) can objectively view and record events as they "really are" and as they "really work." This process does not influence the phenomenon of interest, nor does the phenomenon influence the knower. Situations in which the knower influences the known (or vice versa) represent threats to validity, and the knower implements strategies to reduce or eliminate potential sources of contamination.

Postpositivism is qualified dualist/objectivist. Given the imperfect manner in which the world is viewed and recorded, dualism is de-emphasized: observations are accepted as being prone to error and are always open to critique. Theory is ultimately revisable and open to replacement by a different set of categories and relationships. However, objectivism is still the "regulatory ideal" to which the scientist strives (Lincoln et al., 2011). Scientific analyses are considered to be "true" or "valid" insofar as they allow us to converge on an accurate (if imperfect) understanding of reality (i.e., truth is correspondence). Such analyses are based on the idea that (a) knowledge can be best obtained through the identification of regularities and causal relationships between the component mechanisms that constitute reality; that (b) these regularities and relationships will be easier to identify when the scientist and phenomenon do not contaminate one another; and that (c) the scientific method is the best tool the scientist has to minimize such contamination. Thus, the purpose of models and theories is to provide general explanations that are logically organized and that have clearly established links with the observable world. These explanations extend beyond the observation of individual events and have a heuristic and predictive function.

Finally, constructivism is transactional and subjective. It argues that findings are obtained through the interaction of the knower and the known, and as such they are literally created as the scientific enterprise unfolds. In this way knowledge is subjective insofar as there is no objective location from which to view or obtain knowledge (and even if there was, we have no way of accessing it). Thus, the knower is an active participant rather than a passive observer in the knowledge acquisition and justification process. Truth is not correspondence with some underlying reality but rather the extent to which a particular analysis occasions "successful working" or is considered "viable." As Von Glasersfeld puts it, "To the constructivist, concepts, models, theories…are viable if they prove adequate in the contexts in which they were created" (1995, p. 4). From the constructivist perspective, science can be viewed as "a corpus of rules for effective action, and there is a special sense in which it could be 'true' if it yields the most effective action possible" (Skinner, 1974, p. 235; see also Barnes-Holmes, 2000).

**The axiology question.** *Axiology* refers to the relationship between knowledge and human values. When applied to science, it involves questions such as "How do values relate to (scientific) facts?" and "What role, if any, do the researcher's values play in the scientific process?" According to positivism, the scientist views reality through a one-sided mirror: objectively and impartially. Values and biases have no place in the scientific process and should be prevented from influencing one's activity at all costs. Implementing appropriate methodologies and conceptual controls ensures that scientific products are value free.

Postpositivism takes a similar if qualified stance: all observations are assumed to be theory laden. The search for absolute truth is abandoned and the researcher accepts that analyses are guided by the cultural, social, historical, and personal expectancies she brings to the enterprise (i.e., science is value laden). Nevertheless, progress can be best achieved if the scientist does her utmost to minimize the impact of such contaminating factors on theoretical arguments and empirical findings.

Finally, constructivism is dialectical: given the variable and personal nature of the constructed world, there is no objective location from which reality can be independently observed or recorded. The scientist cannot be separated from subject matter, nor can theory be separated from practice. Thus, values are considered an integral element of the interactions between scientist and the phenomenon being studied.

**The methodology question.** Once the knower (scientist) has determined what can be known, she must then identify a set of tools that are appropriate for generating that knowledge. Not just *any* methodology will suffice. For positivists, methodology should be experimental and manipulative. A mind-independent reality that can be objectively known requires methodologies that can tap into such a reality free from the control of confounding factors. A mind-independent reality also requires that "questions and/or hypotheses be stated in propositional form and subjected to empirical tests to verify them; possible confounding conditions must be carefully controlled [manipulated] to prevent outcomes from being improperly influenced" (Guba & Lincoln, 1994, p. 110).

Postpositivists share a similar view. However, given that all measurement is subject to error, the researcher must engage in a process of *critical multiplism*, in which she takes multiple observations and measurements (that are each subject to different types of error), in order to identify potential sources of error, and then creates control for them, thus better approximating reality. Through independent replication the scientist learns more about the ontological validity of her model. This in turn enables her to engage in the falsification (rather than verification) of hypotheses and theories.

Constructivism challenges the idea that knowledge exists freely in the world and that objective measurement procedures can be designed to capture such a world. All information is subject to interpretation by the researcher and, as such, the relationship between the researcher and subject matter is a central focus of methodology.

**Philosophical assumptions are interactive.** Note that questions about episte-mology, ontology, axiology, and methodology are deeply connected with one another. "Views of the nature of knowledge interact with views of the nature of reality: what there is affects what can be known, and what we think can be known often affects what we think exists" (Thagard, 2007, p. xi). For instance, if one subscribes to the belief that there is a reality independent of the researcher, then scientific inquiry should be conducted in a way that is objectively detached. This will enable the researcher to discover "how things really are" and "how things really work." This in turn requires that the researcher identifies a set of method-ologies that are capable of reflecting objective reality in a pure or relatively uncon-taminated manner. From this perspective, questions that concern axiology (values) fall outside the realm of legitimate scientific inquiry.

**Conclusion.** When we articulate our philosophical assumptions, we are articulat-ing the set of decisions we have made prior to engaging in scientific or therapeutic practice. These decisions involve asking and answering questions that are not empirical but rather preanalytic in nature (e.g., What type of knowledge do we want to accumulate and why? How will we organize and construct that system of knowledge? What qualifies as "real or genuine evidence," and how should it be interpreted?). The answers to these questions form the foundation upon which empirical work is carried out. Just as we need to lay a foundation before we can build a stable house, so too do we need to lay down our philosophical assumptions before we can engage in scientific activity that is consistent and coherent.

# Part 2: Pepper's Four Worldviews and Their Relation to Clinical Psychology

Although worldviews can and have been categorized in many different ways, Pepper's (1942) classification scheme is useful in reflecting upon the components, assumptions, and concerns that drive theory and research in different areas of clinical and applied psychology.

The core of Pepper's thesis is that humans are not prone to engaging in complex, abstract thought, and they tend to rely on commonsense guides or "root metaphors" to keep their intellectual bearings. He argued that the major, relatively adequate philosophical positions can be clustered into one of four core models ("world hypotheses"): formism, mechanism, organicism, and contextualism. Each uses a different root metaphor as a kind of thumbnail guide that suggests how knowledge ought to be justified or represented, how new knowledge should be obtained, and how truth can be evaluated (for more, see Berry, 1984; Hayes et al., 1988; Hayes, 1993).

These worldviews are autonomous (because their basic assumptions are incommensurable) and allow content in different domains of knowledge to be described with precision (i.e., applying a restricted set of principles to specific events) and scope (i.e., analyses that explain a comprehensive range of events across a variety of situations). Their truth criteria provide a way of evaluating the validity of scientific analyses that emerge from a particular worldview. In the following section I consider each of these worldviews and then discuss how they set the stage for particular kinds of clinical research and practice.

## Formism

The root metaphor of formism is the recurrence of recognizable forms. An easy way to think of formism is that it is a form of philosophy based on the action of naming—that is, knowing how to characterize a particular event. For instance, smartphones constitute a class or category in which many particulars are said to "participate." The truth or validity of an analysis is based on simple correspondence: an individual member possesses characteristics that correspond to the characteristics of the class. A brick is not a smartphone because it is not electronic and you cannot make calls with it; a desktop computer is electronic and you can make calls with it, but it is not a smartphone, in part, because it is not portable; and so on. The task of scientists is to create a comprehensive set of categories or names, and the truth or value of their actions can be determined from the exhaustive nature of this categorical system. "If the system has a category for all kinds of things, and things for all categories, then the categorical system is deemed to correspond with the *a priori* assumed world of things and events" (Wilson, Whiteman, & Bordieri, 2013, p. 29). When applied to psychology, formism suggests that phenomena can be understood by assigning them to specific classes or types, and for that reason some nosologies or personality theories provide good examples of formism.

## *Mechanism*

Mechanism is a more sophisticated variant of formism and arguably the position that underpins most empirical work in contemporary psychology. Its root metaphor is the commonsense "machine." This approach "assumes the *a priori* status of parts, but goes on to build models involving parts, relations, and forces animating such a system" (Wilson et al., 2013, p. 29). When applied to psychology, the purpose of science is to identify the parts and their relationships (e.g., mental constructs, neurological connections) that mediate between input (environment) and output (behavior), and to identify the operating conditions or forces that are necessary and sufficient for mechanisms to successfully function (e.g., attention, motivation, cognitive capacity, information). (Note that "mechanism" has sometimes been used within applied psychology as an epithet, meaning "robot-like" or "unfeeling." This is not its meaning in philosophy of science, and I don't suggest any negative connotations when I use the term.)

Within a mechanistic worldview, causation is contiguous: "one step in the mechanism (e.g., a mental state) puts in motion the next step (e.g., another mental state)" (De Houwer, Barnes-Holmes, & Barnes-Holmes, 2016; chapter 7 of this volume, p. 122). Stated more precisely, mechanism argues that mental processes operate under a restricted set of conditions, and these are separate from, but co-vary with, the environmental context under which behavior is observed. Thus, the unit of analysis for mechanisms (mental or physiological) is the component element of the machine (e.g., a process, entity, or construct). Although some of these elements are directly observable in principle (e.g., neurons), in psychology they often are inferred from changes in behavior due to organismic interactions with the environment (see Bechtel, 2008).

Note that the root metaphor of a machine applies both to the knower and what is known. "The knower relates to the world by producing an internal copy of it, through mechanical transformation. This epistemological stance preserves both the knower and the known intact and basically unchanged by their relation" (Hayes et al., 1988, p. 99). Analyses are considered "true" or "valid" when the internal copy of reality (the hypothesized model or theory) maps onto the world as it is. This is a more elaborated version of the correspondence-based truth criterion of formism. How well a particular system reflects reality is evaluated by the extent to which other independent knowers corroborate it through predictive verification or falsification.

Because mechanists view complexity as being built up from parts, they tend to be reductionistic. The goal of science is to identify the most basic units that fill the temporal gaps between one event and another (e.g., mental representations, past behaviors, neural activity, emotions). This is typically achieved by building facsimiles of reality (internal copies) in which truth or validity is determined from its objective correspondence with that reality (e.g., mental models). Description and theoretical prediction constitute satisfactory forms of scientific explanation, given that they allow one to evaluate correspondence between theory and reality. The result (at least in psychology) is a largely hypothetico-deductive and theory-driven research agenda, one that downplays distal factors (histories of learning) and emphasizes behavior as the product of internal, independent causal agents or systems.

**Clinical implications.** The most common extension of mechanistic thinking in clinical psychology is the formulation of theories and models that detail the component elements and operating conditions of the mental machine, which mediates between environment and dysfunctional behavior. In either case, the source and solution to clinical problems can be found in the elements that compose the system: through the addition, revision, and elimination of mechanisms and/or operating conditions, one can impact the probability of clinical outcomes. Given a truth criteria based on the elaborated correspondence between the proposed system and reality, the mechanist considers the predictive verification of theories and therapies essential.

These philosophical assumptions are inherent in many cognitive and behavioral therapies. For example, the impact of stimulus pairings or operant contingencies in early behavior therapy might be explained by the formation and revision of stimulus-response or stimulus-stimulus associations (e.g., see Foa, Steketee, & Rothbaum, 1989). Similarly, the impact of cognitive therapy (Beck, 1993; Mahoney, 1974) might be explained by the cognitive schemas, faulty information-processing styles, irrational cognitions, or automatic thoughts that are believed to mediate the relationship between environmental input and behavioral/emotional output. As a result of these explanations, the target of intervention would be a change in the occurrence of these events, through restructuring, reappraisal, the modification of core beliefs, and so on (e.g., Hofmann, 2011; see chapters 21 and 22).

## *Organicism*

The root metaphor at the core of organicism is that of the growing organism. Organicists view organic development as beginning in one form, growing and transitioning in an expected pattern, and then ultimately culminating in another form that was inherent in what came before. Consider, for example, the organic process through which a seed turns into a tree. There are rules of transition between states or phases, and stability between periods of change, but once rules are identified and explained, the states, phases, and stability are seen as part of a single coherent process. In order to explain the present and predict the future, we must understand the basic rules that govern development and how these rules operate across both time and context (Reese & Overton, 1970; Super & Harkness, 2003).

Organicism is teleological. Just as a seed may be "meant to be" a tree, stages of development make sense only by knowing where they are headed. The truth criterion of organicism is coherence. "When a network of interrelated facts converges on a conclusion, the coherence of this network renders this conclusion 'true.' All contradictions of understanding originate in incomplete knowledge of the whole organic process. When the whole is known, the contradictions are removed and the 'organic whole…is found to have been implicit in the fragments'" (Hayes et al., 1988, p. 100).

Organicists reject the idea of simple, linear cause-effect explanations, preferring a more synthetic (interactional) approach. They argue that a system cannot be understood by breaking it down into its component elements. The whole is not a combination of individual parts; rather, the whole is basic, with parts having meaning only with regard to the whole. The identification of parts or stages is to some degree an arbitrary exercise for the purpose of investigation, but the order of those stages is not. For instance, "where the line is drawn marking the difference between an infant and a toddler may be arbitrary, but that infancy precedes toddlerhood is nonarbitrary and is presumed to reflect the *a priori* organization of development" (Wilson et al., 2013, p. 30).

## Contextualism

The root metaphor of contextualism is the ongoing "act in context." Acts can be anything done in and with a current and historical context and are defined by their purpose and meaning. Contexts can "proceed outward spatially to include all of the universe…[or] backward in time infinitely to include the remotest antecedent, or forward in time to include the most delayed consequence" (Hayes & Brownstein, 1986, p. 178). The act in context is not a description of some static event that occurred in the past. Instead it is a purposeful activity that takes place here and now within physical, social, and temporal contexts. Thus, in contextualism (as in mechanism and organicism), relations and forces may be described. However, the described organization of those forces and relations is not assumed to reflect some a priori organization of the world (as is the case with formism or mechanism) nor some progression toward an "ideal form" (as is the case with organicism). Rather, speaking of the parts and relations is itself the action of scientists who operate in and with their own contexts and for their own purposes (Hayes, 1993). Consequently, scientific activity based on contextualistic thinking (within psychology) is not concerned with descriptions of the "real world" but rather "verbal analyses that permit basic and applied researchers, and practitioners, to predict and influence the behavior of individuals and groups" (De Houwer, Barnes-Holmes, & Barnes-Holmes; chapter 7 of this volume, p. 124).

Note that an act in context can vary from the most proximal behavioral instance (e.g., social anxiety as one interacts with colleagues here and now) to temporally distal and remote behavioral sequences (e.g., the impact a particular experience two years ago has on choosing whether to attend a social gathering in several days' time). What brings order to this spread of possibility is the pragmatic goal of an analyst (see Barnes-Holmes, 2000; Morris, 1988; Wilson et al., 2013). The metric of truth is neither correspondence nor coherence with a mind-independent reality but simply anything that facilitates successful working (this is the same truth criterion previously mentioned in the section on constructivism, and indeed constructivists are often contextualists).

There are, however, varieties of scientific contextualism. In order to know what successfully works, one must know what one is working toward: there must be a clear a priori statement of the scientist's or practitioner's goal or intent (Hayes, 1993). Descriptive contextualists (dramaturgists, narrative psychologists, post-modernists, social constructionists) are focused on analyses that help them appreciate the participation of history and circumstance in the whole; functional contextualists are trying to predict and influence behavior with precision, scope, and depth (Hayes, 1993). Because of this, contextualism is relativistic—what is considered true differs from one scientist to another based on respective goals.

**Clinical implications.** Contextualism focuses the clinical researcher and practitioner on the meaning and purpose of a person's thoughts, feelings, and actions in a given context. Humanistic psychology tends toward a descriptive contextualistic position in which therapists seek to appreciate the wholeness of a psychological event (Schneider, 2011). Many forms of modern cognitive and behavioral methods, such as acceptance and commitment therapy (ACT; Hayes et al., 1999), functional analytic psychotherapy (Kanter, Tsai, & Kohlenberg, 2010), integrative behavioral couples therapy (Jacobson & Christensen, 1998), and behavioral activation (Jacobson, Martell, & Dimidjian, 2001), consciously adopt the core of a functional-contextual position. Others, such as dialectical behavior therapy (Linehan, 1993; Lynch, Chapman, Rosenthal, Kuo, & Linehan, 2006), mindfulness-based cognitive therapy (Segal et al., 2001), and rational-emotive behavior therapy (Ellis & Dryden, 2007), mix the contextual perspective with elements of mechanistic thinking.

ACT can be used as a brief example to help show how contextualistic thinking takes the scientist or practitioner down a different pathway than mechanistic perspectives. Broadly speaking, ACT does not focus on the content of a thought, attempt to manipulate its form or frequency, or concern itself with the extent to which it is "real." Instead it pays close attention to what *function* the thought, feeling, or behavior has for the client in a given context. Consider the example of a public speaker who encounters the thought *I'm going to have a panic attack* as she walks toward a podium. An ACT therapist might not assume that this thought is necessarily harmful or that it has to be eradicated or revised. Rather he might ask, "How can you relate to this thought in a way that will foster what you want?"

The therapist adopts this approach because he views cognitions, emotions, beliefs, and dispositions as dependent variables (actions) and not as (the ultimate) contiguous causes of other dependent variables, such as overt behavior. In order to predict and influence the relationship between, say, thoughts and overt behavior, the therapist needs to identify the independent variables that can be directly manipulated in order to alter that relationship, and—from the therapist's perspective—only contextual variables are open to direct manipulation (Hayes & Brownstein, 1986). Mental mechanisms (e.g., associations in memory, schemas, semantic networks, or propositions) and the hypothesized forces that bind them are (at best) more dependent variables—they are not functional causes. That same truth criterion (successful working) also applies to clients who are "encouraged to abandon any interest in the literal truth of their own thoughts or evaluations…[and] instead…are encouraged to embrace a passionate and ongoing interest in how to live according to their values" (Hayes, 2004, p. 647).

# Part 3: Selection, Evaluation, and Communication Among Worldviews

Now that I've discussed a number of worldviews and how they inform clinical thinking and practice, you may be asking yourself a new set of questions about selection, evaluation, and communication. For instance, exactly how, when, and why did you decide to subscribe to a particular worldview, and is your belief system any better or more useful than that of your peers? Given their fundamental differences, can proponents of one worldview ever communicate and interact with those adopting another perspective? It is to these questions that I now turn.

## *Worldview Selection*

People may find themselves adhering to a particular worldview for several reasons. First, their philosophical orientation (and thus theoretical predilections) may be partially determined by individual differences, such as temperament and personality attributes (e.g., Babbage & Ronan, 2000; Johnson, Germer, Efran, & Overton, 1988). Second, worldviews may not be consciously selected but rather implicitly thrust upon us by the prevailing scientific, cultural, historical, and social contexts in which we find ourselves embedded. In other words, scientists may assimilate or inherit the philosophical framework that underpins the dominant zeitgeist of their field during their training. Thus worldview selection may be to some extent irrational (Pepper, 1942; Feyerabend, 2010; Kuhn, 1962; although see Lakatos, 1978, for arguments centered on rational research-program selection). For instance, once prediction is implicitly adopted as a scientific aim, then (mental) mechanistic explanations may be simpler and "commonsense." If your goal is to predict and influence behavior, a contextual position may seem more valuable. Third, people can evaluate the different types of scientific outcomes that are produced when different worldviews are adopted and effectively "vote with their feet" (Hayes, 1993, p. 18). The popularity of worldviews seems to shift across time, both within and between scientific communities (Kuhn, 1962). Psychological science is no exception, with a variety of metatheoretical paradigms, theories, and empirical issues gaining prominence at one time or another.

## Worldview Evaluation

Although popular convention, personality disposition, or matters of taste may guide the selection of any particular worldview, the standards of evaluation applied to that worldview are specified. When we evaluate a particular product of scientific activity (e.g., a finding, theory, or therapy) as being either good or satisfactory, we are basically asking whether that activity is consistent or coherent with the internal requirements of a worldview and with the consumers of new knowledge.

**Evaluating one's own worldview.** One reason to clarify your own philosophical assumptions is that it allows you to evaluate your own scientific activity. For instance, if one adopts a positivist (realist) position, theories are "mirrors" that vary in the extent to which they reflect the world "as it really is." Evaluation and progress therefore require that standards be applied to scientific inquiry that lead to the development of mirrors that best reflect reality. Postpositivists (critical realists) take a similar (if qualified) position, wherein researchers develop theories that are akin to dirty mirrors contaminated by error and bias. Standards of evaluation and progress involve polishing theoretical mirrors so as to remove distortion in order to represent reality as closely as possible. A researcher can best test a knowledge claim of this kind with a hypothetico-deductive model of theory development, in which highly precise predictions are extended to relatively unexplored domains (see Bechtel, 2008; Gawronski & Bodenhausen, 2015).

Theory testing looks quite different if one takes a contextualistic or constructivist stance. In these worldviews, theories are merely tools with which to achieve some end. Consider how a commonsense tool, say a hammer, could be evaluated: "A hammer is a good 'hammer' if it allows the carpenter to drive a nail. It would not make sense to say that the hammer does so because it accurately refers to the nail or reflects the nail" (Wilson et al., 2013, p. 30). Similarly, a theory is considered a good theory if it allows the scientist to achieve some desired outcome. In this case, theory evaluation involves determining the consistency with which models or theories can be shown to lead to useful interventions across a range of situations (e.g., see Hayes, Barnes-Holmes, & Wilson, 2012; Long, 2013).

**Evaluating the worldview of others.** When evaluating research programs based on a worldview other than your own, it is inherently dogmatic to apply criteria that emerge from your own worldview. A great deal of useless and counterproductive energy has been spent doing so in both basic and applied psychological science. For instance, researchers and therapists adhering to a functional-contextual perspective might question why their colleagues are so preoccupied with pieces of the mental machinery and their operating conditions, when doing so may depreciate the role that histories of learning and contextual variables play in how thoughts lead to other actions. Mechanists may counter that contextualists are not interested in scientific understanding—they are mere "technicians" or "problem solvers" who manipulate the environment in order to produce changes in behavior without any appreciation of the mechanisms that mediate those changes.

What should be clear, however, is that these arguments are pseudoconflicts—an attempt by proponents of one worldview to position their own philosophical assumptions (and thus scientific goals and values) as ultimately right and the worldview of others as wrong. Yet philosophical assumptions cannot be proven to be right or wrong because they are not the result of evidence—they define what is to be considered "evidence." The standards developed within a given worldview can be applied only to the products that emerge from that approach (in much the same way that the rules that make sense within one sport (soccer) cannot be used to govern the activity of another (say, basketball). Furthermore, no worldview is strengthened by showing the weaknesses of other positions.

There are four legitimate forms of evaluation. One is to improve your own scientific products as measured against the criteria appropriate to your approach. A second is less obvious but professionally helpful and collegial: enter into the assumptions of colleagues that differ from your own and then help them improve the scientific products as measured against the criteria that are appropriate to those assumptions. A third is to clearly articulate the assumptions and purposes that underpin your scientific activity and note (nonevaluatively) how they differ from others. For instance, you can describe the root metaphor and truth criterion that you've adopted, and how your analyses are carried out from this perspective, without insisting that others with different assumptions do the same. A fourth approach is to note the goals and uses of science by consumers (e.g., government funders, clients) and to objectively assess whether research programs serve those ends.

## Communication and Collaboration Among Proponents of Different Worldviews

In light of the above, you might wonder if it's possible for adherents of one worldview to communicate and collaborate with those from another without sacrificing their respective goals and values in the process. The received wisdom in psychology is that communication across worldviews is *not* possible. A concrete example is the way researchers use the same words to refer to different concepts (e.g., "cognition" means very different things for mental-mechanistic and functional-contextual researchers; see chapter 7) or use different words to refer to a similar idea (e.g., "attentional allocation" or "stimulus discrimination"). The most common result of these difficulties appears to be either fights over perceived scientific legitimacy or an ignoring of the fruits of colleagues' labors.

There is a radically different way to think of this situation, however, and it helps explain why training in philosophy of science is now expected of practitioners. If scientific goals of different worldviews are orthogonal, it also means they cannot be in direct conflict with one another. Thus, there is no reason why developments within one tradition cannot be used to further the scientific agenda of the other. This book is organized around that core idea. Process-based therapy can be linked to evidence from different traditions. By appreciating legitimate differences, the different wings or waves of evidence-based therapy can complement each other.

One way that individuals from different traditions can achieve scientific cooperation is by adopting a metatheoretical perspective known as the functional-cognitive (FC) framework (see chapter 7 for a detailed treatment). According to this perspective, psychological science can be conducted at two different but supportive levels of analysis: a functional level that aims to explain behavior in terms of elements in the environment, and a cognitive level that aims to understand the mental mechanisms by which elements in the environment influence behavior. The FC framework does not interfere with the individual researcher's goals, nor does it pass judgment on those goals or the reasons behind them. Instead, it seeks a mutually supportive interaction. Research at the functional (contextual) level, for example, can provide knowledge about the environmental determinants of behavior, which can also be used to drive mental research and/or to constrain mental theorizing. So long as each approach remains committed to its form of explanation, knowledge gained at one level can be used to advance progress at the other (De Houwer, 2011). This metatheoretical framework has yielded benefits in several areas of research (for a recent review see Hughes, De Houwer, & Perugini, 2016), and there appears to be no reason not to extend it to clinical psychology and such issues as the differences among wings of behavioral and cognitive therapy (De Houwer, Barnes-Holmes, & Barnes-Holmes, 2016; see also chapter 7 of this volume).

## Conclusion

The main goal of this chapter was to introduce the topic of philosophy of science as it applies to clinical and applied psychology. Philosophical assumptions silently shape and guide our scientific activity and therapeutic practice. "Assumptions or 'world-views' are like the place one stands. What one sees and does is greatly determined by the place from which one views. In this way, assumptions are neither true nor false, but rather provide different views of different landscapes" (Ciarrochi, Robb, & Godsell, 2005, p. 81). Appreciating the role of philosophical assumptions tempers and guides collegial interaction within the field and is an important context for research evaluation, communication, and collaboration. Philosophical assumptions make a difference, whether in the laboratory or the therapy room.

## References

Babbage, D. R., & Ronan, K. R. (2000). Philosophical worldview and personality factors in traditional and social scientists: Studying the world in our own image. *Personality and Individual Differences, 28*(2), 405–420.

Barnes-Holmes, D. (2000). Behavioral pragmatism: No place for reality and truth. *Behavior Analyst, 23*(2), 191–202.

Bechtel, W. (2008). *Mental mechanisms: Philosophical perspectives on cognitive neuroscience.* New York: Routledge.

Beck, A. T. (1993). Cognitive therapy: Past, present, and future. *Journal of Consulting and Clinical Psychology, 61*(2), 194–198.

Berry, F. M. (1984). An introduction to Stephen C. Pepper's philosophical system via world hypotheses: A study in evidence. *Bulletin of the Psychonomic Society, 22*(5), 446–448.

Blaikie, N. (2007). *Approaches to social enquiry: Advancing knowledge.* Cambridge, UK: Polity Press.

Ciarrochi, J., Robb, H., & Godsell, C. (2005). Letting a little nonverbal air into the room: Insights from acceptance and commitment therapy part 1: Philosophical and theoretical underpinnings. *Journal of Rational-Emotive and Cognitive-Behavior Therapy, 23*(2), 79–106.

De Houwer, J. (2011). Why the cognitive approach in psychology would profit from a functional approach and vice versa. *Perspectives on Psychological Science, 6*(2), 202–209.

De Houwer, J., Barnes-Holmes, Y., & Barnes-Holmes, D. (2016). Riding the waves: A functional-cognitive perspective on the relations among behaviour therapy, cognitive behaviour therapy and acceptance and commitment therapy. *International Journal of Psychology, 51*(1), 40–44.

Dougher, M. J. (1995). A bigger picture: Cause and cognition in relation to differing scientific frameworks. *Journal of Behavior Therapy and Experimental Psychiatry, 26*(3), 215–219.

Ellis, A., & Dryden, W. (2007). *The practice of rational emotive behavior therapy* (2nd ed.). New York: Springer.

Feyerabend, P. (2010). *Against method* (4th ed.). New York: Verso Books.

Foa, E. B., Steketee, G., & Rothbaum, B. O. (1989). Behavioral/cognitive conceptualizations of post-traumatic stress disorder. *Behavior Therapy, 20*(2), 155–176.

Forsyth, B. R. (2016). Students' epistemic worldview preferences predict selective recall across history and physics texts. *Educational Psychology, 36*(1), 73–94.

Gawronski, B., & Bodenhausen, G. V. (2015). Theory evaluation. In B. Gawronski & G. V. Bodenhausen (Eds.), *Theory and explanation in social psychology* (pp. 3–23). New York: Guilford Press.

Guba, E. G., & Lincoln, Y. S. (1994). Competing paradigms in qualitative research. In N. K. Denzin & Y. S. Lincoln (Eds.), *The Sage handbook of qualitative research* (pp. 105–117). Thousand Oaks, CA: Sage Publications.

Hayes, S. C. (1993). Analytic goals and the varieties of scientific contextualism. In S. C. Hayes, L. J., Hayes, H. W., Reese, & T. R., Sarbin (Eds.), *Varieties of scientific contextualism* (pp. 11–27). Oakland, CA: New Harbinger Publications.

Hayes, S. C. (1997). Behavioral epistemology includes nonverbal knowing. In L. J. Hayes & P. M. Ghezzi (Eds.), *Investigations in behavioral epistemology* (pp. 35–43). Oakland, CA: New Harbinger Publications.

Hayes, S. C. (2004). Acceptance and commitment therapy, relational frame theory, and the third wave of behavioral and cognitive therapies. *Behavior Therapy, 35*(4), 639–665.

Hayes, S. C., Barnes-Holmes, D., & Wilson, K. G. (2012). Contextual behavioral science: Creating a science more adequate to the challenge of the human condition. *Journal of Contextual Behavioral Science, 1*(1–2), 1–16.

Hayes, S. C., & Brownstein, A. J. (1986). Mentalism, behavior-behavior relations, and a behavior-analytic view of the purposes of science. *Behavior Analyst, 9*(2), 175–190.

Hayes, S. C., Hayes, L. J., & Reese, H. W. (1988). Finding the philosophical core: A review of Stephen C. Pepper's world hypotheses: A study in evidence. *Journal of the Experimental Analysis of Behavior, 50*(1), 97–111.

Hayes, S. C., Strosahl, K. D., & Wilson, K. G. (1999). *Acceptance and commitment therapy: An experiential approach to behavior change.* New York: Guilford Press.

Hofmann, S. G. (2011). *An introduction to modern CBT: Psychological solutions to mental health problems.* Oxford, UK: Wiley.

Hughes, S., De Houwer, J., & Perugini, M. (2016). The functional-cognitive framework for psychological research: Controversies and resolutions. *International Journal of Psychology, 51*(1), 4–14.

Jacobson, N. S., & Christensen, A. (1998). *Acceptance and change in couple therapy: A therapist's guide to transforming relationships.* New York: W. W. Norton.

Jacobson, N. S., Martell, C. R., & Dimidjian, S. (2001). Behavioral activation treatment for depression: Returning to contextual roots. *Clinical Psychology: Science and Practice, 8*(3), 255–270.

Johnson, J. A., Germer, C. K., Efran, J. S., & Overton, W. F. (1988). Personality as the basis for theoretical predilections. *Journal of Personality and Social Psychology, 55*(5), 824–835.

Kanter, J., Tsai, M., & Kohlenberg, R. J. (2010). *The practice of functional analytic psychotherapy.* New York: Springer.

Klepac, R. K., Ronan, G. F., Andrasik, F., Arnold, K. D., Belar, C. D., Berry, S. L., et al. (2012). Guidelines for cognitive behavioral training within doctoral psychology programs in the United States: Report of the Inter-Organizational Task Force on Cognitive and Behavioral Psychology Doctoral Education. *Behavior Therapy, 43*(4), 687–697.

Kuhn, T. S. (1962). *The structure of scientific revolutions.* Chicago: University of Chicago Press.

Lakatos, I. (1978). *The methodology of scientific research programmes.* Philosophical papers (Vol. 1). Cambridge, UK: Cambridge University Press.

Laudan, L. (1978). *Progress and its problems: Toward a theory of scientific growth.* Berkeley: University of California Press.

Lerner, R. M., & Damon, W. E. (Eds.). (2006). *Handbook of child psychology* (Vol. 1, theoretical models of human development, 6th ed.). Hoboken, NJ: Wiley.

Lincoln, Y. S., Lynham, S. A., & Guba, E. G. (2011). Paradigmatic controversies, contradictions, and emerging confluences, revisited. In N. K. Denzin & Y. S. Lincoln (Eds.), *The Sage handbook of qualitative research* (4th ed., pp. 97–128). Thousand Oaks, CA: Sage Publications.

Linehan, M. M. (1993). *Cognitive behavioral treatment of borderline personality disorder.* New York: Guilford Press.

Long, D. M. (2013). Pragmatism, realism, and psychology: Understanding theory selection criteria. *Journal of Contextual Behavioral Science, 2*(3–4), 61–67.

Lynch, T. R., Chapman, A. L., Rosenthal, M. Z., Kuo, J. R., & Linehan, M. M. (2006). Mechanisms of change in dialectical behavior therapy: Theoretical and empirical observations. *Journal of Clinical Psychology, 62*(4), 459–480.

Mahoney, M. J. (1974). *Cognition and behavior modification.* Cambridge, MA: Ballinger.

Morris, E. K. (1988). Contextualism: The world view of behavior analysis. *Journal of Experimental Child Psychology, 46*(3), 289–323.

Pepper, S. C. (1942). *World hypotheses: A study in evidence.* Berkeley: University of California Press.

Reese, H. W., & Overton, W. F. (1970). Models of development and theories of development. In L. R. Goulet & B. P. Baltes (Eds.), *Life-span developmental psychology: Research and theory* (pp. 115–145). New York: Academic Press.

Reyna, L. J. (1995). Cognition, behavior, and causality: A board exchange of views stemming from the debate on the causal efficacy of human thought. *Journal of Behavior Therapy and Experimental Psychiatry, 26*(3), 177.

Schneider, K. J. (2011). *Existential-integrative psychotherapy: Guideposts to the core of practice.* New York: Routledge.

Segal, Z. V., Williams, J. M. G., & Teasdale, J. D. (2001). *Mindfulness-based cognitive therapy for depression: A new approach to preventing relapse.* New York: Guilford Press.

Skinner, B. F. (1974). *About behaviorism.* New York: Alfred A. Knopf.

Super, C. M., & Harkness, S. (2003). The metaphors of development. *Human Development, 46*(1), 3–23.

Thagard, P. (2007). *Philosophy of psychology and cognitive science.* Amsterdam: Elsevier.

Von Glasersfeld, E. (1995). A constructivist approach to teaching. In L. P. Steffe & J. E. Gale (Eds.), *Constructivism in education* (pp. 3–15). Hillsdale, NJ: Lawrence Erlbaum.

Von Glasersfeld, E. (2001). The radical constructivist view of science. *Foundations of Science, 6*(1–3), 31–43.

Wilson, K. G., Whiteman, K., & Bordieri, M. (2013). The pragmatic truth criterion and values in contextual behavioral science. In S. Dymond and B. Roche (Eds.), *Advances in relational frame theory: Research and application* (pp. 27–47). Oakland, CA: New Harbinger Publications.

# CHAPTER 3

# Science in Practice

### Kelly Koerner, PhD
*Evidence-Based Practice Institute*

Evidence-based practice (EBP) originated in medicine to prevent errors and to improve health care outcomes (Sackett, Rosenberg, Gray, Haynes, & Richardson, 1996). In psychology EBP is defined as "the integration of the best available research with clinical expertise in the context of patient characteristics, culture, and preferences" (American Psychological Association Presidential Task Force on Evidence-Based Practice, 2006). In an evidence-based approach to decision making (Spring, 2007a, 2007b), the practitioner should:

1. Ask important questions about the care of individuals, communities, or populations.

2. Acquire the best available evidence regarding the question.

3. Critically appraise the evidence for validity and applicability to the problem at hand.

4. Apply the evidence by engaging in collaborative decision making regarding health with the affected individual(s) and/or group(s). (Appropriate decision making integrates the context, values, and preferences of the care recipient, as well as available resources, including professional expertise.)

5. Assess the outcome and disseminate the results.

EBP seems to be a straightforward process: get the relevant evidence, discuss it with the client, and then carry out the best practice. Yet doing so requires overcoming two sets of significant challenges: (1) finding and appraising evidence relevant to many clinical decisions is difficult, and (2) clinical judgment is notoriously fallible.

# Challenges with Using the Evidence Base to Inform Clinical Decisions

To adopt an evidence-based approach to treat a client's specific problems, practitioners should prepare by reviewing relevant research literature to identify the most effective assessment and treatment options and evaluate evidence claims as scientific knowledge accumulates and evolves. Yet doing so can be difficult or impossible.

Research evidence comes to us more easily than ever before: passively through the day-to-day use of social media or actively when we use a search engine for a specific client-related question. In both cases, however, it's not the quality or merits of the research evidence that drive what we see. Regularly cited articles become ever more likely to be cited, creating an impression of greater quality and masking other evidence (the Matthew effect; see Merton, 1968). Search engines grant higher page positions based on algorithms unrelated to evidence quality.

Consequently, for a balanced evaluation of evidence, practitioners must increasingly rely on experts to distill scientific findings into rigorously curated, aggregated formats, such as practice guidelines, lists of empirically supported treatments, evidence-based procedure registries, and the like. Expert aggregations use an evidentiary hierarchy: meta-analyses and other systematic reviews of randomized controlled trials (RCTs) at the top; followed by individual RCTs; followed by weaker forms of evidence, such as nonrandomized trials, observational studies, case series reports, and qualitative research.

Not only is this fixed evidentiary hierarchy itself controversial (Tucker & Roth, 2006), the existing literature provides little evidence to guide the selection of conditional plans that have a high chance of success: If a client presents marker A, will intervention B predictably and consistently produce change C? For example, say a late-twenties professionally employed Latina woman seeks treatment for depression. Based on the evidence, behavioral activation could be a good choice (Collado, Calderón, MacPherson, & Lejuez, 2016; Kanter et al., 2015). However, if in addition to depression the client has common co-occurring problems such as insomnia or marital conflict, the guidance is either absent or confusing: some evidence guides the practitioner to treat insomnia and depression concurrently (Manber et al., 2008; Stepanksi & Rybarczyk, 2006), while other evidence supports combining depression treatment and marital therapy to help with depression and marital satisfaction (Jacobson, Dobson, Fruzzetti, Schmaling, & Salusky, 1991). If additional common problems are added, such as problem drinking or child behavior problems in the home, the literature provides little or no guidance. Evidence to directly inform decision making for even common branches, such as those regarding sequencing versus combining treatments, is scarce.

In part, the lack of data to inform clinical decisions is an unavoidable consequence of research challenges. Science takes time. The study of psychopathology and psychotherapeutic change is complex. The practitioner's need for nuanced evidence may always outstrip what is practically possible in even the most practice-focused research agenda. But in important ways, the lack of evidence to guide routine clinical decisions is due to more pernicious problems with the methods used to conduct psychotherapy research.

For historical reasons, the research methods used to study behavioral interventions borrowed heavily from methods and metaphors used to develop and test pharmaceuticals. In this predominant psychotherapy-as-technology stage model, stage I consists of basic science being translated into clinical applications. Pilot testing and feasibility trials begin on new and untested treatments, and treatment manuals, training programs, and adherence and competence measures are developed. In stage II, RCTs that emphasize internal validity evaluate the efficacy of promising treatments. In stage III, efficacious treatments are subjected to effectiveness trials and are evaluated with regard to their external validity and transportability to community settings (Rounsaville, Carroll, & Onken, 2001). Important updates have reinvigorated the stage model (Onken, Carroll, Shoham, Cuthbert, & Riddle, 2014), but methodological choices guided by the model have led to unintended consequences for the evidence base that interfere with its utility in guiding routine clinical decisions.

A core problem is that the independent variable to be studied and delivered in psychotherapy has come to be defined almost solely as the unit of the treatment manual, and the problem focus at the level of the psychiatric syndrome. The treatment manual codifies clinical procedures and their order into a protocol to be standardly repeated across therapists and clients by disorder. Manuals that specify protocols for treating depression, insomnia, problem drinking, couple distress, and parenting skills deficits, for example, could be relevant to the case example presented earlier, but each manualized protocol comprises many component strategies. Psychoeducation, self-monitoring, motivation enhancement, problem solving, activation assignments, values clarification, contingency management, shaping, self-management, and so on appear in nearly every manual. Most component strategies are not unique to a single manual but instead are common and duplicated across manuals. Specific protocols may vary in how they emphasize or coordinate these component elements (Chorpita & Daleiden, 2010)—the way procedures are chosen, repeated, or selectively applied, or their delivery format—even if the basic ingredients remain the same. Because researchers and therapists predominantly consider manuals as *the* unit of analysis, they ignore the fact that various manuals contain mostly the same ingredients. Each manual is treated as a distinct intervention with its own siloed research base (Chorpita, Daleiden, & Weisz, 2005; Rotheram-Borus, Swendeman, & Chorpita, 2012).

Strictly privileging manuals as *the* unit of intervention and analysis by disorder leads to unintended problems. Any change made to a manualized protocol could be a substantive departure. Even making a modification to better fit clients' needs or setting constraints may wipe out the relevance of existing evidence. For the researcher, this "ever-expanding list of multi-component manuals designed to treat a dizzying array of topographically defined syndromes and sub-syndromes creates a factorial research problem that is scientifically impossible to mount… [and] makes it increasingly difficult to teach what is known or to focus on what is essential" (Hayes, Luoma, Bond, Masuda, & Lillis, 2006, p. 2). For the practitioner, the choice becomes to either follow manuals to the T regardless of setting or client presentations and preferences, or accept responsibility for not knowing what outcomes can be expected if tailored treatment deviates from the manual.

Packaging knowledge and science at the unit of a "manual for a disorder" emphasizes differences among manuals even if there are overlapping common components. Researchers are incentivized for innovation, but as reimbursement becomes contingent on delivering evidence-based protocols, practitioners become incentivized to claim they are doing treatments with fidelity whether they are or not. Treatment developers then face pressure to develop quality control methods to protect client access to the bona fide version of the treatment, leading to protective steps, such as proprietary trademarking or therapist certification. Such steps then align the professional identities and allegiances of researchers and practitioners with particular branded protocols rather than with effective components linked to client need.

The rationale for rigid adherence to specific manuals is that the greater the therapist's adherence and competence in delivering the standardized, validated protocol, the more likely it is that clients will receive the treatment's active ingredients and thereby obtain the desired outcomes. If this assumption is true, then adherence and competence should be powerful predictors of outcome, and larger packages and protocols should in general show unique, theory-related curative ingredients.

The available research evidence only weakly supports this assumption. With some exceptions, researchers don't consistently find correlations between adherence or competence and treatment outcome (Branson, Shafran, & Myles, 2015; Webb, DeRubeis, & Barber, 2010). And while there are many successful theory-consistent meditational studies, there are also many large, well-designed studies that have failed to find unique, distinct, theory-related processes of change

(Morgenstern & McKay, 2007). If more focus was made on specific components and procedures, a focus on change processes could well be more successful, but using large manuals as the unit of analysis interferes with that possibility.

Adopting concepts and methods from pharmacotherapy research and development has produced other problems. The dose-response idea that a dosage of active ingredients produces uniform and linear patterns of client change does not fit the large individual differences in client responsivity observed in psychotherapy research. Clients differ in whether they are in fact absorbing the material and achieving desired changes in cognitions, emotions, and skills and whether these changes in turn lead to desired outcomes. As a result, large individual differences in client response occur even in treatments that have been standardized and with therapists who show high adherence to the treatment manual (Morgenstern & McKay, 2007).

Similarly, therapists aren't uniform in the same ways that pills are uniform. Nonspecific factors that are common across protocols, such as therapeutic alliance, have been viewed as being "akin to the binding on a pill, i.e., a minimum level of engagement is needed between therapist and patient in order to provide an avenue to transmit the specific curative elements of the approach" (Morgenstern & McKay, 2007, p. 102). Instead, therapists show significant variability rather than homogeneity (Laska, Smith, Wislocki, Minami, & Wampold, 2013), which may impact outcomes in specific ways.

To illustrate, consider work by Bedics, Atkins, Comtois, and Linehan (2012a, 2012b). They studied the relationship between therapeutic alliance and nonsuicidal self-injury in treatment delivered by expert behavioral and nonbehavioral therapists (2012a). Overall ratings of the therapeutic relationship did not predict reduced nonsuicidal self-injury. Instead, reductions were associated with the client's perception that the therapist blended specific aspects—affirming, controlling, and protecting—of the relationship. In a companion study (2012b), they found that among clients with expert nonbehavioral therapists, higher perceived levels of therapist affirmation were associated with *increased* nonsuicidal self-injury. They speculate that the affirmations of nonbehavioral therapists might have inadvertently been timed to reinforce nonsuicidal self-injury, whereas behavior therapists contingently provided warmth and autonomy for improvement. These findings illustrate the kinds of interplay between specific and nonspecific factors that may impact outcome. Treatment effects of even carefully standardized treatments aren't uniform or homogeneous, and research methods that force oversimplified understandings may limit scientific advancement.

Finally, social processes drive the crucial factors related to an EBP's reach, adoption, implementation, and sustainability at the organizational level (Glasgow, Vogt, & Boles, 1999). Historically, the stages of the psychotherapy-as-technology model move sequentially from efficacy trials to effectiveness evaluations, and only then to dissemination and implementation research. As a result, the research on crucial factors that influence external validity, clinical utility, and the intervention's reach, adoption, implementation, and sustainability in routine settings is conducted far too late in the development process (Glasgow et al., 1999). Little evidence is available to guide decision makers who face setting constraints about what they can and cannot change as they implement an EBP.

# The Challenges of Relying on Clinical Judgment

Evidence-based practice, by definition, includes clinical judgment, but gaps in the evidence mean that many clinical decisions are based solely on clinical judgment with little data to inform them. Unfortunately there are known weaknesses of clinical judgment.

Daniel Kahneman's book *Thinking, Fast and Slow* (2011) has popularized our understanding of these weaknesses. According to Kahneman's dual processing theory, we have two modes of processing information: system 1, a fast, associative, low-effort mode that uses heuristic shortcuts to simplify information and reach good-enough solutions, and system 2, a slower rule-based mode that relies on high-effort systematic reasoning.

The fast and frugal system 1 heuristics that help us quickly simplify complex situations leave us prone to a multitude of perception and reasoning biases and errors. Kahneman conceptualizes the two systems as hierarchical and discrete, and he posits that the more rational, conscious system 2 can constrain the irrational, unconscious system 1 to save us from biases and errors. However, experimental data show that these systems are integrated, not discrete or hierarchical, with both prone to "motivated reasoning" (Kunda, 1990; Kahan, 2012, 2013a). If quick, impressionistic thinking doesn't yield the answer we expect or want, we are prone to use our slower reasoning skills to fend off disconfirming evidence and seek data that fit our motivations rather than to reconsider our position (Kahan, 2013b).

In some professions, the work environment itself can correct these problems with judgment because work routines calibrate the unconscious processes of system 1 and train them to select suspected patterns for the attention of system 2's deliberate analysis. Kahneman and Klein (2009) give the example of experienced fire commanders and nurses in neonatal intensive care units who, over years of observing, studying, and debriefing, tacitly learn to detect cues that indicate subtle and complex patterns related to outcomes, such as signs that a building will collapse or an infant will develop an infection. The cues in their work environments signal the probable relationships among causes and outcomes of behavior (valid cues). In such high-validity or "kind" environments, there are stable relationships between objectively identifiable cues and subsequent events, or between cues and the outcomes of possible actions. Standard methods, clear feedback, and direct consequences for error make it possible to tacitly learn the rules of these environments. Hunches based on invalid cues are likely to be detected and assessed for error. Pattern recognition improves. According to Kahneman and Klein (2009), we can develop excellent, expert decision-making abilities, but only when two conditions are met:

1. The environment itself is characterized by stable relationships between objectively identifiable cues and subsequent events or between cues and the outcomes of possible actions (i.e., a high-validity environment).

2. There are opportunities to learn the rules of the environment.

In contrast, the environments in which most psychotherapy is practiced are low-validity or "wicked" environments that make tacit learning difficult (Hogarth, 2001). Cues are dynamic rather than static, predictability of outcomes is poor, and feedback is delayed, sparse, and ambiguous. Psychotherapy practice environments lack standard methods, clear feedback, and direct consequences and therefore provide few opportunities to learn the rules about the relation between clinical judgment, interventions, and outcomes. As a result, the tacit learning and development of intuitive expertise is blocked, which is a recipe for overconfidence (Kahneman & Klein, 2009). Within such low-validity environments, clinical judgment performs more poorly than linear algorithms based on statistical analysis. Even though often wrong, algorithms maintain above-chance accuracy by detecting and using weakly valid cues consistently, which accounts for much of an algorithm's advantage over people (Karelaia & Hogarth, 2008). Without structured routines, heuristic biases outside of our awareness function like an automatic spotlight, unconsciously simplifying complex situations. Perception, attention, and problem solving are caught by a subset of the elements right in front of us. In particular, without the right conditions we are likely to fall prey to the motivated reasoning and predictable biases defined by Heath and Heath (2013):

- Narrow framing—binary do/don't do rather than "What are the ways I could make X better?"

- Confirmation bias—we pretend we want "truth," but all we want is reassurance.

- Short-term emotion—we churn but the facts don't change.

- Overconfidence—we think we know more about how things in the future will unfold than we do.

# Disciplined Improvisation: Create Kind Environments with Heuristic Frameworks

What may be needed is to create the kind environments Kahneman and Klein (2009) and Hogarth (2001) describe: improved conditions in routine practice settings that support learning the relationship between clinical judgment, interventions, and outcomes. By doing so, practitioners can engage in disciplined improvisation as applied scientists, thereby improving the probability of good client outcomes. This requires practitioners to have not only functional scientific literacy but also structured routines that correct for the most common problems with clinical judgment. "Functional scientific literacy" means specialized knowledge related to probability and chance; the tools to think scientifically, and the propensity to do so; the tendency to exhaustively examine possibilities; the tendency to avoid my-side thinking; knowledge of some rules of formal and informal reasoning; and good argument-evaluation skills (Stanovich, West, & Toplak, 2011). This "mindware" is typically haphazardly acquired in professional training.

The rest of this chapter details a short set of structured routines the practitioner can use to correct for the most common problems with clinical judgment and thereby better calibrate the decision-making process and make it possible to do meaningful EBP. In general, each proposed routine helps to generate valid cues in order to detect and learn about stable relationships between objectively identifiable cues and subsequent events, or between cues and the outcomes of possible actions.

Many of the routines involve using a heuristic in a deliberate, structured work routine. Instead of an unconscious spotlight, the heuristic works like a manually controlled spotlight (Heath & Heath, 2013) or a checklist that improves performance (Gawande, 2010). Heuristics, when used deliberately, offer general strategies about how to find an answer or produce a solution in a reasonable time frame that is "good enough" for solving the problem at hand. They help the practitioner find the sweet spot of optimality, completeness, accuracy, precision, and execution time. The following list of routine practices, easily done in a typical workflow, suggests ways to standardize methods and obtain clear feedback that increase the opportunities to learn the rules about the relation between clinical judgment, interventions, and outcomes.

## *Standardize Key Work Routines*

Consider these three steps to standardize key work routines in order to transform a wicked environment into a kinder one that is disciplined enough to help you better detect valid cues and maximize your ability to learn from them.

### 1. USE PROGRESS MONITORING AND OTHER ASSESSMENT METHODS

Monitoring progress—regularly collecting data on the client's functioning, quality of life, and change regarding problems and symptoms—is the most important step in creating an environment with valid cues that make learning possible. Whether this step is called progress monitoring, client-reported outcomes, measurement-based care, or practice-based evidence, it has been demonstrated that tracking client change prevents dropout and treatment failure, reduces treatment length, and improves outcomes (e.g., Carlier et al., 2012; Goodman, McKay, & DePhilippis, 2013).

Where possible, use measures with standardized norms. When idiographic assessment is needed (i.e., comparing people with themselves), consider tools such as goal attainment scaling (Kiresuk, Smith, & Cardillo, 2014) or a "top problems" approach, in which clients identify the top three problems that matter to them and rate the severity of the problems on a scale of 0 to 10 weekly (Weisz et al., 2011). Further, consider standardizing any idiographic functional assessment used. Such standard assessment heuristics (if target problem is X, then use assessment method Y) may increase the speed and consistency with which problems are defined, providing a counter to the limitations of clinical judgment.

In particular, adopt heuristic rules about how to use progress-monitoring data to guide decisions in which bias is likely to be highest. For example, consider a routine such as requiring a change in the treatment plan every ten to twelve weeks if the client has not had at least a 50 percent improvement in symptoms using a validated measure (Unützer & Park, 2012).

More generally, routinely obtain high-quality standardized data to inform decisions. Consider creating invariant routines using evidence-based assessment methods, such as broad symptom rating scales, to identify presenting problems and maintaining factors; followed by more in-depth, specific rating scales; and then standardized clinical interviews (see Christon, McLeod, & Jensen-Doss, 2015, for more on evidence-based assessment). The key is to build routines that stay more or less stable and standardized to reduce method variability and thereby allow for the detection of valid signals identifying relationships between clinical judgment, interventions, and client outcome.

## 2. CONSIDER EXISTING EBPS FOR THE CLIENT'S TOP PROBLEM FIRST

Whenever possible, begin with a standardized treatment protocol for the most important problem. Beginning with a standard protocol offers many advantages. First, treating the most important problem may resolve others. Second, a standardized protocol gives you a benchmark against which to evaluate outcomes. Finally, following an evidence-based protocol allows you to limit your own inconsistency and my-side bias.

Again, although the evidence for protocols isn't strong enough to treat them as algorithms (step-by-step instructions that predictably and reliably yield the correct answer every time), protocols do offer heuristics that usefully simplify complex situations. Therapy protocols can be thought of as means-ends analyses. Means-ends analysis is a heuristic in which the ends are defined, and means to those ends are identified. If no workable means can be found, then the problem is broken into a hierarchy of subproblems, which may in turn be further broken into smaller subproblems until means are found to solve the problem.

The structured if-then guidelines that protocols provide help simplify complex clinical situations into a series of systematic prompts to think or act. Some protocols specify what problems the therapist should analyze and how to analyze them, and they provide further heuristics on how to combine component treatment strategies based on the nature and severity of a client's problems. In these ways, structuring clinical intervention with a protocol can help you detect valid cues and create a structured environment to promote learning.

Another useful standard routine is to systematically consider alternative, relevant treatment protocols as part of shared decision-making and consent-to-treatment conversations with clients. The more a practitioner clearly and deliberately considers alternative courses of action (Heath & Heath, 2013) and creates structured if-then tests, the more such feedback loops can help the practitioner detect whether the expected outcome happened (or didn't) and the more learnable the environment becomes. The PICO acronym is a way to frame a clinical question for a literature search that works well for shared decision making. *P* stands for "patient," "problem," or "population"; *I* for "intervention"; *C* for "comparison," "control," or "comparator"; and *O* for "outcomes" (Huang, Lin, & Demner-Fushman, 2006).

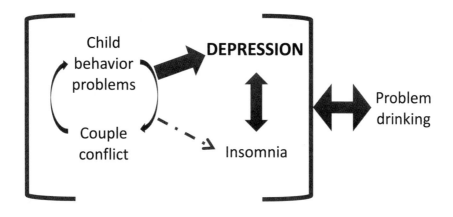

FIGURE 1. Visual diagram conceptualizing the relationship among client problems

For example, figure 1 returns to the earlier client example and shows the visual diagram the client and therapist made to capture the relationship among the client's problems. The client was most troubled by low mood, low energy, fatigue, difficulty concentrating, and feelings of intense guilt and hopelessness scoring in the severe range on the depression scale of the Depression Anxiety Stress Scales (Lovibond & Lovibond, 1995). In her view, her children's behavior problems, and the conflicts she and her husband had over parenting, made each problem worse and greatly impacted her mood, and sometimes her sleep. She turned to alcohol to escape painful emotions. Using PICO, the therapist can explain treatment options and likely outcomes for each of these problems (see table 1 for details).

# Table 1.  Modular component treatment plan

| Patient, Problem, Population | Intervention | Comparison and Outcome |
|---|---|---|
| #1 Depression | Behavioral activation (BA):<br><br>• 50–60% recover (Dimidjian et al., 2006)<br>• Try BA for 8 to 10 sessions, then reevaluate and consider alternative treatment if there is less than 50% change in depression on the Depression Anxiety Stress Scales. | Other options to consider:<br><br>• Natural recovery<br>• Antidepressant medication (ADM): ~1/3 respond, 1/3 partial response, relapse rate high when discontinuing<br>• Combine ADM and psychotherapy: ~53% report symptom reduction<br>• Interpersonal therapy and other active treatment: ~50% symptom reduction<br>• Behavioral couples therapy (Jacobson et al., 1991): 87% recover from depression; couples' distress also reduced |
| #2 Problem drinking | Brief intervention for problem drinking; one of the first activation assignments of BA (O'Donnell et al., 2014) | Reduces amount and frequency for many; less studied with women. Self-help or CBT, if brief, doesn't produce desired change on Alcohol Use Disorders Identification Test (AUDIT). |
| #3 Insomnia | CBT for insomnia (CBT-I); sleep log one of the first activation assignments of BA | CBT-I over medications; effectively improving insomnia may reduce other problems, especially depression. |
| #3 Parenting for child behavior problems | Self-help: Review *The Incredible Years: A Trouble-Shooting Guide for Parents of Children Aged 2–8* (Webster-Stratton, 2006) as an activation assignment. | If self-help doesn't achieve enough gains, consider an evidence-based parent-training program. |
| #3 Couples conflict | Devise activation assignments to strengthen conflict resolution and marital satisfaction. | If individual changes fail to produce sufficient desired changes, consider couples counseling. |

## 3. USE EXPLICIT CASE FORMULATION FOR HYPOTHESIS TESTING

When a standard treatment isn't available or doesn't yield desired results, practitioners use case formulation to tailor interventions, based on the assumption that tailored intervention will outperform the imperfect fit of standardized protocols for the individual. Unfortunately, case formulation has a meager evidence base. Kuyken's thorough and fair-minded review concludes that the evidence for case formulation's

reliability is "supportive of descriptive but not inferential hypotheses,"

validity is "very limited but promising," and

acceptability and usefulness are "mixed" (2006, p. 31).

Kuyken concludes, "There is no compelling evidence that [cognitive behavioral therapy] CBT formulation enhances therapy processes or outcomes" (p. 31).

While there is a lack of strong evidence to suggest that tailored interventions based on case formulations are superior, when used systematically case formulation can serve as a disciplined method to apply the scientific method to clinical work (Persons, 2008). When the therapist must go beyond existing protocols, purposefully specifying dependent and independent variables, combined with progress monitoring, can create conditions for the therapist to learn the stable relationships between judgment, interventions, and outcome; and this method can counter problems with bias and unconsciously applied heuristics. Persons (2008) and Padesky, Kuyken, and Dudley (2011) have articulated systematic approaches to case formulation. At a minimum, the heuristic to apply with case formulation is to specify the treatment targets (dependent variables) and robust change processes (independent variables).

## *Use a Treatment Target Hierarchy Informed by Science*

A treatment target hierarchy provides if-then guidelines that prescribe what to treat when. The target hierarchy constrains therapist variability and thereby makes it more likely that the most essential problems are addressed first, as a checklist does in an emergency room (Gawande, 2010). For example, Linehan (1999) has argued for organizing treatment targets into stages of treatment based on the severity of disorders. In pretreatment, her model directs the therapist to target maximizing initial motivation and commitment to treatment, thereby increasing engagement, and research (Norcross, 2002) supports this common factor. When behavioral dyscontrol is predominant, the therapist is to prioritize target behaviors in a commonsense way by their severity: life-threatening behaviors first, followed by therapy-interfering behavior, quality-of-life-interfering behavior, and improvement of skills.

Defined stages with target hierarchies provide a *process* to organize the allocation of session time, aiding the therapist's ability to think consistently and coherently; sort the relevant from irrelevant; and manage cognitive load. As discussed earlier, these types of checklists or decision-support tools are exactly what humans need in order to detect and respond consistently to valid cues. Treatment target hierarchies may be particularly helpful or needed when a client has multiple disorders and multiple crises that make it difficult to intervene consistently.

Using a treatment target hierarchy may also have effects, because the specific targeted *content* produces client change. For example, it appears that directly targeting suicidal behavior as a problem in itself (rather than seeing it as a sign or symptom that will resolve when the underlying disorder is treated) is associated with better outcomes (Comtois & Linehan, 2006). Treatment target hierarchies provide a practice-friendly way to consolidate scientific knowledge.

A target hierarchy can be constructed from disorder-specific processes or transdiagnostic processes drawn from psychopathology or treatment research. For example, in adapting disorder-specific targets to treat substance abuse, McMain, Sayrs, Dimeff, and Linehan (2007) didn't target stopping the use of illegal drugs and the abuse of prescribed drugs alone; they also targeted the physical and psychological discomfort associated with withdrawal and the urges to use, because withdrawal symptoms, urge intensity from the previous day, duration of urge, and urge intensity upon awakening predict relapse.

Additionally or alternatively, targets can be *transdiagnostic* (i.e., fundamental processes that contribute to or maintain disorders across what current diagnostic nomenclature label as distinct). Mansell, Harvey, Watkins, and Shafran (2009) categorize four views on transdiagnostic processes:

1. **Universal multiple processes maintain all or the majority of psychological disorders.** For example, processes include problematic self-focused attention, explicit memory bias, interpretational biases, and safety behaviors (e.g., Harvey, Watkins, Mansell, & Shafran, 2004).

2. **A range of cognitive and behavioral processes maintain a limited range of disorders, but one that is wider than traditional disorder-specific models.** For example, researchers propose that common processes of maladaptive cognitive appraisals, poor emotion regulation,

emotional avoidance, and emotionally driven behavior are related to anxiety and depression (Barlow, Allen, & Choate, 2004) or clinical perfectionism, core low self-esteem, mood intolerance, and interpersonal difficulties with eating disorder (Fairburn, Cooper, & Shafran, 2003).

3. **Symptom or psychological phenomena themselves, rather than diagnostic categories or labels, should be targeted.** For example, rather than thinking of bipolar disorder and schizophrenia as distinct entities, Reininghaus, Priebe, and Bentall (2013) argue that the data show not only a superordinate psychosis syndrome, but also five independent symptom dimensions: positive symptoms (hallucinations and delusions), negative symptoms (social withdrawal and the inability to experience pleasure), cognitive disorganization, depression, and mania. These dimensions can be treated as targets.

4. **A universal, single process is largely responsible for the maintenance of psychological distress across all or the majority of psychological disorders.** For example, Watkins (2008) proposes the importance of repetitive thinking: the process of thinking attentively, repetitively, or frequently about oneself or one's world. Hayes and colleagues (2006, p. 6) propose the importance of psychological inflexibility: the way "language and cognition interact with direct contingencies to produce an inability to persist or change behavior in the service of long-term valued ends."

## *Link Targets to Robust Change Processes*

Finally, when disciplined improvisation is needed because a client's problems don't match well with an established protocol, or they have failed to respond to an established protocol, try modular components of evidence-based protocols. Chorpita and colleagues (e.g., Chorpita & Daleiden, 2010; Chorpita et al., 2005) have led the effort to create a standardized lexicon of interventions to define the discrete therapy technique or strategy that can serve as an independent variable rather than use the treatment manual as the unit of analysis. In the chapters in section 3 of this book, and in the works of others (e.g., Roth & Pilling, 2008), components of evidence-based protocols are packaged into self-contained modules that contain all the knowledge and competencies needed to deliver a particular intervention.

Such modular approaches may prove to be more scientifically useful and practice oriented than relying on manuals as the unit of analysis. They remove duplication due to overspecification and could offer a way to reliably aggregate findings across studies and distill prescriptive heuristics (Chorpita & Daleiden, 2010). Rotheram-Borus and colleagues (2012) have suggested that reengineering evidence-based therapeutic and preventive-intervention programs based on their most robust features will make it simpler and less expensive to meet the needs of the majority of people, making effective help more accessible, scalable, replicable, and sustainable.

Few prescriptive heuristics are available to guide the matching of component interventions to targets. Further, because available data have yet to demonstrate the unequivocal superiority of the common factors model or psychotherapy-as-technology model, perhaps the best path for practitioners is to be informed by both models.

According to the common factors model, five ingredients produce change. The practitioner should create an (1) emotionally charged bond between the therapist and the client and a (2) confiding, healing setting in which therapy can take place; provide a (3) psychologically derived and culturally embedded explanation for emotional distress that is (4) adaptive (i.e., provides viable and believable options for overcoming specific difficulties) and accepted by the client; and engage in a (5) set of procedures or rituals that lead the client to enact something that is positive, helpful, or adaptive (Laska et al., 2013). From this common factors viewpoint, any therapy that contains all five of these ingredients will be efficacious for most disorders.

From a cognitive behavioral perspective, general means-ends problem-solving strategies offer guidance about how to select component elements for treatment targets. First, assess whether the absence of effective behavior is due to a capability deficit (i.e., the client doesn't know how to do the needed behavior) and, if so, then use skills training procedures. If the client does have the skills but emotions, contingencies, or cognitive processes and content interfere with the ability to behave skillfully, then use the procedures and principles from exposure, contingency management, and cognitive modification to remove the hindrances to skillful behavior. Pull disorder-specific procedures and principles from relevant protocols as needed.

Table 1 uses PICO to illustrate how a modular component treatment plan might look. Behavioral activation (BA) serves as the basic template and starting point. BA is based on the premise that depression results from a lack of reinforcement. Consequently, you can treat multiple targets, such as problematic drinking, insomnia, parenting strategies, and the marital relationship, through the robust common procedure of activation assignments to reduce avoidance (which interferes with reinforcing contingencies) and improve mastery and satisfaction (to improve reinforcement). You can use disorder-specific principles and strategies drawn from specific evidence-based protocols (e.g., for insomnia, problem drinking, or parent training) in a modular fashion to treat specific targets.

# Beyond the Therapy Room: Organizations and Practice-Based Science

Diagnostic categories, with current procedural terminology (CPT) codes for diagnoses and service arms for specific disorders, still organize the world of service delivery and reimbursement. This organization is not adequate to implement the vision discussed in this chapter. In order to move into a new era of EBP, organizational changes must be made to facilitate and support these practices.

Evidence-informed heuristics are emerging to guide these changes, including identifying key variables that determine and sustain "good enough" implementation (e.g., Damschroder et al., 2009; Proctor et al., 2009) and verify the utility of modular components models (Chorpita et al., 2015; Weisz et al., 2012). By instituting progress monitoring as part of standard practice, practitioners and organizations may be able to answer for themselves what is necessary to obtain good outcomes within their quality improvement efforts (Steinfeld et al., 2015). As barriers to practice-based research appear to be surmountable (Barkham, Hardy, & Mellor-Clark, 2010; Koerner & Castonguay, 2015), and newer single-case methods make it possible to aggregate data in meaningful ways to draw generalizable conclusions (Barlow, Nock, & Hersen, 2008; Iwakabe & Gazzola, 2009), practice-based research can offer significant contributions to the scientific literature.

# Conclusion

The ubiquity of EBP implies that it is a straightforward process. However, significant challenges due to weaknesses in both the evidence base and clinical judgment suggest that practitioners and organizations create "kind" environments that will facilitate EBP. By implementing standard work routines, including the systematic use of heuristics that integrate the best current science, it becomes possible to train and better calibrate clinical judgment to detect valid cues and learn the relationships between clinical judgment, interventions, and outcomes. It also becomes possible to answer practice-based questions and to make significant contributions to the wider research literature. Many hands are going to be needed to advance the goal of science in practice.

# References

American Psychological Association Presidential Task Force on Evidence-Based Practice (2006). Evidence-based practice in psychology. *American Psychologist, 61*(4), 271–285.

Barkham, M., Hardy, G. E., & Mellor-Clark, J. (2010). Improving practice and enhancing evidence. In M. Barkham, G. E. Hardy, & J. Mellor-Clark (Eds.), *Developing and delivering practice-based evidence: A guide for the psychological therapies* (pp. 3–20). Chichester, UK: Wiley-Blackwell.

Barlow, D. H., Allen, L. B., & Choate, M. L. (2004). Toward a unified treatment for emotional disorders. *Behavior Therapy, 35*(2), 205–230.

Barlow, D. H., Nock, M. K., & Hersen, M. (2008). *Single case experimental designs: Strategies for studying behavior change* (3rd ed.). Boston: Pearson Allyn and Bacon.

Bedics, J. D., Atkins, D. C., Comtois, K. A., & Linehan, M. M. (2012a). Treatment differences in the therapeutic relationship and introject during a 2-year randomized controlled trial of dialectical behavior therapy versus nonbehavioral psychotherapy experts for borderline personality disorder. *Journal of Consulting Clinical Psychology, 80*(1), 66–77.

Bedics, J. D., Atkins, D. C., Comtois, K. A., & Linehan, M. M. (2012b). Weekly therapist ratings of the therapeutic relationship and patient introject during the course of dialectical behavioral therapy for the treatment of borderline personality disorder. *Psychotherapy (Chicago), 49*(2), 231–240.

Branson, A., Shafran, R., & Myles, P. (2015). Investigating the relationship between competence and patient outcome with CBT. *Behaviour Research and Therapy, 68*, 19–26.

Carlier, I. V., Meuldijk, D., van Vliet, I. M., van Fenema, E., van der Wee, N. J., & Zitman, F. G. (2012). Routine outcome monitoring and feedback on physical or mental health status: Evidence and theory. *Journal of Evaluation in Clinical Practice, 18*(1), 104–110.

Chorpita, B. F., & Daleiden, E. L. (2010). Building evidence-based systems in children's mental health. In J. R. Weisz & A. E. Kazdin (Eds.), *Evidence-based psychotherapies for children and adolescents* (2nd ed., pp. 482–499). New York: Guilford Press.

Chorpita, B. F., Daleiden, E. L., & Weisz, J. R. (2005). Modularity in the design and application of therapeutic interventions. *Applied and Preventive Psychology, 11*(3), 141–156.

Chorpita, B. F., Park, A., Tsai, K., Korathu-Larson, P., Higa-McMillan, C. K., Nakamura, B. J., et al. (2015). Balancing effectiveness with responsiveness: Therapist satisfaction across different treatment designs in the Child STEPs randomized effectiveness trial. *Journal of Consulting and Clinical Psychology, 83*(4), 709–718.

Christon, L. M., McLeod, B. D., & Jensen-Doss, A. (2015). Evidence-based assessment meets evidence-based treatment: An approach to science-informed case conceptualization. *Cognitive and Behavioral Practice, 22*(1), 36–48.

Collado, A., Calderón, M., MacPherson, L., & Lejuez, C. (2016). The efficacy of behavioral activation treatment among depressed Spanish-speaking Latinos. *Journal of Consulting and Clinical Psychology, 84*(7), 651–657.

Comtois, K. A., & Linehan, M. M. (2006). Psychosocial treatments of suicidal behaviors: A practice-friendly review. *Journal of Clinical Psychology, 62*(2), 161–170.

Damschroder, L. J., Aron, D. C., Keith, R. E., Kirsh, S. R., Alexander, J. A., & Lowery, J. C. (2009). Fostering implementation of health services research findings into practice: A consolidated framework for advancing implementation science. *Implementation Science, 4*, 50.

Dimidjian, S., Hollon, S. D., Dobson, K. S., Schmaling, K. B., Kohlenberg, R. J., Addis, M. E., et al. (2006). Randomized trial of behavioral activation, cognitive therapy, and antidepressant medication in the acute treatment of adults with major depression. *Journal of Consulting and Clinical Psychology, 74*(4), 658–670.

Fairburn, C. G., Cooper, Z., & Shafran, R. (2003). Cognitive behaviour therapy for eating disorders: A "transdiagnostic" theory and treatment. *Behaviour Research and Therapy, 41*(5), 509–528.

Gawande, A. (2010). *The checklist manifesto: How to get things right.* New York: Metropolitan Books.

Glasgow, R. E., Vogt, T. M., & Boles, S. M. (1999). Evaluating the public health impact of health promotion interventions: The RE-AIM framework. *American Journal of Public Health, 89*(9), 1322–1327.

Goodman, J. D., McKay, J. R., & DePhilippis, D. (2013). Progress monitoring in mental health and addiction treatment: A means of improving care. *Professional Psychology: Research and Practice, 44*(4), 231–246.

Harvey, A. G., Watkins, E., Mansell, W., & Shafran, R. (2004). *Cognitive behavioural processes across psychological disorders: A transdiagnostic approach to research and treatment.* Oxford: Oxford University Press.

Hayes, S. C., Luoma, J. B., Bond, F. W., Masuda, A., & Lillis, J. (2006) Acceptance and commitment therapy: Model, processes, and outcomes. *Behaviour Research and Therapy, 44*(1), 1–25.

Heath, C., & Heath, D. (2013). *Decisive: How to make better choices in life and work.* New York: Random House.

Hogarth, R. M. (2001). *Educating intuition.* Chicago: University of Chicago Press.

Huang X., Lin J., & Demner-Fushman D. (2006). Evaluation of PICO as a knowledge representation for clinical questions. *AMIA Annual Symposium Proceedings Archive,* 359–363.

Iwakabe, S., & Gazzola, N. (2009). From single-case studies to practice-based knowledge: Aggregating and synthesizing case studies. *Psychotherapy Research, 19*(4–5), 601–611.

Jacobson, N. S., Dobson, K., Fruzzetti, A. E., Schmaling, K. B., & Salusky, S. (1991). Marital therapy as a treatment for depression. *Journal of Consulting and Clinical Psychology, 59*(4), 547–557.

Kahan, D. (2012). Two common (and recent) mistakes about dual process reasoning and cognitive bias. February 3. http://www.culturalcognition.net/blog/2012/2/3/two-common-recent-mistakes-about-dual-process-reasoning-cogn.html.

Kahan, D. M. (2013a). Ideology, motivated reasoning, and cognitive reflection. *Judgment and Decision Making, 8*(4), 407–424.

Kahan, D. M. (2013b). "Integrated and reciprocal": Dual process reasoning and science communication part 2. July 24. http://www.culturalcognition.net/blog/2013/7/24/integrated-reciprocal-dual-process-reasoning-and-science-com.html.

Kahneman, D. (2011). *Thinking, fast and slow.* New York: Farrar, Straus and Giroux.

Kahneman, D., & Klein, G. (2009). Conditions for intuitive expertise: A failure to disagree. *American Psychologist, 64*(6), 515–526.

Kanter, J. W., Santiago-Rivera, A. L., Santos, M. M., Nagy, G., López, M., Hurtado, G. D., et al. (2015). A randomized hybrid efficacy and effectiveness trial of behavioral activation for Latinos with depression. *Behavior therapy, 46*(2), 177–192.

Karelaia, N., & Hogarth, R. M. (2008). Determinants of linear judgment: A meta-analysis of lens model studies. *Psychological Bulletin, 134*(3), 404–426.

Kiresuk, T. J., Smith, A., & Cardillo, J. E. (2014). *Goal attainment scaling: Applications, theory, and measurement.* London: Psychology Press.

Koerner, K., & Castonguay, L. G. (2015). Practice-oriented research: What it takes to do collaborative research in private practice. *Psychotherapy Research, 25*(1), 67–83.

Kunda, Z. (1990). The case for motivated reasoning. *Psychological Bulletin, 108*(3), 480–498.

Kuyken, W. (2006). Evidence-based case formulation: Is the emperor clothed? In N. Tarrier & J. Johnson (Eds.), *Case formulation in cognitive behaviour therapy: The treatment of challenging and complex cases* (pp. 12–35). New York: Routledge.

Laska, K. M., Smith, T. L., Wislocki, A. P., Minami, T., & Wampold, B. E. (2013). Uniformity of evidence-based treatments in practice? Therapist effects in the delivery of cognitive processing therapy for PTSD. *Journal of Counseling Psychology, 60*(1), 31–41.

Linehan, M. M. (1999). Development, evaluation, and dissemination of effective psychosocial treatments: Levels of disorder, stages of care, and stages of treatment research. In M. D. Glantz & C. R. Hartel (Eds.), *Drug abuse: Origins and interventions* (pp. 367–394). Washington, DC: American Psychological Association.

Lovibond, P. F., & Lovibond, S. H. (1995). The structure of negative emotional states: Comparison of the Depression Anxiety Stress Scales (DASS) with the Beck Depression and Anxiety Inventories. *Behaviour Research and Therapy, 33*(3), 335–343.

Manber, R., Edinger, J. D., Gress, J. L., San Pedro-Salcedo, M. G., Kuo, T. F., & Kalista, T. (2008). Cognitive behavioral therapy for insomnia enhances depression outcome in patients with comorbid major depressive disorder and insomnia. *Sleep, 31*(4), 489–495.

Mansell, W., Harvey, A., Watkins, E., & Shafran, R. (2009). Conceptual foundations of the transdiagnostic approach to CBT. *Journal of Cognitive Psychotherapy, 23*(1), 6–19.

McMain, S., Sayrs, J. H., Dimeff, L. A., & Linehan, M. M. (2007). Dialectical behavior therapy for individuals with borderline personality disorder and substance dependence. In L. A. Dimeff & K. Koerner (Eds.), *Dialectical behavior therapy in clinical practice: Applications across disorders and settings* (pp. 145–173). New York: Guilford Press.

Merton, R. K. (1968). The Matthew effect in science. *Science, 159*, 56–63.

Morgenstern, J., & McKay, J. R. (2007). Rethinking the paradigms that inform behavioral treatment research for substance use disorders. *Addiction, 102*(9), 1377–1389.

Norcross, J. C. (2002). *Psychotherapy relationships that work: Therapist contributions and responsiveness to patients.* New York: Oxford University Press.

O'Donnell, A., Anderson, P., Newbury-Birch, D., Schulte, B., Schmidt, C., Reimer, J., et al. (2014). The impact of brief alcohol interventions in primary healthcare: A systematic review of reviews. *Alcohol and Alcoholism, 49*(1), 66–78.

Onken, L. S., Carroll, K. M., Shoham, V., Cuthbert, B. N., & Riddle, M. (2014). Reenvisioning clinical science: Unifying the discipline to improve the public health. *Clinical Psychological Science, 2*(1), 22–34.

Padesky, C. A., Kuyken, W., & Dudley, R. (2011). *Collaborative case conceptualization rating scale and coding manual.* Vol. 5, July 19. Unpublished manual retrieved from http://padesky.com/pdf_padesky/CCCRS_Coding_Manual_v5_web.pdf.

Persons, J. B. (2008). *The case formulation approach to cognitive-behavior therapy.* New York: Guildford Press.

Proctor, E. K., Landsverk, J., Aarons, G., Chambers, D., Glisson, C., & Mittman, B. (2009). Implementation research in mental health services: An emerging science with conceptual, methodological, and training challenges. *Administration and Policy in Mental Health and Mental Health Services Research, 36*(1), 24–34.

Reininghaus, U., Priebe, S., & Bentall, R. P. (2013). Testing the psychopathology of psychosis: Evidence for a general psychosis dimension. *Schizophrenia Bulletin, 39*(4), 884–895.

Roth, A. D., & Pilling, S. (2008). Using an evidence-based methodology to identify the competences required to deliver effective cognitive and behavioral therapy for depression and anxiety disorders. *Behavioral and Cognitive Psychotherapy, 36*(2), 129–147.

Rotheram-Borus, M. J., Swendeman, D., & Chorpita, B. F. (2012). Disruptive innovations for designing and diffusing evidence-based interventions. *American Psychologist, 67*(6), 463–476.

Rounsaville, B. J, Carroll K. M., & Onken L. S. (2001). A stage model of behavioral therapies research: Getting started and moving on from stage 1. *Clinical Psychology: Science and Practice, 8*(2):133–142.

Sackett, D. L., Rosenberg, W. M., Gray, J. M., Haynes, R. B., & Richardson, W. S. (1996). Evidence based medicine: What it is and what it isn't. *BMJ, 312*(7023), 72–73.

Spring, B. (2007a). Steps for evidence-based behavioral practice. http://www.ebbp.org/steps.html.

Spring, B. (2007b). Evidence-based practice in clinical psychology: What it is, why it matters; what you need to know. *Journal of Clinical Psychology, 63*(7), 611–631.

Stanovich, K. E., West, R. F., & Toplak, M. E. (2011). Individual differences as essential components of heuristics and biases research. In K. Manktelow, D. Over, & S. Elqayam (Eds.), *The Science of reason: A Festschrift for Jonathan St. B. T. Evans* (pp. 355–396). New York: Psychology Press.

Steinfeld, B., Scott, J., Vilander, G., Marx, L., Quirk, M., Lindberg, J., et al. (2015). The role of lean process improvement in implementation of evidence-based practices in behavioral health care. *Journal of Behavioral Health Services & Research, 42*(4), 504–518.

Stepanski, E. J., & Rybarczyk, B. (2006). Emerging research on the treatment and etiology of secondary or comorbid insomnia. *Sleep Medicine Reviews, 10*(1), 7–18.

Tucker, J. A., & Roth, D. L. (2006). Extending the evidence hierarchy to enhance evidence based practice for substance use disorders. *Addiction, 101*(7), 918–932.

Unützer, J., & Park, M. (2012). Strategies to improve the management of depression in primary care. *Primary Care: Clinics in Office Practice, 39*(2), 415–431.

Watkins, E. R. (2008). Constructive and unconstructive repetitive thought. *Psychological Bulletin, 134*(2),163–206.

Webb, C. A., DeRubeis, R. J., & Barber, J. P. (2010). Therapist adherence/competence and treatment outcome: A meta-analytic review. *Journal of Consulting and Clinical Psychology, 78*(2), 200–211.

Webster-Stratton, C. (2006). *The incredible years: A trouble-shooting guide for parents of children aged 2–8* (rev. ed.). Seattle: The Incredible Years.

Weisz, J. R., Chorpita, B. F., Frye, A., Ng, M. Y., Lau, N., Bearman, S. K., et al. (2011). Youth top problems: using idiographic, consumer-guided assessment to identify treatment needs and to track change during psychotherapy. *Journal of consulting and clinical psychology, 79*(3), 369–380.

Weisz, J. R., Chorpita, B. F., Palinkas, L. A., Schoenwald, S. K., Miranda, J., Bearman, S. K., et al. (2012). Testing standard and modular designs for psychotherapy treating depression, anxiety, and conduct problems in youth: A randomized effectiveness trial. *Archives of General Psychiatry, 69*(3), 274–282.

# CHAPTER 4

# Information Technology and the Changing Role of Practice

Gerhard Andersson, PhD

*Department of Behavioral Sciences and Learning,*
*Linköping University, and Karolinska Institute*

Psychotherapy has gradually changed from a mainly individual face-to-face practice to various alternative forms of treatment delivery. Examples include group treatment, information materials, class-based interventions, unguided prevention programs, and guided self-help programs using either books or computerized interventions based on different platforms (e.g., computers, via the Internet, and smartphones). Not all of these changes in the practitioner's role are recent, nor have they been caused by modern information technology, but my focus in this chapter is on those that have been.

Although controversy about group and class-based interventions remains (Morrison, 2001), the changes produced by these methods have been with the field for some time, these methods are already part of regular practice, and they have empirical support with at least some conditions (Cuijpers, van Straten, & Warmerdam, 2008; White, Keenan, & Brooks, 1992). The same is true with some forms of information technology as well, such as using a text-based intervention in the form of books and leaflets as a stand-alone treatment, often referred to as bibliotherapy (Keeley, Williams, & Shapiro, 2002). Some newer forms of intervention, such as seeking out web-based information material or online support groups, fall outside of the scope of this chapter (G. Andersson, 2014) because they are rarely integrated with practice per se. In this chapter I will instead comment on the changes in the role of practice in which modern information technology has been introduced to *complement* and sometimes even *replace* traditional formats of service delivery.

# Internet-Based Treatments with No Clinician Contact

There are many Internet-based self-help programs that are automated and involve no contact with a human being. These programs can have different purposes, ranging from prevention to early intervention in a stepped-care process (Nordgreen et al., 2016) to full psychological treatment.

Treatments with no contact with a clinician are often presented under a name other than "treatment," and they tend to target specific symptoms rather than mental health disorders and syndromes (Leykin, Muñoz, Contreras, & Latham, 2014). This may partly be the result of legal restrictions in some countries and professional and ethical regulations. For example, in the United States it isn't possible for a clinician to treat a person via the Internet if the person lives in a state in which the clinician is not licensed.

Magnitude of need and lack of face-to-face services are motivators for the creation of self-guided programs (Muñoz, 2010), but such programs face problems, such as the fact that many who register fail to complete the interventions (Christensen, Griffiths, Groves, & Korten, 2006). Automated reminders and other programmed ways to foster adherence may boost treatments with no human support. Recent studies suggest that this form of augmented, unguided Internet treatment can be effective, with fewer dropouts than in previous studies (Titov et al., 2013).

The level of human involvement tends to be higher when online interventions are used as part of the health care system. Online interventions often automatically include at least some human support, such as a prescribing primary-care clinician or research staff member who sees a research participant for assessment (Ritterband et al., 2009). The level of human involvement can increase when clinicians are part of the process of supportive engagement.

# Internet-Based Treatments with Clinician Support

Internet-based treatments with some form of clinician support have emerged as an evidence-based approach to deliver psychological treatments for several conditions, including anxiety (Olthuis, Watt, Bailey, Hayden, & Stewart, 2015), depression, and somatic disorders (G. Andersson, 2014). These programs are often full-scale treatments that span five to fifteen weeks and include many of the components of face-to-face interventions. Several features of guided Internet treatments are likely to influence how psychological treatments will be practiced in the future.

First, guided Internet-based treatments generally include online assessment procedures. Many researchers and clinicians see value in the repeated assessment of outcome during treatment (Lambert, 2015), but this is often not possible in clinical practice given time constraints, and the administration and coding involved with questionnaires. Modern information technology can facilitate outcome monitoring. Clinicians can administer self-report questionnaires with maintained psychometric properties via the Internet (Van Ballegooijen, Riper, Cuijpers, van Oppen, & Smit, 2016), and with the help of mobile phones they can collect data in real time from clients (Luxton, McCann, Bush, Mishkind, & Reger, 2011). This is useful not only in research but also in regular treatment. For example, smartphones can be used instead of paper and pencil to collect distress ratings during exposure therapy. Gustafson and colleagues (2014) used a smartphone app to support the treatment of drug abuse. Yet another possibility is to use video chat when interviewing clients. Of course, this requires secure online solutions, making ordinary programs for social media less suitable, even if clinicians increasingly use common systems such as Skype (Armfield, Gray, & Smith, 2012).

Second, how guided Internet-based treatments are scheduled and the content they use (for a recent review of Internet versions of evidence-based treatment, see G. Andersson, Carlbring, & Lindefors, 2016) are also likely to influence future psychological practice. Overall, the scheduling of online programs tends to mimic face-to-face scheduling, and these programs provide weekly homework assignments. Moreover, the treatments have a total length similar to that of face-to-face manuals. The content of online treatment programs varies, but most are based on cognitive behavioral therapy (CBT) (G. Andersson, 2014); others are informed by interpersonal psychotherapy (Dagöö et al., 2014) or psychodynamic psychotherapy (Johansson, Frederick, & Andersson, 2013) and so on.

While many treatment programs have been derived from evidence-based protocols for specific disorders, such as panic disorder and depression, evidence-based treatments tend to overlap across disorders and problems, and it is important to give end users freedom regarding treatment preferences. Two different and partly overlapping solutions to this dilemma have been developed.

A focus on transdiagnostic mechanisms is the first solution. Examples are Barlow's unified protocol for mood and anxiety disorders (Barlow, Allen, & Choate, 2004) and acceptance and commitment therapy's focus on psychological flexibility across different forms of mental and behavioral health (Hayes, Strosahl, & Wilson, 2012). Titov, Andrews, Johnston, Robinson, and Spence (2010) have developed and tested a transdiagnostic Internet treatment for anxiety and depression, with good results. Researchers have tested other transdiagnostic approaches, such as mindfulness (Boettcher et al., 2014), affect-focused psychodynamic treatment (Johansson, Björklund, et al., 2013), and acceptance and commitment therapy (Levin, Pistorello, Hayes, Seeley, & Levin, 2015), using the Internet format. In addition, researchers have used the Internet to test generic treatments, such as applied relaxation, and for specific disorders, such as social anxiety disorder (Carlbring, Ekselius, & Andersson, 2003).

Without additional tailoring, even transdiagnostic approaches are not capable of handling client preferences, and case-formulated treatments, which clinicians often favor, are not possible if treatment content is more or less fixed. One exception is the transdiagnostic approach by Titov and colleagues (2011), which offers clients material in addition to that of the fixed program. Similarly, the program described by Levin and colleagues (2015) provides for "flavors" of acceptance and commitment therapy to fit the client problem area.

Another approach to giving end users freedom regarding treatment preferences, developed by our research group in Sweden, consists of tailoring Internet treatment according to a diagnostic interview; a case formulation; and, to some extent, client preferences (Carlbring et al., 2010). In practice, tailoring might consist of set modules and flexible modules. A client may be prescribed a ten-week program consisting of psychoeducation (fixed), tailored modules based on case presentation and preferences (for example, modules on social anxiety and stress management), and then a fixed ending (relapse prevention). This transdiagnostic approach can address comorbidity for cases in which problems, such as insomnia, relationship issues, and psychiatric conditions (e.g., generalized anxiety), coexist. Evidence to date suggests that tailored Internet treatment probably is as effective as disorder-specific treatments (Berger, Boettcher, & Caspar, 2014), and in one study on depression, tailored treatment was found to be superior to standard Internet treatment for more severe cases (Johansson et al., 2012).

An advantage of treatment programs delivered via the Internet is that they can go beyond text to include audio files, animations, videos, chat rooms, texting, automated reminders, and other technological solutions that, in principle, can guide the client through a behavior change process in a seamless manner that would be difficult to fully replicate in face-to-face therapy. Text is still a major part of most interventions, and many people are used to processing text, but in most programs different presentation formats are mixed with, for example, an introductory video from a therapist, text-based instructions and psychoeducation, interactive homework instructions, and pictures to illustrate concepts. Indeed, researchers have developed treatments that use illustrations extensively; for example, there is a depression treatment in manga format (Imamura et al., 2014), and programs from Australia use pictures drawn by former artists at Disney (Mewton, Sachdev, & Andrews, 2013).

Another strength of Internet-based therapy is that it can be modified to fit people who speak different languages and have different cultural backgrounds. Figure 1 presents an example. It's a screenshot of a treatment study for depression used in a trial with people speaking the Kurdish language Sorani. The depression manual was originally written in Swedish, as you can see from the video's title. The figure shows that Internet interventions can easily be translated and adapted for use in other languages. In a similar way, Internet-based therapy can change program examples, names, or photos to fit cultural expectations (e.g., a picture showing a man and a woman shaking hands can be changed to two women shaking hands for an Internet protocol presented in Farsi).

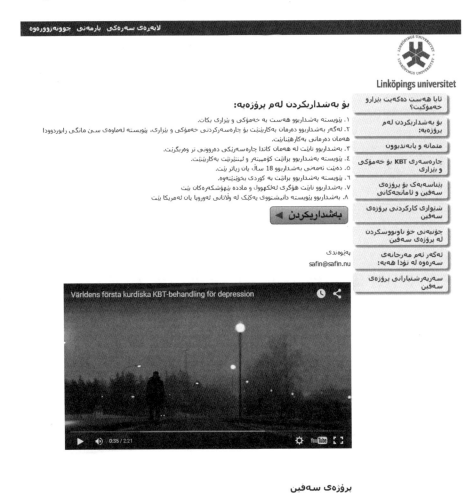

FIGURE 1. A screenshot from a depression treatment presented in the Kurdish language Sorani (copyright © 2017 Department of Behavioral Sciences and Learning, Linköping University, and used by permission)

The third feature of guided Internet-based treatments likely to affect future psychology practices is the role of the clinician. Most reviews and meta-analyses have found that clinical support boosts treatment outcomes for online programs and reduces dropout (Baumeister, Reichler, Munzinger, & Lin, 2014), but more work is needed regarding the role and training of therapists guiding Internet-based treatments (G. Andersson, 2014). However, support may be differentially associated with outcome; for example, depression treatments may be more dependent on support (Johansson & Andersson, 2012), and some other conditions potentially require less clinical support (Berger et al., 2011). Both clinicians and clients may prefer to have some form of clinical contact, but the amount and form of support needed is not yet known empirically. It may be that on-demand support, similar to help lines, could be sufficient for some clients (Rheker, Andersson, & Weise, 2015). Other clients may need scheduled support and tailored reminders. A challenge for future research will be to identify outcome moderators that will help clinicians decide what form of support a client needs.

Overall, the effects of Internet-based treatments challenge the assumption that a therapeutic alliance is a necessary feature behind effective psychosocial treatments (Horvath, del Re, Fluckiger, & Symonds, 2011). Several studies (e.g., Sucala et al., 2012) have looked at the therapeutic alliance between the client and the online therapist, and in most, clients have rated the alliance as high (using measures such as the working alliance inventory), but these ratings have rarely correlated with outcome.

# Are We Ready to Implement Internet Treatment?

In this chapter I focus on guided Internet-based treatment because the evidence base is large for a range of problems and clinical conditions (G. Andersson, 2014). However, there are barriers to clinicians incorporating modern information technology in daily clinical practice. First, clients may not view Internet treatment as a firsthand treatment (Mohr et al., 2010), even if some surveys suggest that clients may be more positive than clinicians (Gun, Titov, & Andrews, 2011; Wootton, Titov, Dear, Spence, & Kemp, 2011). Second, attitudes may differ depending on target group; for example, clinicians may be less willing to use Internet treatment with younger clients (Vigerland et al., 2014).

Third, providers may fear that Internet treatments will come to be regarded as being equally effective as face-to-face treatments. Direct comparative studies suggest that this may be the case when it comes to guided Internet treatments (G. Andersson, Cuijpers, Carlbring, Riper, & Hedman, 2014), with the caveat that no treatment is likely to be suitable for all clients and outcomes may vary across clinicians. From a clinical point of view, it is highly likely (given the overall equivalence in studies) that there are some clients and some clinicians for whom face-to-face treatment is superior, but there are also clients and clinicians for whom Internet treatment is more effective. Unfortunately, the literature on predictors of outcome does not send a clear message, as there are few consistent findings on what works for whom.

Fourth, clinicians are concerned about whether they can trust the findings from efficacy studies in which participants are recruited via advertisements. Given the rapid speed of research on guided Internet treatments (with the help of technology), there are now several effectiveness studies (those that are clinically representative, with ordinary clients seen in regular settings and not recruited via advertisements) showing that such treatments (so far, without exception, those based on CBT) work well when delivered in regular care (G. Andersson & Hedman, 2013), with some recent studies performed with very large samples (e.g., ~2,000 clients; Titov et al., 2015). Finally, ethical concerns and restrictions may also limit the reach of Internet treatments (Dever Fitzgerald, Hunter, Hadjistavropoulos, & Koocher, 2010), as may service delivery models and funding.

In sum, in spite of the fast-growing empirical support for guided Internet treatments, changes in the structure of practice are slow. There are examples of established Internet-treatment facilities (e.g., one has been treating tinnitus distress in Uppsala, Sweden, since 1999; Kaldo et al., 2013) and implementations in countries such as Australia, the Netherlands, Germany, and Norway, but many treatment programs are not used yet in regular care.

# Guided Self-Help As an Adjunct to Standard Therapy

Self-help books have already penetrated therapy practices and found use within them. Given the large number of self-help books available on the market, some of which have been supported by controlled treatment trials, it is not surprising that many clinicians use and recommend them. One study on CBT therapists in the United Kingdom found that 88.7 percent of therapists used self-help materials, mostly as a supplement to individual therapy (Keeley et al., 2002). A similar survey found that only 1 percent of practicing clinicians used computerized interventions as an *alternative* to face-to-face services (Whitfield & Williams, 2004), but the blending of face-to-face services and modern information technology is a recent development likely to change how therapists and clinicians practice.

An example of this blending is an online support system for CBT in which all the paperwork (for example, homework assignments, diaries, questionnaires, information material) exists online, but the system is used to complement face-to-face sessions rather than as a replacement (Månsson, Ruiz, Gervind, Dahlin, & Andersson, 2013). An online support system of this kind builds on earlier technological developments, such as the CD-ROM support system for general practice clinicians (Roy-Byrne et al., 2010). Another approach is to use the online treatment program as a base and to complement it with face-to-face meetings (Van der Vaart et al., 2014). A recent depression study in Norway, conducted in general practice, successfully used that approach based on the online MoodGYM program (Høifødt et al., 2013).

With the spread of modern mobile phones (i.e., smartphones), additional opportunities have emerged for blended practice. Practitioners can use the technology in the way they use self-help books, recommending it to clients with the hope of making intervention more effective and efficient. In one recent project, a smartphone app was developed to support behavioral activation. The app was blended with four face-to-face sessions and was tested—against a full behavioral activation arm consisting of ten face-to-face sessions under supervision—in a randomized trial with eighty-eight clients with diagnosed depression (Ly et al., 2015). Results showed no difference between the two treatments and large within-group effects for both treatments.

Trials such as this show that we have now reached a stage at which regular face-to-face services will need to learn how to incorporate modern information technology on empirical grounds. It seems inevitable that Internet-supported interventions using different platforms, such as computers, smartphones, and tablets, will become more common. The blending of these interventions into regular clinical care can occur from two perspectives: regular services, such as evidence-based psychological treatment, can use technology as an adjunct to regular face-to-face sessions, or online treatment programs, smartphone apps, and other devices can be supported by clinicians. Many trials and clinical applications of Internet interventions have used both styles of blending over the years. What is not yet clear is how clinicians are going to adjust their roles to make use of technological developments.

# Ongoing and Future Developments

In light of the rapid spread of modern information technology across the world, it is clear that the practice of psychological assessment and treatment will change. It is hard to predict exactly how. In this section I will comment on a few possible scenarios and make observations about the current state of affairs.

First, it seems likely that some Internet-based interventions will emerge that can *only* be conveniently done in computerized forms, driving their early adoption. Attention modification training, which moved from being mostly laboratory based (Amir et al., 2009) to online delivery, is such an example. Its development shows both promise and risks, since promising findings from laboratory research have not been replicated in programs delivered via the Internet (Boettcher, Berger, & Renneberg, 2012; Carlbring et al., 2012), and paradoxical results have been reported (Boettcher et al., 2013; Kuckertz et al., 2014). However, additional examples seem sure to emerge (especially given point three below).

Second, specific treatment components (e.g., mindfulness and physical exercise) that are sometimes embedded in evidence-based psychological treatments have also been delivered over the Internet in controlled trials. Mindfulness components have been part of treatment protocols in studies on Internet-delivered acceptance-oriented treatments (Hesser et al., 2012). In a study on depression, a physical exercise program was delivered via the Internet with promising results (Ström et al., 2013), again showing that Internet delivery can be a feasible way to test the effects of interventions. There have also been controlled trials on mindfulness (Boettcher et al., 2014; Morledge et al., 2013) and problem solving as treatment components delivered as stand-alone interventions via the Internet (Van Straten, Cuijpers, & Smits, 2008). As these specific components are better developed, their linkage to new forms of functional analysis and program development seem likely, especially if the process-oriented approach in the present volume begins to provide more focus on moderation and processes of change. It is worth noting that Internet studies allow for larger samples and thus can facilitate dismantling studies in which the effects of specific components are isolated.

Third, we are now in the position where it is likely that new interventions will be tested directly in Internet trials rather than first being developed and tested in regular face-to-face trials. One such example is a treatment of procrastination (Rozental, Forsell, Svensson, Andersson, & Carlbring, 2015). The change of focus from psychiatric syndromes to the problems people have and the processes that foster them seems likely to increase Internet trials. This overall trend may narrow the focus of Internet interventions to problem areas (an example is the treatment of perfectionism; Arpin-Cribbie, Irvine, & Ritvo, 2012). It also may broaden the range of problem areas—from mild to moderate psychiatric conditions, where there are now few conditions for which no programs exist (G. Andersson, 2014); to somatic health problems, such as chronic pain; to general health problems, such as stress and insomnia (G. Andersson, 2014).

Fourth, on the process front, Internet treatment research can be a testing ground for new ideas regarding the processes that moderate or mediate treatment outcome. Again, given the larger samples of participants in Internet trials, it is easier to get sufficient statistical power to test outcome predictors but also mediators of outcome in process research (Ljótsson et al., 2013). A large controlled study of two hundred people suffering from social anxiety disorder found that knowledge about social anxiety and confidence in that knowledge increased following treatment (G. Andersson, Carlbring, & Furmark, on behalf of the SOFIE Research Group, 2012). This example in CBT psychoeducation is important, but few studies have investigated what clients actually learn from their therapies, and knowledge acquisition deserves to be studied more as it is an important goal of most psychosocial interventions (Harvey et al., 2014).

Another example of research (Bricker, Wyszynski, Comstock, & Heffner, 2013) done in association with Internet trials had participants accept the physical, cognitive, and emotional cues to smoke. This study attributed 80 percent of the increased level of smoking cessation at follow-up to an acceptance and commitment therapy website and Smokefree.gov, the smoking-cessation website developed by the National Cancer Institute. A study done by Månsson and colleagues (2015), on brain mechanisms as outcomes and predictors of outcome, is yet another example of an Internet-associated trial. Other studies (e.g., E. Andersson et al., 2013) have investigated genetic markers of outcome, but this research has not yet generated any strong findings.

A fifth and final area of interest is the provision of training, supervision, and education via the Internet. There are few studies on online education in CBT (Rakovshik et al., 2013) and even fewer for online supervision. However, university education has changed dramatically, and an increasing number of education programs across the world use modern information technology. Online supervision is probably common even if there are restrictions regarding security and very little research regarding its efficacy. There is a need for systematic research on how we can use the Internet to increase access to education in evidence-based psychological treatments.

## Concluding Remarks

In this chapter I gave several examples of how clinical practice might change due to the introduction of modern information technology in society. In a short time researchers have conducted a large number of Internet-based studies, and it is now common for new treatments targeting new populations to be tested directly with Internet research and not just time-consuming studies with face-to-face sessions. But there are also challenges with Internet-based interventions. Diagnostic procedures and case formulations are generally based on human interaction between clinicians and clients. To date, for Internet treatments these therapy procedures have often been done either in clinic or via telephone. There is a need to improve online screening and diagnostic procedures but also to implement other tests, such as cognitive testing, for online delivery. In this chapter I did not discuss cost-effectiveness and the potential cost savings with Internet interventions (Donker et al., 2015), but it is worth adding that Internet-intervention costs are less than face-to-face services and, perhaps more importantly, clients can be reached more easily and earlier with Internet treatment, which may reduce suffering.

Clinicians being trained today grew up in the Internet era, and they may be better prepared than more senior peers to embrace the bold new world that looms on the horizon. The opportunities are great, but it seems likely that practice changes will proceed gradually. This may be a good thing, as the pace appears to be encouraging the field to begin the change process by blending the best of face-to-face and modern information technology, creating a solid foundation for the additional and perhaps more professionally challenging steps likely to be taken in the future.

# References

Amir, N., Beard, C., Taylor, C. T., Klumpp, H., Elias, J., Burns, M., et. al. (2009). Attention training in individuals with generalized social phobia: A randomized controlled trial. *Journal of Consulting and Clinical Psychology, 77*(5), 961–973.

Andersson, E., Rück, C., Lavebratt, C., Hedman, E., Schalling, M., Lindefors, N., et al. (2013). Genetic polymorphisms in monoamine systems and outcome of cognitive behavior therapy for social anxiety disorder. *PLoS One, 8*(11), e79015.

Andersson, G. (2014). *The internet and CBT: A clinical guide.* Boca Raton, FL: CRC Press.

Andersson, G., Carlbring, P., & Furmark, T., on behalf of the SOFIE Research Group. (2012). Therapist experience and knowledge acquisition in Internet-delivered CBT for social anxiety disorder: A randomized controlled trial. *PLoS One, 7*(5), e37411.

Andersson, G., Carlbring, P., & Lindefors, N. (2016). History and current status of ICBT. In N. Lindefors & G. Andersson (Eds.), *Guided Internet-based treatments in psychiatry* (pp. 1–16). Switzerland: Springer.

Andersson, G., Cuijpers, P., Carlbring, P., Riper, H., & Hedman, E. (2014). Guided Internet-based vs. face-to-face cognitive behavior therapy for psychiatric and somatic disorders: A systematic review and meta-analysis. *World Psychiatry, 13*(3), 288–295.

Andersson, G., & Hedman, E. (2013). Effectiveness of guided Internet-based cognitive behavior therapy in regular clinical settings. *Verhaltenstherapie, 23,* 140–148.

Armfield, N. R., Gray, L. C., & Smith, A. C. (2012). Clinical use of Skype: A review of the evidence base. *Journal of Telemedicine and Telecare, 18*(3), 125–127.

Arpin-Cribbie, C., Irvine, J., & Ritvo, P. (2012). Web-based cognitive-behavioral therapy for perfectionism: A randomized controlled trial. *Psychotherapy Research, 22*(2), 194–207.

Barlow, D. H., Allen, L. B., & Choate, M. L. (2004). Toward a unified treatment for emotional disorders. *Behavior Therapy, 35*(2), 205–230.

Baumeister, H., Reichler, L., Munzinger, M., & Lin, J. (2014). The impact of guidance on Internet-based mental health interventions—A systematic review. *Internet Interventions, 1*(4), 205–215.

Berger, T., Boettcher, J., & Caspar, F. (2014). Internet-based guided self-help for several anxiety disorders: A randomized controlled trial comparing a tailored with a standardized disorder-specific approach. *Psychotherapy (Chicago), 51*(2), 207–219.

Berger, T., Caspar, F., Richardson, R., Kneubühler, B., Sutter, D., & Andersson, G. (2011). Internet-based treatment of social phobia: A randomized controlled trial comparing unguided with two types of guided self-help. *Behaviour Research and Therapy, 49*(3), 158–169.

Boettcher, J., Åström, V., Påhlsson, D., Schenström, O., Andersson, G., & Carlbring, P. (2014). Internet-based mindfulness treatment for anxiety disorders: A randomized controlled trial. *Behavior Therapy, 45*(2), 241–253.

Boettcher, J., Berger, T., & Renneberg, B. (2012). Internet-based attention training for social anxiety: A randomized controlled trial. *Cognitive Therapy and Research, 36*(5), 522–536.

Boettcher, J., Leek, L., Matson, L., Holmes, E. A., Browning, M., MacLeod, C., et al. (2013). Internet-based attention modification for social anxiety: A randomised controlled comparison of training towards negative and training towards positive cues. *PLoS One, 8*(9), e71760.

Bricker, J., Wyszynski, C., Comstock, B., & Heffner, J. L. (2013). Pilot randomized controlled trial of web-based acceptance and commitment therapy for smoking cessation. *Nicotine and Tobacco Research, 15*(10), 1756–1764.

Carlbring, P., Apelstrand, M., Sehlin, H., Amir, N., Rousseau, A., Hofmann, S., et al. (2012). Internet-delivered attention bias modification training in individuals with social anxiety disorder—A double blind randomized controlled trial. *BMC Psychiatry, 12*, 66.

Carlbring, P., Ekselius, L., & Andersson, G. (2003). Treatment of panic disorder via the Internet: A randomized trial of CBT vs. applied relaxation. *Journal of Behavior Therapy and Experimental Psychiatry, 34*(2), 129–140.

Carlbring, P., Maurin, L., Törngren, C., Linna, E., Eriksson, T., Sparthan, E., et al. (2010). Individually-tailored, Internet-based treatment for anxiety disorders: A randomized controlled trial. *Behaviour Research and Therapy, 49*(1), 18–24.

Christensen, H., Griffiths, K., Groves, C., & Korten, A. (2006). Free range users and one hit wonders: Community users of an Internet-based cognitive behaviour therapy program. *Australian and New Zealand Journal of Psychiatry, 40*(1), 59–62.

Cuijpers, P., van Straten, A., & Warmerdam, L. (2008). Are individual and group treatments equally effective in the treatment of depression in adults? A meta-analysis. *European Journal of Psychiatry, 22*(1), 38–51.

Dagöö, J., Asplund, R. P., Bsenko, H. A., Hjerling, S., Holmberg, A., Westh, S., et al. (2014). Cognitive behavior therapy versus interpersonal psychotherapy for social anxiety disorder delivered via smartphone and computer: A randomized controlled trial. *Journal of Anxiety Disorders, 28*(4), 410–417.

Dever Fitzgerald, T., Hunter, P. V., Hadjistavropoulos, T., & Koocher, G. P. (2010). Ethical and legal considerations for Internet-based psychotherapy. *Cognitive Behaviour Therapy, 39*(3), 173–187.

Donker, T., Blankers, M., Hedman, E., Ljótsson, B., Petrie, K., & Christensen, H. (2015). Economic evaluations of Internet interventions for mental health: A systematic review. *Psychological Medicine, 45*(16), 3357–3376.

Gun, S. Y., Titov, N., & Andrews, G. (2011). Acceptability of Internet treatment of anxiety and depression. *Australasian Psychiatry, 19*(3), 259–264.

Gustafson, D. H., McTavish, F. M., Chih, M. Y., Atwood, A. K., Johnson, R. A., Boyle, M. G., et al. (2014). A smartphone application to support recovery from alcoholism: A randomized clinical trial. *JAMA Psychiatry, 71*(5), 566–572.

Harvey, A. G., Lee, J., Williams, J., Hollon, S. D., Walker, M. P., Thompson, M. A., & Smith, R. (2014). Improving outcome of psychosocial treatments by enhancing memory and learning. *Perspectives on Psychological Science, 9*(2), 161–179.

Hayes, S. C., Strosahl, K. D., & Wilson, K. G. (2012). *Acceptance and commitment therapy: The process and practice of mindful change* (2nd ed.). New York: Guilford Press.

Hesser, H., Gustafsson, T., Lundén, C., Henrikson, O., Fattahi, K., Johnsson, E., et al. (2012). A randomized controlled trial of Internet-delivered cognitive behavior therapy and acceptance and commitment therapy in the treatment of tinnitus. *Journal of Consulting and Clinical Psychology, 80*(4), 649–661.

Høifødt, R. S., Lillevoll, K. R., Griffiths, K. M., Wilsgaard, T., Eisemann, M., Waterloo, K., et al. (2013). The clinical effectiveness of web-based cognitive behavioral therapy with face-to-face therapist support for depressed primary care patients: Randomized controlled trial. *Journal of Medical Internet Research, 15*(8), e153.

Horvath, A. O., del Re, A. C., Flückiger, C., & Symonds, D. (2011). Alliance in individual psychotherapy. *Psychotherapy, 48*(1), 9–16.

Imamura, K., Kawakami, N., Furukawa, T. A., Matsuyama, Y., Shimazu, A., Umanodan, R., et al. (2014). Effects of an Internet-based cognitive behavioral therapy (iCBT) program in manga format on improving subthreshold depressive symptoms among healthy workers: A randomized controlled trial. *PLoS One, 9*(5), e97167.

Johansson, R., & Andersson, G. (2012). Internet-based psychological treatments for depression. *Expert Review of Neurotherapeutics, 12*(7), 861–870.

Johansson, R., Björklund, M., Hornborg, C., Karlsson, S., Hesser, H., Ljótsson, B., et al. (2013). Affect-focused psychodynamic psychotherapy for depression and anxiety through the Internet: A randomized controlled trial. *PeerJ, 1*, e102.

Johansson, R., Frederick, R. J., & Andersson, G. (2013). Using the Internet to provide psychodynamic psychotherapy. *Psychodynamic Psychiatry, 41*(4), 385–412.

Johansson, R., Sjöberg, E., Sjögren, M., Johnsson, E., Carlbring, P., Andersson, T., et al. (2012). Tailored vs. standardized Internet-based cognitive behavior therapy for depression and comorbid symptoms: A randomized controlled trial. *PLoS One, 7*(5), e36905.

Kaldo, V., Haak, T., Buhrman, M., Alfonsson, S., Larsen, H. C., & Andersson, G. (2013). Internet-based cognitive behaviour therapy for tinnitus patients delivered in a regular clinical setting: Outcome and analysis of treatment dropout. *Cognitive Behaviour Therapy, 42*(2), 146–158.

Keeley, H., Williams, C., & Shapiro, D. A. (2002). A United Kingdom survey of accredited cognitive behaviour therapists' attitudes towards and use of structured self-help materials. *Behavioural and Cognitive Psychotherapy, 30*(2), 193–203.

Kuckertz, J. M., Gildebrant, E., Liliequist, B., Karlström, P., Väppling, C., Bodlund, O., et al. (2014). Moderation and mediation of the effect of attention training in social anxiety disorder. *Behaviour Research and Therapy, 53*, 30–40.

Lambert, M. J. (2015). Progress feedback and the OQ-system: The past and the future. *Psychotherapy, 52*(4), 381–390.

Levin, M. E., Pistorello, J., Hayes, S. C., Seeley, J. R., & Levin, C. (2015). Feasibility of an acceptance and commitment therapy adjunctive web-based program for counseling centers. *Journal of Counseling Psychology, 62*(3), 529–536.

Leykin, Y., Muñoz, R. F., Contreras, O., & Latham, M. D. (2014). Results from a trial of an unsupported Internet intervention for depressive symptoms. *Internet Interventions, 1*(4), 175–181.

Ljótsson, B., Hesser, H., Andersson, E., Lindfors, P., Hursti, T., Rück, C., et al. (2013). Mechanisms of change in an exposure-based treatment for irritable bowel syndrome. *Journal of Consulting and Clinical Psychology, 81*(6), 1113–1126.

Luxton, D. D., McCann, R. A., Bush, N. E., Mishkind, M. C., & Reger, G. M. (2011). mHealth for mental health: Integrating smartphone technology in behavioral healthcare. *Professional Psychology: Research and Practice, 42*(6), 505–512.

Ly, K. H., Topooco, N., Cederlund, H., Wallin, A., Bergström, J., Molander, O., et al. (2015). Smartphone-supported versus full behavioural activation for depression: A randomised controlled trial. *PLoS One, 10*(5), e0126559.

Månsson, K. N. T., Frick, A., Boraxbekk, C. J., Marquand, A. F., Williams, S. C. R., Carlbring, P., et al. (2015). Predicting long-term outcome of Internet-delivered cognitive behavior therapy for social anxiety disorder using fMRI and support vector machine learning. *Translational Psychiatry, 5*(3), e530.

Månsson, K. N. T., Ruiz, E. S., Gervind, E., Dahlin, M., & Andersson, G. (2013). Development and initial evaluation of an Internet-based support system for face to face cognitive behavior therapy: A proof of concept study. *Journal of Medical Internet Research, 15*(12), e280.

Mewton, L., Sachdev, P. S., & Andrews, G. (2013). A naturalistic study of the acceptability and effectiveness of Internet-delivered cognitive behavioural therapy for psychiatric disorders in older Australians. *PLoS One, 8*(8), e71825.

Mohr, D. C., Siddique, J., Ho, J., Duffecy, J., Jin, L., & Fokuo, J. K. (2010). Interest in behavioral and psychological treatments delivered face-to-face, by telephone, and by Internet. *Annals of Behavioral Medicine, 40*(1), 89–98.

Morledge, T. J., Allexandre, D., Fox, E., Fu, A. Z., Higashi, M. K., Kruzikas, D. T., et al. (2013). Feasibility of an online mindfulness program for stress management—a randomized, controlled trial. *Annals of Behavioral Medicine, 46*(2), 137–148.

Morrison, N. (2001). Group cognitive therapy: Treatment of choice or sub-optimal option? *Behavioural and Cognitive Psychotherapy, 29*(3), 311–332.

Muñoz, R. F. (2010). Using evidence-based Internet interventions to reduce health disparities worldwide. *Journal of Medical Internet Research, 12*(5), e60.

Nordgreen, T., Haug, T., Öst, L.-G., Andersson, G., Carlbring, P., Kvale, G., et al. (2016). Stepped care versus direct face-to-face cognitive behavior therapy for social anxiety disorder and panic disorder: A randomized effectiveness trial. *Behavior Therapy, 47*(2), 166–183.

Olthuis, J. V., Watt, M. C., Bailey, K., Hayden, J. A., & Stewart, S. H. (2015). Therapist-supported Internet cognitive behavioural therapy for anxiety disorders in adults. *Cochrane Database for Systematic Reviews, 3*(CD011565).

Rakovshik, S. G., McManus, F., Westbrook, D., Kholmogorova, A. B., Garanian, N. G., Zvereva, N. V., et al. (2013). Randomized trial comparing Internet-based training in cognitive behavioural therapy theory, assessment and formulation to delayed-training control. *Behaviour Research and Therapy, 51*(6), 231–239.

Rheker, J., Andersson, G., & Weise, C. (2015). The role of "on demand" therapist guidance vs. no support in the treatment of tinnitus via the Internet: A randomized controlled trial. *Internet Interventions, 2*(2), 189–199.

Ritterband, L. M., Thorndike, F. P., Gonder-Frederick, L. A., Magee, J. C., Bailey, E. T., Saylor, D. K., et al. (2009). Efficacy of an Internet-based behavioral intervention for adults with insomnia. *Archives of General Psychiatry, 66*(7), 692–698.

Roy-Byrne, P., Craske, M. G., Sullivan, G., Rose, R. D., Edlund, M. J., Lang, A. J., et al. (2010). Delivery of evidence-based treatment for multiple anxiety disorders in primary care: A randomized controlled trial. *JAMA, 303*(19), 1921–1928.

Rozental, A., Forsell, E., Svensson, A., Andersson, G., & Carlbring, P. (2015). Internet-based cognitive-behavior therapy for procrastination: A randomized controlled trial. *Journal of Consulting and Clinical Psychology, 83*(4), 808–824.

Ström, M., Uckelstam, C.-J., Andersson, G., Hassmén, P., Umefjord, G., & Carlbring, P. (2013). Internet-delivered therapist-guided physical activity for mild to moderate depression: A randomized controlled trial. *PeerJ, 1,* e178.

Sucala, M., Schnur, J. B., Constantino, M. J., Miller, S. J., Brackman, E. H., & Montgomery, G. H. (2012). The therapeutic relationship in e-therapy for mental health: A systematic review. *Journal of Medical Internet Research, 14*(4), e110.

Titov, N., Andrews, G., Johnston, L., Robinson, E., & Spence, J. (2010). Transdiagnostic Internet treatment for anxiety disorders: A randomized controlled trial. *Behaviour Research and Therapy, 48*(9), 890–899.

Titov, N., Dear, B. F., Johnston, L., Lorian, C., Zou, J., Wootton, B., et al. (2013). Improving adherence and clinical outcomes in self-guided Internet treatment for anxiety and depression: Randomised controlled trial. *PLoS One, 8*(7), e62873.

Titov, N., Dear, B. F., Schwencke, G., Andrews, G., Johnston, L., Craske, M. G., et al. (2011). Transdiagnostic Internet treatment for anxiety and depression: A randomised controlled trial. *Behaviour Research and Therapy, 49*(8), 441–452.

Titov, N., Dear, B. F., Staples, L. G., Bennett-Levy, J., Klein, B., Rapee, R. M., et al. (2015). Mind-Spot Clinic: An accessible, efficient, and effective online treatment service for anxiety and depression. *Psychiatric Services, 66*(10), 1043–1050.

Van Ballegooijen, W., Riper, H., Cuijpers, P., van Oppen, P., & Smit, J. H. (2016). Validation of online psychometric instruments for common mental health disorders: A systematic review. *BMC Psychiatry, 16,* 45.

Van der Vaart, R., Witting, M., Riper, H., Kooistra, L., Bohlmeijer, E. T., & van Gemert-Pijnen, L. J. (2014). Blending online therapy into regular face-to-face therapy for depression: Content, ratio and preconditions according to patients and therapists using a Delphi study. *BMC Psychiatry, 14,* 355.

Van Straten, A., Cuijpers, P., & Smits, N. (2008). Effectiveness of a web-based self-help intervention for symptoms of depression, anxiety, and stress: Randomized controlled trial. *Journal of Medical Internet Research, 10*(1), e7.

Vigerland, S., Ljótsson, B., Gustafsson, F. B., Hagert, S., Thulin, U., Andersson, G., et al. (2014). Attitudes towards the use of computerized cognitive behavior therapy (cCBT) with children and adolescents: A survey among Swedish mental health professionals. *Internet Interventions, 1*(3), 111–117.

White, J., Keenan, M., & Brooks, N. (1992). Stress control: A controlled comparative investigation of large group therapy for generalized anxiety disorder. *Behavioural Psychotherapy, 20*(2), 97–113.

Whitfield, G., & Williams, C. (2004). If the evidence is so good—Why doesn't anyone use them? A national survey of the use of computerized cognitive behaviour therapy. *Behavioural and Cognitive Psychotherapy, 32*(1), 57–65

Wootton, B. M., Titov, N., Dear, B. F., Spence, J., & Kemp, A. (2011). The acceptability of Internet-based treatment and characteristics of an adult sample with obsessive compulsive disorder: An Internet survey. *PLoS One, 6*(6), e20548.

# CHAPTER 5

# Ethical Competence in Behavioral and Cognitive Therapies

## Kenneth S. Pope, PhD,

### *Independent Practice, Norwalk, CT*

Ethical competence in cognitive and behavioral therapy confronts us with cognitive and behavioral challenges. Both of these challenges are psychologically difficult.

We must meet the cognitive challenges of using informed judgment to find—or sometimes to create—the most ethical path through constantly changing situations. None of these situations is exactly the same as any other. We may be like many other therapists in all sorts of ways, but each of us is unique in important ways. A client may fall into all sorts of categories that include many other clients, but each is unique in important ways. Therapists, clients, and complex situations are not frozen in time—none is exactly the same as last month, last week, or yesterday. To adapt Heraclitus, over the course of our work with a client, we never step into the identical therapeutic situation with the identical client twice. Coming up with the most ethical response to these unique, constantly changing situations forces us to set aside hopes for easy answers, a cookbook approach, or one-size-fits-all solutions. It calls on us to be alert, open, informed, mindful, and actively questioning.

Ethical competence also confronts us with behavioral challenges, because doing the right thing can sometimes be unpleasant, frightening, costly, or virtually impossible. Consider these examples:

**Example 1: Assessments provided by the CEO.** It's your first day working at a clinic, and your supervisor tells you that clinic policy requires you to conduct all assessments using only those tests created by the clinic's CEO. You do an online search and find there are no peer-reviewed studies of the tests' reliability or validity. The only two publications you can find are a newsletter article by the CEO touting the benefits of the tests and an article in a scientific journal discussing the battery as an example of pseudoscience. What do you do?

**Example 2: Changing diagnoses to get coverage.** Your new client desperately needs therapy, and you desperately need a new client if you're going to be able to pay the office rent in your new practice. But the client's insurance does not cover the client's condition. Of course, if you were to choose a covered diagnosis that doesn't fit the client, the client will get therapy and you can pay your rent. Some might call the false diagnosis route a reasonable (in light of the DSM's lack of adequate scientific basis), ethical (seeking to "do no harm" by not depriving your client of necessary professional help), and humane response to someone who is suffering and in need. Others might call it dishonesty, lying, and insurance fraud. What do you do?

**Example 3: Boarding a cruise, with a client's suicide note in hand.** It's been a grueling week, but you and your spouse will be celebrating your anniversary tonight by departing on a budget-breaking five-day cruise. Just as you're about to hand in your nonrefundable tickets and board the ship, you get an e-mail from a client saying only this: "I can't take it anymore. Nothing can help me. I'm through with therapy and everything else. Don't try to contact me. Soon it'll all be over." What do you do? You have only a few seconds to decide because you're holding up the line.

Doing what we judge to be the right thing can require us to go against our own financial self-interest, earn us the criticism of our colleagues, and be the very last thing we *want* to do. We may have to force ourselves to turn away from overwhelming temptations, face some of our deepest fears, and dig deep within ourselves to summon up moral courage we didn't know we had.

This chapter highlights some of the most important—and often the most troublesome—issues we encounter in meeting the cognitive and behavioral challenges of developing ethical competence and putting it to use in clinical practice. It concludes with a set of suggested steps for thinking through our work's ethical aspects.

# Ethics Codes

Consider the following scenarios:

You're talking with a colleague who uses behavior modification to work with the parents of kids who are disruptive at home and school. He tells you that he finds negative reinforcement most effective, so he instructs the parents to administer a gentle spanking whenever an undesired behavior occurs. This, he says, creates what is called a Pavlovian fading of the unwanted behavior. He confides that although the therapy controls the child's behavior, he is actually covertly conditioning the parents using methods so effective that they produce what Skinner called errorless learning. The more he talks, the more you realize that he has no understanding whatsoever of behavior therapy terms, principles, research, or theory. You grow concerned that he is not competent to do therapy and may be harming his clients. Does the ethics code require you to take any steps? If so, what are they? What do you think you'd wind up doing?

A woman seeking therapy schedules an initial appointment with you. During the appointment, she tells you she is currently seeing a psychologist who uses a psychodynamic approach. She had high hopes for the psychologist initially, but she feels her therapist wastes too much time dredging around in the past, and lately the therapist has started treating her just like her mother used to treat her. She is furious at her therapist and believes she would do much better with someone who uses cognitive behavioral therapy, but she just wants to make sure she has a new therapist in place before she quits her current therapy. Does the ethics code allow you to simply begin treating her right away or are there steps you must take? If there are steps, what are they? What would you actually do in this situation?

You're using cognitive processing therapy to treat a former professional mixed martial arts fighter with post-traumatic stress disorder (PTSD). However, as therapy progresses you go from being uneasy to fearful to terrified that something might trigger a violent—and perhaps lethal—attack against you. Does the ethics code allow you to terminate by phone or letter without seeing the client again? What would you do?

Ethical competence enables us to make hard choices about what to do in such difficult situations using judgment informed by the relevant ethics codes. The American Psychological Association (APA) and the Canadian Psychological Association (CPA) publish two of the most prominent and influential codes.

The APA's (2010) current code includes an introduction, a preamble, five general principles, and eighty-nine specific ethical standards. The preamble and general principles (beneficence and nonmaleficence; fidelity and responsibility; integrity; justice; and respect for people's rights and dignity) are aspirational goals meant to guide psychologists toward psychology's highest ideals. The eighty-nine ethical standards are enforceable rules of conduct.

As of this writing, the CPA was revising its ethics code. The most recent draft revision (February 2015) follows the prior version in presenting four principles to inform ethical judgments. The CPA orders the principles according to the weight each is to be given, beginning with the most important: principle I, respect for the dignity of persons and peoples; principle II, responsible caring; principle III, integrity in relationships; and principle IV, responsibility to society. Each principle is followed by a list of associated values, and each value, in turn, is followed by ethical standards showing how that principle and value apply to what psychologists do (e.g., providing therapy, conducting research, teaching). The draft code emphasizes that "Although the…ordering of principles can be helpful in resolving some ethical questions, issues, or dilemmas, the complexity of many situations requires consideration of other factors and engagement in a creative, self-reflective, and deliberative ethical decision-making process that includes consideration of many other factors" (Canadian Psychological Association, 2015, p. 2). The draft code suggests a set of ten steps for making ethical judgments in such complex situations.

Ethical competence requires us to know what the relevant ethical codes tell us about the work at hand. It also requires us to understand that codes are there to *inform* our professional judgment, not to take the place of an active, thoughtful, questioning, creative approach to our ethical responsibilities. We cannot outsource our judgment or our personal responsibility to a code. A code can guide us away from clearly unethical approaches and awaken our awareness of key values and concerns. But a code cannot tell us how to apply those values and address those concerns in a complex, constantly changing situation involving a unique therapist and client, especially when some of the ethical values may conflict with each other.

# Research

Ethical competence requires us to know what we're doing when we use cognitive and behavioral interventions. There is no way to make sound ethical judgments about our work if we don't understand the work itself and what current research tells us about our intervention's effectiveness, risks, downsides, and contraindications.

The APA ethics code states that "psychologists' work is based upon established scientific and professional knowledge of the discipline" (2010, section 2.04). The 2015 draft of the fourth edition of the CPA ethics code emphasizes that psychologists "keep themselves up to date with a broad range of relevant knowledge, research methods, techniques, and technologies and their impact on individuals and groups (e.g., couples, families, organizations, communities and peoples), through the reading of relevant literature, peer consultation, and continuing education activities, in order that their practice, teaching and research activities will benefit and not harm others" (2015, section II.9).

It is not only our own informed judgment at stake but also our client's. If we cannot explain clearly the current state of the scientific knowledge about the effectiveness, shortcomings, risks, and alternatives to a cognitive or behavioral therapy, we cannot fulfill our ethical and legal responsibilities regarding the client's right to *informed* consent and *informed* refusal.

New research is constantly sharpening—and sometimes completely revising and reshaping—our understanding of cognitive and behavioral approaches. Keeping up is both a responsibility and a challenge. David Barlow emphasizes how fast research can shift our understanding of which interventions are effective, worthless, or even detrimental: "Stunning developments in health care have occurred during the last several years. Widely accepted health-care strategies have been brought into question by research evidence as not only lacking benefit but also, perhaps, as inducing harm" (2004, p. 869; see also Barlow, 2010; Lilienfeld, Marshall, Todd, & Shane, 2014). Neimeyer, Taylor, Rozensky, and Cox (2014) used a Delphi poll to estimate that the current half-life of knowledge in cognitive and behavioral psychology is 9.6 years. Dubin describes the half-life of knowledge in psychology as "the time after completion of professional training when, because of new developments, practicing professionals have become roughly half as competent as they were upon graduation to meet the demands of their profession" (1972, p. 487).

Decades ago many therapists seized on a wonderfully compelling and inexpensive anger management therapy. Clients learned to engage in a simple behavior to deal therapeutically with their anger: they spent time hitting a bag, doll, pillow, or similar target with their fists or a bat. It was easy to come up with theoretical rationales for why the hitting behavior would relieve the anger: it behaviorally discharged the frustration that fueled the anger; it redirected the anger to an acceptable object; it provided a dynamic catharsis; it led to a sense of satisfaction and exhaustion that was incompatible with feeling angry; it created a "vent" for the emotional intensity; and so on. Despite its solid grounding in theory and its popularity, the therapy did have a downside: it didn't work. Not only did it fail to help clients manage their anger, but studies showed that the therapy tended to make clients even angrier than they had been, raised their blood pressure, left them feeling worse, and increased the likelihood of future angry outbursts. (For research and discussions, see Bushman, 2002; Lohr, Olatunji, Baumeister, & Bushman, 2007; and Tavris, 1989.) We bear an essential ethical responsibility to keep our eyes open for evidence that new, popular, promising—or our own favorite—therapies fail to deliver as much benefit as other approaches, produce no improvement whatsoever, or even cause harm. Clients depend on us to avoid wasting their time (and money) or leaving them worse off than they were when they came to us for help. Discussing the ethics of staying current with research—including studies contradicting the use of certain approaches—George Stricker writes, "We all must labor with the absence of affirmative data, but there is no excuse for ignoring contradictory data" (1992, p. 544).

To understand what current research tells us about an intervention's effectiveness, downsides, risks, and contraindications involves understanding the research itself rather than relying on brief summaries like "cognitive behavior therapy was found to be effective in treating PTSD." Understanding a research finding like this includes our ability to answer key questions, such as these: What do we know about the clients and how they were recruited and screened? Was cognitive behavioral therapy (CBT) compared with other treatments, and, if so, were the clients randomly assigned to treatment groups? How was the outcome evaluated? Did the evaluators know which client received which treatment? What percentage of clients, if any, in each treatment group failed to improve? What client characteristics or psychological processes moderated outcomes (e.g., multiple traumas, concurrent social problems, high levels of rumination)? What percentage of clients, if any, in each treatment group were worse off after treatment than at the beginning, and *in what ways* were they worse off? Are any statistically significant differences between treatments also clinically significant (e.g., effect size)? Could funding, sponsorship, or conflicts of interest have unintentionally introduced bias into how the hypotheses were framed, the methodologies chosen, the data analyzed, or the results reported? (See Flacco et al., 2015; Jacobson, 2015.) How long after treatment was the follow-up, and were there any significant changes in the outcome in the months or years after termination?

Knowing the answers to such questions is one key to fulfilling our ethical responsibility to practice with competence. Like ethics codes, research informs our judgment but does not take its place. Competent practice as well as our clients and others impacted by our work depend on us to make informed judgments about how to help without hurting.

Informed judgment will sometimes guide us a bit beyond techniques that are empirically supported for a particular situation, and we must adapt a technique the best we can for a new use. What is crucial is that we understand both what the research tells us *and* the limits of that knowledge. Many research findings, for example, are based on statistical differences between groups of people. Part of the inherent limits of our knowledge is that an intervention strongly supported by statistically and clinically significant findings from these statistically based studies may—or may not—"work" with the client sitting across from us. B. F. Skinner highlighted the fallacy of assuming that statistical differences between groups or other statistical associations will automatically translate to a specific individual: "No one goes to the circus to see the average dog jump through a hoop significantly oftener than untrained dogs raised under the same circumstances" (1956, p. 228). Our work with each client becomes similar to an $N = 1$ study, in which we monitor carefully the effects of our interventions on one particular person.

Littell (2010) adapted Skinner's insight to the therapeutic situation while underscoring the need to understand the research itself rather than settle for secondhand assurances that a particular therapy is "evidence based":

> Most scientific knowledge is tentative and nomothetic, not directly applicable to individual cases. Experts have stepped into this breach by packaging empirical evidence for use in practice. Sometimes this is little more than a ruse to promote favorite theories and therapies. Yet, wrapped in scientific rhetoric, some authoritative pronouncements have become orthodoxy. (pp. 167–168)

# Laws, Licensing Rules, Legal Standards of Care, and Other Governmental Regulations

Imagine yourself in the following situations:

> You are using CBT to treat a woman with PTSD. Aware of experimental and meta-analytic studies suggesting that CBT decreases the heart rate (HR) of clients with PTSD, you show her how to measure her pulse at the beginning and end of each session and suggest that she chart her HR during the week, particularly when she is experiencing the symptoms of PTSD. She shows steady improvement with this intervention and even mentions that it seems to be helping with the occasional heart palpitations, for which she takes cardiac meds.

> Do the laws, licensing rules, legal standards of care, and other governmental regulations consider you to be practicing medicine? Do they require you to be knowledgeable about the physiology, biology, normal functioning, and pathology of the human heart as well as the nature and effects of medications relevant to this client? Do they require you to obtain her medical records prior to initiating interventions that are known to affect the heart or other organs? Do they require you to include information about the possible effects of CBT on people with PTSD in your informed consent process? If yes, can you address this informed consent

requirement by just writing in the chart that you discussed it with the client and that the client provided informed consent for the intervention, or are you legally required to obtain the client's written informed consent? (Note that the relevant regulations vary from jurisdiction to jurisdiction so that what one state or province requires may not be mentioned or even be prohibited by another state or province.)

---

Your client is an elderly man who came to you for help because he's become depressed over his chronic medical problems. He constantly worries that his problems will get worse. His days are filled with rumination. After discussing various treatment options, he decides to try mindfulness-based stress reduction. Both of you see improvement by the second session. Unfortunately, prior to beginning therapy he agreed to leave the following week to spend six weeks with one of his daughters and her husband who live in another state. You and your client agree that the weekly sessions can continue uninterrupted via Skype.

Do the laws, licensing rules, legal standards of care, and other governmental regulations require you to be licensed in the state where his daughter lives? Do the laws, licensing rules, legal standards of care, and other governmental regulations of your own state, of the daughter's state, or both states apply to the therapy (e.g., requirements for competence, informed consent, maintaining records, release of confidential information, exceptions to privilege, and so on)? If the governmental regulations of the daughter's state apply, are you knowledgeable about them? Do either state regulations or those of the federal US Health Insurance Portability and Accountability Act (HIPAA) and its amendments require that the Skype sessions be encrypted? Do they require encryption of phone calls, e-mails, texts, or other electronic communications between you and the client? If you practice in a Canadian province and the client is in another province, do the relevant provincial regulations, the Canadian Privacy Act, or the Canadian Personal Information Protection and Electronic Documents Act (PIPEDA) require encryption of your communications?

---

As you begin the first session with a new client, she informs you that she is sixteen and would like some kind of relaxation therapy for her anxiety attacks. She asks you if therapy is confidential, and you say, "Yes, with certain exceptions," and before you can explain the exceptions she blurts out that she is planning to have an abortion and keep it secret from her parents, and if you tell anyone she will kill herself.

According to the law, is she old enough to provide informed consent, or must a parent or guardian provide consent for her treatment? Does a parent or guardian have a legal right to see her therapy records and to know what she told you? If you have strong religious objections to abortion, does the law allow you to refuse to treat her on that basis?

---

Ethical competence includes knowing the relevant laws, licensing rules, legal standards of care, and other governmental regulations that tell clinicians in a particular jurisdiction what they can, must, or must not do. This information is key not only to making sound professional judgments but also to ensuring clients' right to informed consent. For some clients, deciding whether to give or withhold consent to treatment may hinge on whether the therapist must make a legally mandated report in certain situations or whether there are exceptions to privacy, confidentiality, or privilege.

Like ethics codes and research studies, the power of the state—expressed through legislation, case law, administrative regulations, and so forth and enforced by courts, licensing boards, and other governmental agencies—informs our professional judgments but cannot make those judgments for us. When working with a client who is psychotic, developmentally disabled, or under the influence of drugs, the law may require us to obtain informed consent, but it cannot not tell us the best way to inform this particular client, to assess whether the client is offering an informed agreement for treatment, or even to determine whether the client is capable of freely giving informed consent. The law in our jurisdiction may call for a therapist whose client makes a violent threat against an identifiable third party to take reasonable steps to protect the third party, but the law cannot tell us which steps make the most sense with a particular client and third party.

Ethical competence also includes being alert to instances when the law and ethics may conflict with each other. For example, what the law requires may be at odds, in our professional opinion, with the client's basic rights or with our own belief of what is ethical and "doing the right thing." Facing such conflicts, we can consult with experts and other colleagues and try to come up with creative solutions that bridge the conflict without violating either ethics or the law. If we are unable to resolve the conflict, we must decide what it means to do the right thing in a given situation, to weigh whether we are prepared to accept the costs and risks of that path, and to accept the consequences of whatever path we ultimately choose.

# Contexts

Imagine yourself in the shoes of the following hypothetical therapists:

Your new client had seen on your web page that you help people change their habitual patterns of thinking, alter the way they respond to situations, and get rid of self-defeating behaviors. He tells you that he was very lucky to find a job and wants your help to hold on to it at all costs because that's the only way he can support himself and his elderly father who lives with him. The problem, he explains, is that he is the only one of his race and religion who works there, and the other employees don't respect him, using slurs and telling cruel jokes ridiculing his race and religion. Once he got up the courage to ask a small group of them what they had against him, his race, and his religion, and they all denied ever treating him with anything but great respect or ever using a slur or telling any jokes mentioning race or religion. As soon as he started to walk away, they broke out laughing.

He refuses to consider quitting, bringing up the matter again to his coworkers, making some sort of formal complaint, or suing the company. He just wants you to help him learn not to have such strong emotional reactions at work, to stop dwelling on his coworkers' behavior, and to find alternatives to responses that are maladaptive and self-defeating in that setting. He'd like to learn how to adopt a more positive attitude and be more accepting of fellow employees. He wants to try either pretending that he doesn't hear or laughing along good-naturedly when they tell a cruel joke or use a slur.

Do you provide the therapy he asks for? If not, what do you do? If you imagined a specific race and religion for your client, would your reaction be any different if you imagined a different race and religion for the client?

---

Your soon-to-be new client calls to schedule her first appointment, telling you that she gets anxious and tongue-tied whenever she has to speak to an audience. She wants to learn how to calm herself and be relaxed and at ease when she gets up to talk. During the call you ask how she got your name. She laughs and says that you are the only therapist in her community that is in her insurance coverage network, so it's you or nothing.

During the first session, she asks what sorts of therapy might help her. You mention self-talk, deep breathing exercises, cognitive behavior modification, and a range of other approaches, and then ask if there are any kinds of talks, settings, or audiences that are particularly frightening or difficult. She explains that she is chair of a new political action committee (PAC) and must ask groups of people for money and support. You realize that her PAC works against some of your most deeply held values. You believe—though many would disagree with you—that her policies, if enacted, would violate some basic human rights and harm many people. If you help her become a more effective speaker, she will likely become more able to enlist support and raise large sums of money to pass laws that diametrically oppose your deepest values.

Do you put the tools of cognitive and behavioral therapy to work helping her? If so, do you disclose your own values? Are there any situations in which you would refuse to work with a client because of your own deepest values? Which of your values, if any, would lead you to refuse?

---

None of us works in a vacuum. Our work takes place in a variety of contexts that may affect the work we do. Ethical competence includes remaining aware of these contexts and how they affect us, our clients, and the work we do.

The array of attitudes, beliefs, and values in a society, organization, or other setting is one major source of contextual effects. The two hypothetical scenarios above illustrate the ways in which the interventions we use—which some would view as per se value-neutral—can, when viewed in these contexts, be seen to work for or against certain values, policies, or populations and to raise ethical issues.

Davison, writing in the same decade that homosexuality was finally removed from the DSM as a sociopathic personality disturbance disorder, urged the field to pay attention to these contexts and their ethical implications. He focused on the view of homosexuality prevalent at the time both in general society and the profession:

Behavior therapy is nothing if it does not represent a profound commitment to dispassionate inquiry...I want to voice some concerns I have been wrestling with... Any comprehensive perusal of the...literature in behavior therapy...will confirm...that therapists by and large regard homosexual behavior and attitudes to be undesirable, sometimes pathological, and at any rate in need of change toward a heterosexual orientation. And I do not take special issue with aversion therapy since I suggest that the more positive therapies of homosexuality are similarly to be questioned on ethical grounds. (1976, p. 158)

The concerns he was wrestling with led him to make what was at the time a radical proposal:

> Since professionals are unlikely to work on treatment procedures unless they see a problem, it is probable that the very existence of change-of-orientation programs strengthens societal prejudices against homosexuality and contributes to the self-hate and embarrassment that are determinants of the "voluntary" desire by some homosexuals to become heterosexual. It is therefore proposed that we stop offering therapy to help homosexuals change and concentrate instead on improving the quality of their interpersonal relationships. Alternatively, more energy could be devoted to sexual enhancement procedures in general, regardless of the adult gender mix. (p. 157)

A second major source of contextual effects is culture. A cognitive or behavioral intervention well suited to one culture may violate another culture's norms, customs, assumptions, or values. The research supporting the use of an intervention for a given problem may have been conducted on people from a different culture than the person sitting across from us in our consulting room. We may face difficulties communicating clearly with clients if they are from cultures that are unfamiliar to us.

When considering how the client's culture influences the client and the therapy, it's easy to overlook how our own culture influences us, our approach to clients, and the work we do. *The Spirit Catches You and You Fall Down: A Hmong Child, Her American Doctors, and the Collision of Two Cultures* (Fadiman, 1997) highlights the dangers of overlooking culture's effects on everyone involved. The book describes how the staff of a California hospital tried to help a Hmong child whose American physicians had diagnosed with epilepsy. Her parents, however, viewed her problems as being due to spirits. The staff tried to help the girl, but lack of attention to cultural differences derailed the process. The book chronicles the intervention of the medical community that insisted upon removing the child from her loving parents, with horrible results. The book quotes medical anthropologist Arthur Kleinman:

> As powerful an influence as the culture of the Hmong patient and her family is on this case, the culture of biomedicine is equally powerful. If you can't see that your own culture has its own set of interests, emotions, and biases, how can you expect to deal successfully with someone else's culture? (p. 261)

# Cognitive Biases

The degree to which we can think through the complex array of ethical standards, research, laws and regulations, and contexts and come up with the most ethical way to provide therapy that helps without hurting depends on the quality of our judgment. Unfortunately, human cognition often falls prey to a vast array of mistakes in paying attention, making assumptions, selecting and weighing information, reasoning, using language with precision, navigating safely through pressure and temptations, and arriving at decisions. *All* of us have our vulnerabilities, weaknesses, and blind spots—yes, even you there…you know who you are: the one about to nod off while wondering how many more pages there are in this chapter—along with our skills, strengths, and insights. Ethical competence includes staying abreast of the literature on logical fallacies, pseudoscientific reasoning, heuristics that can lead us astray, ethical rationalizations, and other barriers to critical thinking and sound judgment.

For example, we may find ourselves favoring a particular intervention, relying on studies that support it, while unintentionally ignoring, denying, discounting, or finding ways to discredit evidence of the intervention's downsides, risks, or inability to match the effectiveness of other interventions. Decades of psychological research reveals an almost endless catalog of shared human tendencies—confirmation bias, cognitive dissonance, premature cognitive commitment, the WYSIATI (what you see is all there is) fallacy, false consensus…and on and on—to overlook, avoid, or ignore whatever fails to fit our beliefs and loyalties (Pope, 2016).

Glitches in judgment can affect us on the group, organizational, social, as well as individual level. In 1973, for example, Meehl published an essay—"Why I Do Not Attend Case Conferences"—that quickly went that decade's version of viral. He pointed out variations of the "groupthink process" (1977, p. 228) that sends judgment off course and may be familiar to many of us:

> In one respect the clinical case conference is no different from other academic group phenomena such as committee meetings, in that many intelligent, educated, sane, rational persons seem to undergo a kind of intellectual deterioration when they gather around a table in one room. (1977, p. 227)

The key to benefiting from the literature on judgment pitfalls is to resist the temptation to apply the information only to others instead of starting with ourselves and using it as a mirror to strengthen our ethical competence. Readings in this area include Kahneman (2011); Kleespies (2014); Pinker (2013); Taleb (2010);

Zsambok and Klein (2014); and the chapters "Avoiding Pseudoscience, Fads, and Academic Urban Legends," "Ethical Judgment Under Uncertainty and Pressure: Critical Thinking About Heuristics, Authorities, and Groups," "26 Logical Fallacies in Ethical Reasoning," "Using and Misusing Words to Reveal and Conceal," and "Ethics Placebos, Cons, and Creative Cheating: A User's Guide" in Pope and Vasquez (2016).

# Helpful Steps

The following set of steps (adapted from Pope & Vasquez, 2016) may be useful in thinking through ethical dilemmas in a careful and structured way. Eight of these steps (2, 8, 11, 12, 14, 15, 16, and 17) were adapted from the CPA (2015) ethics code.

Step 1: State the question, dilemma, or concern as clearly as possible.

Step 2: Anticipate who will be affected by the decision.

Step 3: Figure out who, if anyone, is the client.

Step 4: Assess whether our areas of competence—and of missing knowledge, skills, experience, or expertise—fit the situation.

Step 5: Review relevant formal ethical standards.

Step 6: Review relevant legal standards.

Step 7: Review the relevant research and theory.

Step 8: Consider whether personal feelings, biases, or self-interest might shade our ethical judgment.

Step 9: Consider whether social, cultural, religious, or similar factors affect the situation and the search for the best response.

Step 10: Consider consultation.

Step 11: Develop alternative courses of action.

Step 12: Think through the alternative courses of action.

Step 13: Try to adopt the perspective of each person who will be affected.

Step 14: Decide what to do, review or reconsider it, and take action.

Step 15: Document the process and assess the results.

Step 16: Assume personal responsibility for the consequences.

Step 17: Consider implications for preparation, planning, and prevention.

Davison's courageous confronting of social biases against homosexuality, discussed earlier, provides us with an example of thinking through an ethical dilemma. He states the question clearly (step 1). He identifies the clients (step 3). He thinks through how personal or cultural biases can impact the therapy given to these clients (steps 8 and 9). Taking the perspective of the stakeholders (step 13), he considers alternative courses of action (step 11). He recommends a clear course of action (step 14). He makes no attempt to disappear into abstractions, professional jargon, or daunting sentence structures but instead assumes personal responsibility (step 16) for his analysis and recommendations through, for example, his use of the first-person singular (e.g., "I want to voice some concerns I have been wrestling with…I do not take special issue with aversion therapy since I suggest that the more positive therapies of homosexuality are similarly to be questioned on ethical grounds."). He models the kind of careful step-by-step analysis all of us can use to confront difficult ethical dilemmas.

# References

American Psychological Association. (2010). *Ethical principles of psychologists and code of conduct including 2010 and 2016 amendments.* Retrieved from http://www.apa.org/ethics/code/index.aspx.

Barlow, D. H. (2004). Psychological treatments. *American Psychologist, 59*(9), 869–878.

Barlow, D. H. (2010). Negative effects from psychological treatments: A perspective. *American Psychologist, 65*(1), 13–20.

Bushman, B. J. (2002). Does venting anger feed or extinguish the flame? Catharsis, rumination, distraction, anger, and aggressive responding. *Personality and Social Psychology Bulletin, 28*(6), 724–731.

Canadian Psychological Association. (2015). *Canadian code of ethics for psychologists* (4th ed., February 2015 draft). Ottawa, Ontario: Canadian Psychological Association.

Davison, G. C. (1976). Homosexuality: The ethical challenge. *Journal of Consulting and Clinical Psychology, 44*(2), 157–162.

Dubin, S. S. (1972). Obsolescence or lifelong education: A choice for the professional. *American Psychologist, 27*(5), 486–498.

Fadiman, A. (1997). *The spirit catches you and you fall down: A Hmong child, her American doctors, and the collision of two cultures.* New York: Farrar, Straus and Giroux.

Flacco, M. E., Manzoli, L., Boccia, S., Capasso, L., Aleksovska, K., Rosso, A., et al. (2015). Head-to-head randomized trials are mostly industry sponsored and almost always favor the industry sponsor. *Journal of Clinical Epidemiology, 68*(7), 811–820.

Jacobson, R. (2015). Many antidepressant studies found tainted by pharma company influence: A review of studies that assess clinical antidepressants shows hidden conflicts of interest and financial ties to corporate drugmakers. *Scientific American*, October 21. http://www.scientifi-camerican.com/article/many-antidepressant-studies-found-tainted-by-pharma-company-influence.

Kahneman, D. (2011). *Thinking, fast and slow.* New York: Farrar, Straus and Giroux.

Kleespies, P. M. (2014). Decision making under stress: Theoretical and empirical bases. In P. M. Kleespies, *Decision making in behavioral emergencies: Acquiring skill in evaluating and managing high-risk patients* (pp. 31–46). Washington, DC: American Psychological Association.

Lilienfeld, S. O., Marshall, J., Todd, J. T., & Shane, H. C. (2014). The persistence of fad interventions in the face of negative scientific evidence: Facilitated communication for autism as a case example. *Evidence-Based Communication Assessment and Intervention, 8*(2), 62–101.

Littell, J. H. (2010). Evidence-based practice: Evidence or orthodoxy? In B. L. Duncan, S. D. Miller, B. E. Wampold, & M. A. Hubble (Eds.), *The heart and soul of change: Delivering what works in therapy* (2nd ed., pp. 167–198). Washington, DC: American Psychological Association.

Lohr, J. M., Olatunji, B. O., Baumeister, R. F., & Bushman, B. J. (2007). The psychology of anger venting and empirically supported alternatives that do no harm. *Scientific Review of Mental Health Practice, 5*(1), 53–64.

Meehl, P. (1977). Why I do not attend case conferences. In P. Meehl (Ed.), *Psychodiagnosis: Selected papers* (pp. 225–302). New York: W. W. Norton.

Neimeyer, G. J., Taylor, J. M., Rozensky, R. H., & Cox, D. R. (2014). The diminishing durability of knowledge in professional psychology: A second look at specializations. *Professional Psychology: Research and Practice, 45*(2), 92–98.

Pinker, S. (2013). *Language, cognition, and human nature: Selected articles.* New York: Oxford University Press.

Pope, K. S. (2016). The code not taken: The path from guild ethics to torture and our continuing choices—The Canadian Psychological Association John C. Service Member of the Year Award Address. *Canadian Psychology/Psychologie canadienne, 57*(1), 51–59. Retrieved from http://kspope.com/PsychologyEthics.php.

Pope, K. S., & Vasquez, M. J. T. (2016). *Ethics in psychotherapy and counseling: A practical guide* (5th ed.). New York: John Wiley and Sons.

Skinner B. F. (1956). A case history in scientific method. *American Psychologist, 11*(5), 221–233.

Stricker, G. (1992). The relationship of research to clinical practice. *American Psychologist, 47*(4), 543–549.

Taleb, N. N. (2010). *The black swan: The impact of the highly improbable* (2nd ed.). New York: Random House.

Tavris, C. (1989). *Anger: The misunderstood emotion.* New York: Simon and Schuster.

Zsambok, C. E., & Klein, G. A. (Eds.). (2014). *Naturalistic decision making.* New York: Psychology Press.

PART 2

# CHAPTER 6

# Core Behavioral Processes

Mark R. Dixon, PhD
Ruth Anne Rehfeldt, PhD

*Rehabilitation Institute, Southern Illinois University*

The purpose of this chapter is to summarize principles that explain the operation of direct contingencies on behavior, in the form of habituation, operant conditioning, and classical conditioning. We will also explore their impact on the processes of stimulus control and generalization and will briefly mention habituation and the extension of direct contingencies into issues of language and cognition.

## Direct Contingency Learning

Direct contingencies are ancient processes of behavioral regulation. Habituation is present even in slime molds (Boisseau, Vogel, & Dussutour, 2016), nonneural single-cell organisms that evolved about 1.7 billion years ago. Contingency learning—operant and classical conditioning—appears to be about 0.5 billion years old since virtually all complex species that have evolved since the Cambrian Period show these processes, while earlier life-forms do not (Ginsburg & Jablonka, 2010).

Despite the age of these regulatory processes, clinically relevant behavior is often the result, at least in part, of direct-acting contingencies found within the environment. Such conditions either elicit or evoke behavior from the subject of interest and encompass the core principles of classical and operant conditioning. Although operant and classical conditioning principles are typically described in isolation, these learning processes overlap and interact to a degree (Rescorla & Solomon, 1967). In order to gain a basic understanding of them, however, it is most effective to first describe them separately.

## Habituation and Sensitization

One of the oldest and most basic forms of learning (Pierce & Cheney, 2013) is *habituation* (and its less studied opposite, sensitization): when an unconditioned stimulus elicits an unconditioned response, and that stimulus is presented over and over, the response may decline in magnitude to the point that it no longer occurs at all. For example, Bradley, Lang, and Cuthbert (1993) recorded heart rate, electrodermal, and facial corrugator-muscle responses as measures of the startle reflex, finding that the startle responses decreased dramatically with repeated presentations of stimuli that induced them. Researchers often use habituation paradigms to study the physiological bases of different neurological disorders. For instance, Penders and Delwaide (1971) found that patients with Parkinson's disease showed no habituation of the eye-blink response with electromyography relative to individuals without the disease, but they did display normal habituation responses when treated with either L-dopa or amantadine medication.

## Classical Conditioning

Human and nonhuman organisms display many types of reflexive behaviors, many of which are unlearned and may help the organism survive. For example, placing food in one's mouth elicits salivation, and a puff of air into one's eye may elicit a blink. Because such behavior-environment relations are unlearned and of innate origin, the eliciting stimuli are referred to as unconditioned stimuli, while the response is described as an unconditioned response. *Classical conditioning* occurs when a once-neutral stimulus (NS) is paired temporally with an unconditioned stimulus (US) to produce the unconditioned response (UR). Over repeated pairings the US becomes unnecessary and the NS begins to produce an elicited response on its own. This new "automatic" response to a once-neutral stimulus is termed a conditioned response (CR). An example that is commonly provided to illustrate this basic form of classical conditioning consists of a dog that initially has no response to the sound of a bell, yet when the bell (NS) is paired with food (US), which produces a salivation response (UR), the dog salivates at the sound of the bell. After the food (US) is no longer provided with the sound of the bell, the animal still salivates (CR) at the sound of the bell (CS).

In classical conditioning, the eliciting functions of one stimulus transfer to another stimulus due to their contiguity, or pairing. When the neutral stimulus has acquired the eliciting functions of the unconditioned stimulus, it's referred to as a conditioned stimulus, and the response is referred to as a conditioned response. For example, certain poisonous foods may induce nausea as an automatic, reflexive response. A neutral stimulus, such as an odor or sound that has no such effect on behavior, may similarly come to elicit that nausea response after repeated pairings of the unconditioned and neutral stimuli. This "taste aversion" effect can produce havoc with cancer patients, who need to avoid eating unfamiliar food before chemotherapy in order to avoid conditioned nausea with that food. In a more positive example, the smell of coffee alone wakes up coffee drinkers in the morning (Domjan, 2013). Coffee is a stimulant drug, and its taste and smell precede its stimulant effects. The temporal contiguity of stimuli is critical for conditioning to occur; in other words, the two stimuli must be presented close in time to one another in order to establish the conditioned response.

Importantly, in *second-order conditioning*, additional previously neutral stimuli can acquire eliciting functions based on their temporal contiguity with other conditioned stimuli. This means that an organism doesn't always need to have repeated contact with an unconditioned stimulus in order for conditioned responses to new stimuli to develop. Second-order conditioning helps explain how, in the clinical environment, classical conditioning can lead to a client reacting to a stimulus that is only distally related to directly impactful events.

Most general forms of classical conditioning appear to require close proximity in stimulus pairings (generally less than a second), although with taste aversion the delay between the unconditioned stimulus and conditioned stimulus can be as long as a day (Bureš, Bermúdez-Rattoni, & Yamamoto, 1998). Though typically the conditioned stimulus and unconditioned stimulus need to be paired close together in time, they can occur in different temporal arrangements. In *forward conditioning*, the previously described paradigm, the conditioned stimulus is presented first, and the unconditioned stimulus is presented while the conditioned stimulus remains present. In *backward conditioning*, the conditioned stimulus is presented after the unconditioned stimulus has been presented. There has long been a debate as to whether backward conditioning can actually occur, in part due to Pavlov's skepticism about it, but the body of evidence suggests that it does (Spetch, Wilkie, & Pinel, 1981).

*Trace conditioning* involves presenting the unconditioned stimulus and then, after it stops, the conditioned stimulus (conditioning is said to occur because the unconditioned stimulus left a "trace" in the organism's nervous system or memory). *Simultaneous conditioning* involves presenting two stimuli at the same time.

Researchers have proposed that respondent conditioning is the learning process underlying the development of any number of conditioned fear and phobic responses. For example, John B. Watson, the founder of behaviorism, conducted the famous "Little Albert" experiment. In this experiment, a young child was shown a small, furry white animal, the display of which was paired with the sound of a steel bar being struck, which caused a startle response in the child. In a process known as respondent generalization, stimuli that physically resembled the small, furry animal came to elicit the same startle and emotional response. Öhman and Mineka (2001) suggest that the acquisition of such conditioned fear responses has an evolutionary basis, noting that there are typically cues or warning stimuli that signal to an organism that some pending disaster may threaten its survival. The acquisition of such conditioned fear responses, the authors elaborate, may allow an organism to escape or avoid stimuli that could be harmful. These researchers, as well as others, have focused their work on the neural circuitry involved in the acquisition of responses, implicating, for example, the role of the amygdala in classical conditioning.

Behavior therapists have long appealed to respondent conditioning as an explanation for the genesis of anxiety disorders (e.g., Wolpe & Rowan, 1988). In recent years, research of this kind has focused especially on the neural mechanisms involved in fear conditioning. It appears, however, that much of the fear conditioning in humans is based on symbolic and cognitive generalization, not just the formal similarities between aversive experiences and the current situation (Dymond, Dunsmoor, Vervliet, Roche, & Hermans, 2015). We will touch on this issue at the end of this chapter, and the point is expanded on in chapter 7.

## Operant Conditioning

Most nonreflexive forms of learning fall into the operant category of conditioning, a class of response topographies that operate in a similar way upon the environment to produce a consequence. Consider the many different ways one can pass through a doorway: a person can walk, dance, run, roll, summersault, or be dragged by another through the entrance. All these response forms, or topographies, operate in a similar fashion upon the environment: they get the person through the doorway. A focus on responses that have common effects, or classes, has proved useful to researchers and therapists in their understanding of how various conditioning processes strengthen or weaken behavior over time.

The three-term contingency (Skinner, 1953; Sidman, 2009) is the unit of analysis most researchers use to investigate operant conditioning. This contingency of conditioning, often denoted as A-B-C, specifies the contextual conditions that surround and involve the behavior of interest being studied. The A represents the "antecedent," or precursors, that sets the occasion for a behavior; the B represents the "behavior" engaged in by the subject of interest; and the C indicates the "consequences" that follow the behavior (additional terms can be added to this three-term formulation, as we note later). This three-term contingency provides the analyst with information about why an individual exhibits a behavior, as well as how to produce similar behavior in the future.

Given particular antecedent conditions, when the behavior is emitted, the consequence that follows may alter the probability of similar behaviors occurring in the future. If a class of behaviors of interest is followed by a consequence that increases the probability of those behaviors happening in the future, *reinforcement* is said to have occurred (Skinner, 1969); if the consequence that follows suppresses the probability of the behaviors happening again in the future, then *punishment* is said to have occurred (Dinsmoor, 1998).

A real-world example may help illustrate these processes (see also chapters 11–14). Consider a child engaging in a tantrum. In isolation, emotional displays provide us little insight into the *why* of the tantrum or the conditions that may increase or decrease the probability of a tantrum in the future. However, once we examine the antecedents and consequences surrounding this behavior, we can obtain needed information that may help us alter it. Suppose we learn that tantrums happen whenever the child's father makes reasonable task demands (e.g., "It is time to set the table. Remember, you have to do your chores to get your allowance.") but not her mother. We have information needed to deduce the probability of the behavior but still lack information on why it's happening. When examining the consequences of such tantrums, suppose we discover that the father withdraws the task request and goes to the living room to watch TV as soon as a tantrum occurs, but the mother stays with the request and records the tantrum in order to implement the allowance contingency. Together the antecedents and consequences provide us a complete account of why the tantrums occur and the conditions under which they increase in probability. The three-term contingency is complete.

The basic notions of antecedents and consequences become exponentially intricate rather quickly. For example, it matters whether consequences are delayed (Madden, Begotka, Raiff, & Kastern, 2003); are not highly preferred by the subject (DeLeon & Iwata, 1996); stay identical over too long of a period of time (Podlesnik & Shahan, 2009); or require behavior that was too effortful, demanding, or complex (Heyman & Monaghan, 1987). Similar issues exist in antecedent stimulus control (see chapter 12).

One of the most commonly explored modifications to the general process of reinforcement is its delivery cycle. Often termed a "schedule of reinforcement" (Skinner, 1969), this delivery of a consequence can have an important impact on the probability of a behavior occurring. Schedules of reinforcement abound, with perhaps the most common variants using ratio and interval parameters. When a ratio schedule is in place, only a certain number of responses will yield the programmed consequence. The amount can be fixed, as in after every five responses (a fixed ratio–5, or FR-5 schedule) there is a consequence, or it can be variable, as in on average there will be a consequence following every five responses (a variable ratio–5, or VR-5 schedule). When an interval schedule is in place, only the first response will produce the consequence after a period of time has elapsed, and like the ratio schedule, it too can contain a fixed (FI) or variable (VI) period of time that must elapse. Seeing Old Faithful erupt is an example of an FI schedule: no amount of looking will hasten or delay it. Seeing an unoccupied taxi cab to hail is a VI schedule: regular looking will not make the cab arrive, but it could come by at any moment. Logical deductions and empirical data allow us to conclude how these various schedules can produce different behavior patterns. A ratio schedule will yield consequences much quicker if the response is emitted more frequently, and thus it tends to encourage higher rates of responding than an interval schedule.

A great deal of research and analysis has been performed and predictions made regarding these basic schedules of reinforcement (e.g., Zuriff, 1970), and this work has laid a foundation for the clinical application of contingency processes (see chapter 11). One important discovery within the domain of schedules of reinforcement and punishment is that all complex species tend to show very similar patterns of responding under identical schedule contingencies, at least until the arrival of verbal behavior (Lowe & Horne, 1985).

Behavior that is controlled by positive consequence appears to be different from behavior controlled by an aversive consequence being removed following the emission of a response (what is termed escape conditioning), or when a consequence is postponed or prevented by responding (avoidance conditioning; see Dinsmoor, 1977, for more on this distinction); this is a key area of concern for applied workers in clinical psychology. Avoidance learning can be especially troublesome in applied contexts, because it prevents further contact with the environment, which can allow avoidance to continue long after its reasons for being have disappeared.

A clinical example of avoidance conditioning is the avoidance of physiological conditions that typically accompany fear. Classical conditioning may have had a role in establishing these physiological conditions, but operant contingencies can lead to active escape or avoidance, reinforcing the overt behavior. There is a long history of such "two factor" reasoning (e.g., Dinsmoor, 1954) in behavioral and cognitive therapies.

*Negative reinforcement* procedures involve the removal or prevention of a stimulus, whereas *positive reinforcement* procedures involve the presentation of a stimulus. The terms "positive" and "negative" should be thought of more in their additive or subtractive senses than in their good or bad evaluative senses. There are still theoretical arguments about the fundamental nature of this distinction, but as an applied matter it is an important one both practically and ethically. For example, the deliberate utilization of aversive stimuli as part of a negative reinforcement procedure may introduce ethical considerations, especially when procedures based on a more positive consequence may yield very similar outcomes (Bailey & Burch, 2013).

One of the most crucial factors that should not be overlooked when implementing behavior change procedures using direct contingencies, regardless of the schedule or type of reinforcement, is the passage of time. Time between the emission of the behavior and the delivery of the consequence has a radical impact on the future probability of behavior emission (Ainslie & Herrnstein, 1981). To produce optimal effects, delays should be kept to a minimum. As time increases from behavior emission to consequence delivery, the ability to influence future behavior weakens (Mazur, 2000). If a child stops a tantrum at 1 p.m. and special privileges are delivered at 3 p.m., there are many other behaviors that may have occurred during this two-hour interval of time. As such, the delayed consequence may inadvertently strengthen the behavior occurring at 2:59 p.m., whatever that may be. Many cultural practices are based on the idea that delayed consequence linked to temporally distant prior behavior will be effective. Examples include a yearly bonus at work or report card grades. These delayed consequences are more likely to be operational, if at all, through verbal rules than through direct contingency control.

The perversely weak effect of delayed consequences can be seen in the many clinically significant self-control problems people face. Behavior surrounding obesity, for example, is difficult to address because of the long delay between eating or proper exercise and the actual consequences of weight gain or weight loss.

Although delayed consequences are inherently weak for controlling behavior, therapists can improve on their effectiveness through a variety of contingency manipulation techniques (see chapter 14). First, the therapist can initially make the delayed consequences available immediately and then gradually delay them over time, resulting in much higher rates of sustained behavior (Logue & Peña-Correal, 1984). Second, therapists can provide clients with a concurrent activity to engage in during a delay to reinforce delivery, leading to more-sustained behavior than when no activities are present (Grosch & Neuringer, 1981). People who are asked to speak about the eventual delivery of delayed consequences perform better at tasks requiring a delayed consequence compared with those who do not make such verbalizations (Binder, Dixon, & Ghezzi, 2000). Delay to consequence delivery is an inherent challenge when attempting to increase or decrease a behavior of interest. When clinical situations necessitate delays, therapists should take concrete steps to improve the effectiveness of delayed consequences.

When consequences that previously maintained a behavior are no longer provided, the principle of extinction is considered to be in place. *Extinction* is the elimination of the previously delivered consequence in the A-B-C contingency, and it has a somewhat predictable effect on behavior over time. Eliminating positive consequences will eventually suppress a response until it's terminated completely, and the elimination of aversive consequences will reinstate the response. A variety of other effects are commonly seen in extinction: previously reinforced and then extinguished behavior is likely to show resurgence (Shahan & Sweeney, 2011); the rates of a particular behavior are likely to temporarily increase in an "extinction burst" (Lerman & Iwata, 1995); and aggression or other potentially problematic behaviors, such as self-harm, may occur (Lerman, Iwata, & Wallace, 1999). In part, to reduce these negative side effects, when attempting to eliminate an undesired behavior with extinction, typically therapists concurrently reinforce an alternative behavior that is incompatible or simply more appropriate (for a review, see Petscher, Rey, & Bailey, 2009). Sometimes therapists pair extinction with time-based reinforcement schedules that deliver noncontingent consequences—irrespective of alternative behavior—in an attempt to eliminate an undesirable contingency without also instigating the emotional or aggressive results of a sudden decrease in reinforcement (Lalli, Casey, & Kates, 1997). Over the past few decades, these combinations have considerably increased the ability of applied psychologists to use extinction to promote more socially appropriate behaviors in clinical settings.

## Observational Learning

Some basic forms of social learning occur by just observing others. Observational learning exists across the animal kingdom: in very young children, nonhuman animals, and fully developed adult humans (Zentall, 1996). Consider this example from animal cognition research: A food-deprived target subject is allowed to observe a rival model obtain food consequences when it engages in a behavior for which the target subject has not been trained. Following a few observations, when the antecedents are presented to the target animal it presents accurate emissions of the behavior. Researchers have observed learning of this kind in a wide variety of animals (Fiorito & Scotto, 1992; McKinley & Young, 2003), suggesting that many complex organisms come into the world evolutionarily prepared to learn from the actions, successes, and failures of others.

Other learning processes then build upon basic observational learning. For example, normal human neonates will imitate a small number of specific behaviors, such as smiling or tongue thrusting (Meltzoff & Moore, 1977), but later they will use these gestures to regulate others socially (Nagy & Molnar, 2004), leading to a self-sustaining learning process and the acquisition of imitation as a generalized class of behavior (Poulson, Kymissis, Reeve, Andreatos, & Reeve, 1991).

The social nature of human beings makes observational learning especially important in applied programs. It can be a force for good or ill. For example, research has shown that group therapy in the area of youth addiction has iatrogenic effects due to social learning within the group (Dishion, McCord, & Poulin, 1999). Properly managed, however, learning in a social context can have profound and even lifelong effects. The "good behavior game," in which classes compete to show good behavior, provides an example of these effects. Even brief exposure to this game in elementary school affects violence, drug use, and other outcomes over many years (Embry, 2002).

# Discrimination Learning and Stimulus and Response Generalization

As practitioners develop optimal responding using principles of direct contingency learning, they should place emphasis on refining the precision with which actions are elicited or evoked. For example, clients may fail to respond because they do not detect antecedent conditions that signal the availability of reinforcement. Conversely, they may respond even though stimuli indicating that reinforcement could occur are not present, and the predictable but unexpected subsequent absence of reinforcement may weaken the operant response over time. Similar issues can occur with classical conditioning processes when conditioned stimuli are weak in salience or vague across a variety of stimulus dimensions (volume, tone, color, temperature), such that conditioned responses are not elicited.

## Discrimination

Not only is it important for people to learn when reinforcement will be available and what pattern of responding will produce it, it is also important to learn the contextual conditions under which responding will be reinforced (see chapter 12). A *discriminative stimulus*, or Sd, is a stimulus event that predicts reinforcement is likely if a behavior occurs; an event that predicts that reinforcement is not likely even if a behavior occurs is called S-delta, or SΔ. It is often clinically important to ensure that responding occurs only in some contexts but not others; when responding is regulated in that way it is said to be under stimulus control. Generally, alternate contingencies are used to train such discriminations. A *multiple schedule* (MULT for short) consists of a reinforcement-dense schedule for specific action when an Sd is present, and a reinforcement-lean schedule (or even extinction) when an SΔ is present. *Differential reinforcement* is the difference in access to preferred consequences, and it is the foundation for the development of stimulus control.

By simply bringing needed actions under good stimulus control, people can sometimes make appropriate behavior more likely. For example, Fisher, Greer, Fuhrman, and Querim (2015) used a multiple schedule that alternated a reinforcement schedule with extinction (EXT) to teach individuals with severe, challenging behaviors simple requests. The schedule resulted in rapid stimulus control over requests and decreases in challenging behaviors as the environment itself became more predictable to the individuals.

Discrimination training of this kind can be used in another way; for example, it can be used to help an existing consequence become more effective. In one study, a MULT VI-VI schedule was changed to a MULT VI-EXT schedule. As a result, responding during the unchanged component of the schedule increased substantially, a phenomenon known as *behavioral contrast* (Pierce & Cheney, 2013).

In everyday behavior, much of discrimination learning involves learning to do the right thing in the right time and place. For example, children learn that certain jokes may be reinforced in the presence of peers but not adults, or that quiet, still behavior is expected in the school classroom but loud behavior may be differentially reinforced on the school playground. Osborne, Rudrud, and Zezoney (1990) used a creative example of discrimination teaching to enhance the ability of collegiate baseball players to hit curve balls. In an alternating fashion, in some periods balls were unmarked, while in others the seams of the balls were marked with ¼-inch or ⅛-inch orange stripes. Players hit a greater percentage of the balls that included the visually discriminative stimuli. Discrimination learning is also involved when individuals are taught functional communication skills. The Picture Exchange Communication System, for example, is a widely used alternative and augmentative communication system for individuals with severe language impairments due to autism or other developmental disabilities (e.g., Bondy & Frost, 2001). When an individual selects the picture of a preferred item in an array of pictures and exchanges it with a caregiver, the individual is granted access to that preferred item, differentially reinforcing the picture presentation with the real item.

Challenging behaviors among people with developmental or psychiatric disabilities often occur in the presence of particular stimuli, and knowledge of stimulus control processes can help undermine the detrimental regulation of behavior. Touchette, MacDonald, and Langer (1985) used a tool known as a scatter plot to help identify temporal periods throughout the day during which a severe challenging behavior never occurs or occurs with near certainty. This tool is especially appropriate for severe problem behavior, for which there may be only two practically important rates: zero and unacceptable. If a practitioner finds that challenging behavior occurs most frequently when certain work tasks or chores are presented to an individual, or when particular staff members are present, these stimulus situations can be targeted for change.

Many academic tasks involve discrimination learning. For example, teaching a child to receptively identify letters is an example of a discrimination task: a child's selection of the letter *b* is occasioned by the presentation of the letter *b*. Advanced reading is also considered a form of discrimination learning, as reading aloud comes under the discriminative control of the print stimuli and eventually recedes to the covert level (i.e., not reading aloud). Many individuals with autism spectrum disorder and other developmental disabilities display a phenomenon known as stimulus overselectivity, which occurs when restricted properties of stimuli control responding (Ploog, 2010). In the case of the letter-labeling task mentioned before, stimulus overselectivity occurs when an individual inaccurately identifies every letter with a closed loop as the letter *b*. Dube and colleagues (2010) suggest that when a reinforcement contingency is in place for the emission of an observing response to all of the relevant features of a stimulus (i.e., not only the closed loop but the stem on the letter), difficulties with overselectivity can be remedied. In other words, if attending to all of the important features of a stimulus is reinforced, all of the relevant properties of a stimulus are likely to occasion correct responses.

While discrimination learning is regarded as an example of a three-term contingency, a fourth term, a conditional stimulus, may come to control the three-term contingency. For example, Catania (1998) notes that an individual stating "apple" in the presence of an apple is only differentially reinforced if another person has asked "What is that?" while pointing at the apple. In this scenario, the question ("What is that?") is regarded as a conditional stimulus. The apple serves as a discriminative stimulus, meaning that labeling it "apple" in its presence will only be reinforced on the condition that the question "What is that?" is asked.

## Generalization

Some practitioners view stimulus generalization as the opposite process of discrimination. In stimulus generalization, responding occurs in the presence of stimuli that have not been directly reinforced but are physically similar (e.g., color, shape, and so on) to an original conditioned or discriminative stimulus. A generalization gradient shows the relationship between the probability of a response occurring and the value of a stimulus along that physical dimension. For example, if a child learns to say "it's blue" in the presence of a specific wavelength of light, the probability of that response will steadily decrease when the child is presented with lights of more and more dissimilar wavelengths.

Practitioners typically view stimulus generalization as a desirable intervention outcome in applied settings. They often implement behavioral interventions in very structured, tightly controlled settings, only to find that intervention effects may not generalize to novel but important contexts. Stokes and Baer (1977) proposed a technology for promoting stimulus generalization, including the following strategies: teaching with sufficient examples, teaching loosely, using indiscriminable stimuli between the teaching and generalization settings, programming common stimuli between the teaching and generalization environments, and sequentially modifying the teaching environment until it more closely resembles generalization settings. Teaching with multiple examples involves using different stimuli so that an individual is likely to respond correctly in the presence of stimuli that may be dissimilar from the one used during instruction. For example, a child may be likely to correctly label all dogs as "dog" if he or she has been taught to label many varieties, sizes, breeds, and colors of dogs as "dog."

*Response generalization* involves the spread of the effects of reinforcement to other responses not correlated with reinforcement. For example, if the target behavior of smiling at peers is differentially reinforced, making eye contact with and initiating conversation with peers may also begin to increase in probability even though these actions were not directly reinforced. When this occurs, the behaviors are said to compose a response class or functional class (Catania, 1998).

# Interaction of Behavioral Principles with Language and Cognition

The implementation of the basic principles of learning in applied settings needs to be tempered by the known interaction between them and human symbolic processes. Basic behavioral and cognitive approaches to the study of human cognition will be explored in the next chapter, but it is worth noting that when language abilities emerge in human beings, more than direct contingencies and simple forms of observational learning regulate behavior. For example, we have all been told to not touch a hot stove, but not all of us have had a history of being burned by a stove. Our ability to avoid the stove when it's hot seems to be under a different sort of stimulus control than the stove itself. Cognitive perspectives have long claimed this to be the case, but in the context of this chapter (and the theme of this volume) it seems worth the effort to briefly note that the behavioral wings of the behavioral and cognitive therapy traditions have studied this phenomenon for several decades in an attempt to understand it.

More than thirty years ago behavioral psychologists concluded that, at times, verbal stimuli in the form of instructions, commands, or rules stated by an individual or another person come to control responding in ways that alter the operation of direct contingencies (Catania, Matthews, & Shimoff, 1982). Describing contingencies (Catania, Shimoff, & Matthews, 1989), or motivating behavior, verbally (Schlinger & Blakely, 1987) can alter how direct contingencies operate. A number of laboratory studies have shown that when experimenter-provided rules conflict with programmed contingencies, the responding of normal adult participants tends to remain under instructional control rather than adapt to changing contingencies, even when doing so has a cost (e.g., Catania, Lowe, & Horne, 1990); and when adaption to the environment does take place, that effect too can be due to the presence of verbal rules, which can alter sensitivity to subsequent environmental changes (e.g., Hayes, Brownstein, Haas, & Greenway, 1986).

The increasing dominance of symbolic processes over the processes of direct contingency learning has a developmental trajectory. For example, on similar reinforcement schedules, young, preverbal children show patterns of responding that mirror those of nonhumans, but as verbal repertoires develop, the patterns of reinforcement schedule performance in older children and adults differ from those commonly seen in textbooks (Bentall & Lowe, 1987). In particular, the literature on derived relational responding (Hayes, Barnes-Holmes, & Roche, 2001) has provided behavioral psychologists with a way to forge common ground with the traditional concerns of cognitive therapists and theorists, and it has done so in ways that appear to be empowering practitioners to develop new methods to facilitate flexible cognitive repertoires (see Rehfeldt & Barnes-Holmes, 2009; Rehfeldt & Root, 2005; Rosales & Rehfeldt, 2007).

A study by Dougher, Hamilton, Fink, and Harrington (2007) provides a basic example of how symbolic processes interact with operant and classical conditioning. One group of subjects learned that three arbitrary events (squiggles on a screen) were related comparatively, such that $X < Y < Z$. Another group learned nothing about how X, Y, and Z were related. Both groups were then shocked repeatedly in the presence of Y until that graphic form elicited anxiety as measured by a galvanic skin response. Participants in both groups were not much aroused by the stimulus X, and in the group that had not been trained how to relate X, Y, and Z, participants showed little arousal to Z. In the relationally trained group, however, participants were more aroused by Z *than they were by* Y. This response cannot be stimulus generalization, because the stimuli were arbitrary. Instead the symbolic relation of "Z is bigger than Y" created more arousal to a stimulus that had never been paired with shock than one that had repeatedly been paired.

These same basic findings extend to self-rules as well. For example, Taylor and O'Reilly (1997) and Faloon and Rehfeldt (2008) found that the stating of overt self-rules by participants with developmental disabilities facilitated the acquisition of a chained task, and the participants maintained their performance when they were taught to state such self-rules at the covert level. When participants in both studies were required to recite random numbers backward, blocking the emission of self-rules, performance declined, thus showing a functional relationship between the emission of overt and covert self-rules and the performing of a task.

In these cases, self-verbalization had a facilitative effect, but in many clinical situations the opposite is true. For example, a person having an anxiety attack in one situation may respond even more powerfully to another situation merely because it is thought to be "bigger" regardless of its actual physical properties, such as in the study by Dougher and colleagues (2007). This is a problem empirical clinicians often find themselves trying to solve with clients, as will be explored in section 3 of this volume. However, such effects do not eliminate the relevance of the principles of direct contingency learning; rather, they draw the field into a more process-oriented focus in which older and more recently acquired processes interact to produce behavior.

# Conclusion

Core behavioral processes provide practitioners with precise principles to generate treatment options for individuals with behavioral, emotional, or physical concerns. Regardless of the appearance of the behavior, treatment needs to be individualized based on the processes impacting it. Selecting an inaccurate cause of behavior will most typically prevent the client from experiencing positive change. The principles of direct contingency learning are among the best established in all of psychology and have the great benefit of orienting the practitioner toward contextual events that can be changed. Empirical clinicians need to rest their actions on core processes that have the most proven scientific merit, because people have placed their lives in our hands.

# References

Ainslie, G., & Herrnstein, R. J. (1981). Preference reversal and delayed reinforcement. *Animal Learning and Behavior, 9*(4), 476–482.

Bailey, J. S., & Burch, M. R. (2013). *Ethics for behavior analysts* (2nd expanded ed.). Abingdon, UK: Taylor and Francis.

Bentall, R. P., & Lowe, C. F. (1987). The role of verbal behavior in human learning: III. Instructional effects in children. *Journal of the Experimental Analysis of Behavior, 47*(2), 177–190.

Binder, L. M., Dixon, M. R., & Ghezzi, P. M. (2000). A procedure to teach self-control to children with attention deficit hyperactivity disorder. *Journal of Applied Behavior Analysis, 33*(2), 233–237.

Boisseau, R. P., Vogel, D., & Dussutour, A. (2016). Habituation in non-neural organisms: Evidence from slime moulds. *Proceedings of the Royal Society B, 283*(1829), n.p.

Bondy, A. S., & Frost, L. A. (2001). The Picture Exchange Communication System. *Behavior Modification, 25*(5), 725–744.

Bradley, M. M., Lang, P. J., & Cuthbert, B. N. (1993). Emotion, novelty, and the startle reflex: Habituation in humans. *Behavioral Neuroscience, 107*(6), 970–980.

Bureš, J., Bermúdez-Rattoni, F., & Yamamoto, T. (1998). *Conditioned taste aversion: Memory of a special kind.* Oxford: Oxford University Press.

Catania, A. C. (1998). *Learning* (4th ed.). Upper Saddle River, NJ: Prentice Hall.

Catania, A. C., Lowe, C. F., & Horne, P. (1990). Nonverbal behavior correlated with the shaped verbal behavior of children. *Analysis of Verbal Behavior, 8*, 43–55.

Catania, A. C., Matthews, B. A., & Shimoff, E. (1982). Instructed versus shaped human verbal behavior: Interactions with nonverbal responding. *Journal of the Experimental Analysis of Behavior, 38*(3), 233–248.

Catania, A. C., Shimoff, E., & Matthews, B. A. (1989). An experimental analysis of rule-governed behavior. In S. C. Hayes (Ed.), *Rule-governed behavior: Cognition, contingencies, and instructional control* (pp. 119–150). New York: Springer.

DeLeon, I. G., & Iwata, B. A. (1996). Evaluation of a multiple-stimulus presentation format for assessing reinforcer preferences. *Journal of Applied Behavior Analysis, 29*(4), 519–533.

Dinsmoor, J. A. (1954). Punishment: I. The avoidance hypothesis. *Psychological Review, 61*(1), 34–46.

Dinsmoor, J. A. (1977). Escape, avoidance, punishment: Where do we stand? *Journal of the Experimental Analysis of Behavior, 28*(1), 83–95.

Dinsmoor, J. A. (1998). Punishment. In W. T. O'Donohue (Ed.), *Learning and behavior therapy* (pp. 188–204). Needham Heights, MA: Allyn and Bacon

Dishion, T. J., McCord, J., & Poulin, F. (1999). When interventions harm: Peer groups and problem behavior. *American Psychologist, 54*(9), 755–764.

Domjan, M. (2013). Pavlovian conditioning. In A. L. C. Runehov & L. Oviedo (Eds.), *Encyclopedia of sciences and religions* (pp. 1608–1608). Netherlands: Springer.

Dougher, M. J., Hamilton, D. A., Fink, B. C., & Harrington, J. (2007). Transformation of the discriminative and eliciting functions of generalized relational stimuli. *Journal of the Experimental Analysis of Behavior, 88*(2), 179–197.

Dube, W. V., Dickson, C. A., Balsamo, L. M., O'Donnell, K. L., Tomanari, G. Y., Farren, K. M., et al. (2010). Observing behavior and atypically restricted stimulus control. *Journal of the Experimental Analysis of Behavior, 94*(3), 297–313.

Dymond, S., Dunsmoor, J. E., Vervliet, B., Roche, B., & Hermans, D. (2015). Fear generalization in humans: Systematic review and implications for anxiety disorder research. *Behavior Therapy, 46*(5), 561–582.

Embry, D. D. (2002). The good behavior game: A best practice candidate as a universal behavioral vaccine. *Clinical Child and Family Psychology Review, 5*(4), 273–297.

Faloon, B. J., & Rehfeldt, R. A. (2008). The role of overt and covert self-rules in establishing a daily living skill in adults with mild developmental disabilities. *Journal of Applied Behavior Analysis, 41*(3), 393–404.

Fiorito, G., & Scotto, P. (1992). Observational learning in *Octopus vulgaris. Science, 256*(5056), 545–547.

Fisher, W. W., Greer, B. D., Fuhrman, A. M., & Querim, A. C. (2015). Using multiple schedules during functional communication training to promote rapid transfer of treatment effects. *Journal of Applied Behavior Analysis, 48*(4), 713–733.

Ginsburg, S., & Jablonka, E. (2010). The evolution of associative learning: A factor in the Cambrian explosion. *Journal of Theoretical Biology, 266*(1), 11–20.

Grosch, J., & Neuringer, A. (1981). Self-control in pigeons under the Mischel paradigm. *Journal of the Experimental Analysis of Behavior, 35*(1), 3–21.

Hayes, S. C., Barnes-Holmes, D., & Roche, B. (Eds.). (2001). *Relational frame theory: A post-Skinnerian account of human language and cognition.* New York: Kluwer Academic/Plenum Publishers.

Hayes, S. C., Brownstein, A. J., Haas, J. R., & Greenway, D. E. (1986). Instructions, multiple schedules, and extinction: Distinguishing rule-governed from schedule-controlled behavior. *Journal of the Experimental Analysis of Behavior, 46*(2), 137–147.

Heyman, G. M., & Monaghan, M. M. (1987). Effects of changes in response requirement and deprivation on the parameters of the matching law equation: New data and review. *Journal of Experimental Psychology: Animal Behavior Processes, 13*(4), 384–394.

Lalli, J. S., Casey, S. D., & Kates, K. (1997). Noncontingent reinforcement as treatment for severe problem behavior: Some procedural variations. *Journal of Applied Behavior Analysis, 30*(1), 127–137.

Lerman, D. C., & Iwata, B. A. (1995). Prevalence of the extinction burst and its attenuation during treatment. *Journal of Applied Behavior Analysis, 28*(1), 93–94.

Lerman, D. C., Iwata, B. A., & Wallace, M. D. (1999). Side effects of extinction: Prevalence of bursting and aggression during the treatment of self-injurious behavior. *Journal of Applied Behavior Analysis, 32*(1), 1–8.

Logue, A. W., & Peña-Correal, T. E. (1984). Responding during reinforcement delay in a self-control paradigm. *Journal of the Experimental Analysis of Behavior, 41*(3), 267–277.

Lowe, C. F., & Horne, P. J. (1985). On the generality of behavioural principles: Human choice and the matching law. In C. F. Lowe (Ed.), *Behaviour analysis and contemporary psychology* (pp. 97–115). London: Lawrence Erlbaum.

Madden, G. J., Begotka, A. M., Raiff, B. R., & Kastern, L. L. (2003). Delay discounting of real and hypothetical rewards. *Experimental and Clinical Psychopharmacology, 11*(2), 139–145.

Mazur, J. E. (2000). Tradeoffs among delay, rate, and amount of reinforcement. *Behavioural Processes, 49*(1), 1–10.

McKinley, S., & Young, R. J. (2003). The efficacy of the model-rival method when compared with operant conditioning for training domestic dogs to perform a retrieval-selection task. *Applied Animal Behaviour Science, 81*(4), 357–365.

Meltzoff, A. N., & Moore, M. K. (1977). Imitation of facial and manual gestures by human neonates. *Science, 198*(4312), 75–78.

Nagy, E., & Molnar, P. (2004). Homo imitans or homo provocans? Human imprinting model of neonatal imitation. *Infant Behavior and Development, 27*(1), 54–63.

Öhman, A., & Mineka, S. (2001). Fears, phobias, and preparedness: Toward an evolved module of fear and fear learning. *Psychological Review, 108*(3), 483–522.

Osborne, K., Rudrud, E., & Zezoney, F. (1990). Improved curveball hitting through the enhancement of visual cues. *Journal of Applied Behavior Analysis, 23*(3), 371–377.

Penders, C. A., & Delwaide, P. J. (1971). Blink reflex studies in patients with Parkinsonism before and during therapy. *Journal of Neurology, Neurosurgery and Psychiatry, 34*(6), 674–678.

Petscher, E. S., Rey, C., & Bailey, J. S. (2009). A review of empirical support for differential reinforcement of alternative behavior. *Research in Developmental Disabilities, 30*(3), 409–425.

Pierce, W. D., & Cheney, C. D. (2013). *Behavior analysis and learning* (5th ed.). Oxon, UK: Psychology Press.

Ploog, B. O. (2010). Stimulus overselectivity four decades later: A review of the literature and its implications for current research in autism spectrum disorder. *Journal of Autism and Developmental Disorders, 40*(11), 1332–1349.

Podlesnik, C. A., & Shahan, T. A. (2009). Behavioral momentum and relapse of extinguished operant responding. *Learning and Behavior, 37*(4), 357–364.

Poulson, C. L., Kymissis, E., Reeve, K. F., Andreatos, M., & Reeve, L. (1991). Generalized vocal imitation in infants. *Journal of Experimental Child Psychology, 51*(2), 267–279.

Rehfeldt, R. A., & Barnes-Holmes, Y. (2009). *Derived relational responding: Applications for learners with autism and other developmental disabilities: A progressive guide to change.* Oakland, CA: New Harbinger Publications.

Rehfeldt, R. A., & Root, S. L. (2005). Establishing derived requesting skills in adults with severe developmental disabilities. *Journal of Applied Behavior Analysis, 38*(1), 101–105.

Rescorla, R. A., & Solomon, R. L. (1967). Two-process learning theory: Relationships between Pavlovian conditioning and instrumental learning. *Psychological Review, 74*(3), 151–182.

Rosales, R. R., & Rehfeldt, R. A. (2007). Contriving transitive conditioned establishing operations to establish derived manding skills in adults with severe developmental disabilities. *Journal of Applied Behavior Analysis, 40*(1), 105–121.

Schlinger, H., & Blakely, E. (1987). Function-altering effects of contingency-specifying stimuli. *Behavior Analyst, 10*(1), 41–45.

Shahan, T. A., & Sweeney, M. M. (2011). A model of resurgence based on behavioral momentum theory. *Journal of the Experimental Analysis of Behavior, 95*(1), 91–108.

Sidman, M. (2009). The measurement of behavioral development. In N. A. Krasnegor, D. B. Gray, & T. Thompson (Eds.), *Advances in behavioral pharmacology* (vol. 5, pp. 43–52). Abingdon, UK: Routledge.

Skinner, B. F. (1953). *Science and human behavior.* New York: Free Press.

Skinner, B. F. (1969). *Contingencies of reinforcement: A theoretical analysis.* Englewood Cliffs, NJ: Prentice Hall.

Spetch, M. L., Wilkie, D. M., & Pinel, J. P. J. (1981). Backward conditioning: A reevaluation of the empirical evidence. *Psychological Bulletin, 89*(1), 163–175.

Stokes, T. F., & Baer, D. M. (1977). An implicit technology of generalization. *Journal of Applied Behavior Analysis, 10*(2), 349–367.

Taylor, I., & O'Reilly, M. F. (1997). Toward a functional analysis of private verbal self-regulation. *Journal of Applied Behavior Analysis, 30*(1), 43–58.

Touchette, P. E., MacDonald, R. F., & Langer, S. N. (1985). A scatter plot for identifying stimulus control of problem behavior. *Journal of Applied Behavior Analysis, 18*(4), 343–351.

Wolpe, J., & Rowan, V. C. (1988). Panic disorder: A product of classical conditioning. *Behaviour Research and Therapy, 26*(6), 441–450.

Zentall, T. R. (1996). An analysis of imitative learning in animals. In C. M. Heyes & B. G. Galef Jr. (Eds.), *Social learning in animals: The roots of culture* (pp. 221–243). San Diego: Academic Press.

Zuriff, G. E. (1970). A comparison of variable-ratio and variable-interval schedules of reinforcement. *Journal of the Experimental Analysis of Behavior, 13*(3), 369–374.

# CHAPTER 7

# What Is Cognition?
# A Functional-Cognitive Perspective

Jan De Houwer, PhD
Dermot Barnes-Holmes, DPhil
Yvonne Barnes-Holmes, PhD

*Department of Experimental Clinical and Health Psychology,
Ghent University*

It is fair to say that the concepts "cognition" and "cognitive" are pivotal in modern-day psychology, and that is no less true in empirical clinical psychology. To illustrate, a search on Web of Science performed on September 19, 2016, generated 468,850 hits when using "cognition OR cognitive" as a search term. As a (less-than-perfect but not trivial) comparison, consider the fact that the search term "emotion OR emotional" generated less than half that number of hits (209,087). A similar ratio was found when these searches were limited to articles dealing with clinical psychology or psychotherapy.

Despite its pivotal role, it is often not entirely clear what "cognition" (and thus "cognitive" as involving cognition) exactly means. In the first two sections of this chapter, we discuss two different perspectives on the nature of cognition. First, within cognitive psychology, cognition is typically defined in terms of information processing. Second, within functional psychology, cognition is conceptualized in terms of behavior. We then point out that both perspectives are not mutually

Ghent University Grant BOF16/MET_V/002, awarded to Jan De Houwer, made the preparation of this chapter possible. Dermot Barnes-Holmes is supported by an Odysseus Group 1 Award (2015–2020) from the Scientific Research Foundation, Flanders (FWO-Vlaanderen). Correspondence can be addressed to Jan De Houwer, Ghent University, Henri Dunantlaan 2, B-9000 Ghent, Belgium, or Jan.DeHouwer@UGent.be.

exclusive. More specifically, they can be reconciled within a functional-cognitive framework for psychological research that recognizes two interdependent levels of explanation in psychology: a functional level that aims to explain behavior in terms of elements in the environment, and a cognitive level that is directed at understanding the mental mechanisms by which elements in the environment influence behavior. We end the chapter by highlighting some of the implications of this functional-cognitive perspective on cognition for evidence-based psychotherapy.

# Cognition as Information Processing

Although the term *cognition* has a long history dating back to the ancient Greeks (see Chaney, 2013, for a review), Neisser provided one of the currently most influential definitions about fifty years ago in his seminal textbook on cognitive psychology:

> As used here, the term "cognition" refers to all the processes by which the sensory input is transformed, reduced, elaborated, stored, recovered, and used. It is concerned with these processes even when they operate in the absence of relevant stimulation, as in images and hallucinations… Given such a sweeping definition, it is apparent that cognition is involved in everything a human being might possibly do; that every psychological phenomenon is a cognitive phenomenon. (1967, p. 4)

Neisser went on to compare cognition with information processing in a computer:

> The task of a psychologist trying to understand human cognition is analogous to that of a man trying to discover how a computer has been programmed. In particular, if the program seems to store and reuse information, he would like to know by what "routines" or "procedures" this is done. (1967, p. 6)

Despite the fact that few contemporary cognitive psychologists still adhere to the idea of serial computers as a model for the mind, three aspects of Neisser's definition have remained influential. First and foremost, Neisser views cognition as information processing. This is a mental perspective insofar as the mind is considered to be informational in nature. As noted by Gardner (1987), linking cognition and the mind to information carves out a new level of explanation at which cognitive psychologists can operate. To fully appreciate the importance of this idea, one has to realize that information can be conceived of as nonphysical in nature. Wiener, one of the founders of information theory, put it as follows: "Information is information, not matter or energy" (1961, p. 132). The assumption that information is nonphysical fits with the idea that the same piece of information (i.e., the same content) can, in principle, be instantiated in entirely different physical substrates (i.e., different vehicles such as desktop computers, magnetic tapes, brains; see Bechtel, 2008, for an insightful discussion of the distinction between the content and vehicles of information).

Consider the growth rings of a tree. These rings carry information about the climate during the years that the tree grew, but that same information can also be captured by glacial ice layers or meteorological records. Moreover, the physical tree is only a vehicle for this content; it is not the content itself. This becomes apparent from the fact that growth rings reveal their content about climate only to entities that can read the information (e.g., a climate scientist who, by combining observations of growth rings with her knowledge about the effects of climate on tree growth, can extract information about climate from the size of the growth rings). Importantly, because of the nonphysical nature of information, the study of information content can never be reduced to a mere study of the vehicles that contain the physical information. Hence, cognitive psychology as the study of information content in humans can never be reduced to a study of the physical brain, nor to a study of the whole organism (but see Bechtel, 2008, for the idea that at a very detailed level of analysis, there might be a unique overlap between content and vehicle and thus the potential to understand content by understanding the vehicle). In sum, Neisser's definition of cognition as information processing legitimized cognitive psychology as a separate science of the mental world (also see Brysbaert & Rastle, 2013, for an excellent discussion).

A second interesting feature of Neisser's definition is that it very much focuses on cognition as a dynamic process. This dynamic process can be described as a mental mechanism, that is, a chain of information-processing steps (Bechtel, 2008). Cognition is thus akin to a physical mechanism that consists of parts and operations in which one part operates on another part (e.g., one cogwheel puts in motion another cogwheel and so forth). The main difference is that the parts and operations in mental mechanisms are informational in nature rather than physical. Because of their informational nature, these mental mechanisms are assumed to allow organisms to add meaning to the physical world. Like physical mechanisms, cognition involves contiguous causation—that is, mental states that operate on each other. Put simply, one step in the mechanism (e.g., a mental state) puts in motion the next step (e.g., another mental state).[1]

The fundamental assumption of contiguous causation becomes apparent in how cognitive psychologists deal with the phenomenon of latent learning—that is, the impact that experiences at Time 1 (e.g., a rat exploring a maze with no food in it; a person experiencing a traumatic event) have on behavior during a later Time 2 (e.g., the speed at which the rat locates food that has been placed in the same maze; panic attacks that occur days, weeks, or years after the traumatic event; Tolman & Honzik, 1930; see Chiesa, 1992, and De Houwer, Barnes-Holmes, & Moors, 2013, for a related discussion of latent learning). Working with the assumption that each thought and behavior needs a contiguous cause—that is, something here and now that causes the thoughts and behaviors at that time—cognitive psychologists deduce that the change in behavior at Time 2 must be due to information that is present at Time 2. This contiguous cause cannot be the experience with the maze at Time 1 because this event has already passed at Time 2, when the behavior is observed. If one accepts the basic assumption that mental mechanisms necessarily drive behavior, then the only possible explanation for latent learning is that (a) the original experience at Time 1 produced some kind of mental representation at Time 1, (b) this representation was retained in memory until Time 2, and (c) it functioned as a contiguous cause of the thoughts and behaviors at Time 2. Hence, from a cognitive perspective (i.e., based on the assumption that mental mechanisms drive all behavior), latent learning can be said to demonstrate the existence of mental representations in memory.

A third important feature of Neisser's definition is that it does not refer to consciousness. Hence, the definition is compatible with the idea that mental mechanisms can operate not only consciously but also unconsciously. In a sense, cognitive psychologists must accept a role for unconscious cognition if they want to maintain the assumption that "cognition is involved in everything a human being might possibly do" (Neisser, 1967, p. 4). Often, people seem completely unaware of what is driving their behavior. Cognitive psychologists can attribute such behaviors to the operation of unconscious cognition—that is, to information processing that is inaccessible to conscious introspection. In fact, some have

---

1    Note that we have simplified our description of mental mechanisms for presentational purposes. First, the metaphor of cogwheels suggests a strictly linear mechanism, whereas mental mechanisms can operate also in a parallel or recursive manner. Second, in principle, it is possible that mental states arise spontaneously—that is, without being caused in a contiguous manner (although it would be difficult to demonstrate that a mental state is not caused by environmental input or other mental states). However, all mechanisms have in common that they consist of parts that operate on each other, even when those mechanisms operate in a parallel or recursive manner and even if the state of some parts can sometimes also change spontaneously.

argued that in most situations in daily life, unconscious rather than conscious cognition drives human behavior, a claim often illustrated with a picture of an iceberg that is situated mostly underwater (e.g., Bargh, 2014).

Of course, Neisser's definition is not the only definition of cognition within the cognitive psychology literature, nor has it gone uncontested (see Moors, 2007, for an excellent analysis of the various definitions that have been put forward in the literature). Some researchers specify criteria that single out some instances of information processing as "true" instances of cognition (e.g., criteria regarding the type of representations on which information processes operate or regarding the output of the processes; see Moors, 2007). Other cognitive psychologists use the term "cognition" to refer to a subset of mental states. For instance, when contrasting cognition and emotion, cognitive researchers sometimes imply that cognitive states are nonemotional in that they involve "cold" beliefs rather than "hot" emotional experiences. Still others even exclude all phenomenological, conscious experience from the realm of cognitive states (see Moors, 2007).

Finally, whereas Neisser's reference to cognition as the operation of a computer program implies disembodied, serial information processing, others propose that humans process information in a parallel manner using subsymbolic representations (e.g., McClelland & Rumelhart, 1985) or in ways that are closely tied into the biological nature of the human body (i.e., "embodied"; e.g., Barsalou, 2008). Despite these important differences in opinion, most if not all cognitive psychologists retain both the *assumption* that humans (and nonhuman animals) process information and the *goal* to try to uncover how humans process information. Hence, we can safely conclude that, from the perspective of cognitive psychology, information processing lies at the heart of cognition. Cognitive work in psychotherapy is often not formally based on specific theories in cognitive science, but most of these perspectives retain an information-processing focus as specific types of schemas, core beliefs, irrational cognitions, and the like are examined.

# A Functional-Analytic Approach to Human Language and Cognition

During the past fifty years, cognitive psychology has been so dominant in the field of psychology that many psychologists will be surprised to discover that one can also think of cognition in a way that does not involve information processing. This is particularly important for the current volume, because some of the psychotherapy work in acceptance and mindfulness is based on a functional-analytic approach that adopts a noninformational perspective on language and thinking.

This approach describes relations between environment and behavior in a way that serves to predict and influence behavior (see Chiesa 1994; Hayes & Brownstein, 1986). We are not arguing that the functional approach is inherently better or superior to the traditional or "mainstream" approach, but rather that psychologists and clinical psychologists, in particular, should not be presented with an either-or choice with regard to the approach that they adopt.

## A Functional-Analytic Approach

A functional approach to cognition begins with a functional-contextual orientation to behavior (see the section "Contextualism" in chapter 2, or Zettle, Hayes, Barnes-Holmes, & Biglan, 2016, for a recent book-length treatment). In a functional-contextual approach, functional relations can be "spread out" between and among events across both time and space. Let us return to the example of latent learning. For a functional psychologist, it suffices to say that a change in behavior at Time 2 is a function of an experience at Time 1. While what Skinner called "the physiologist of the future" (1974, p. 236) may one day provide additional information about that gap, the concept of the functional relation itself is in no way incomplete merely because it is spread out across time and space. For functional contextualists, descriptions of this kind are considered adequate because they generate scientific verbal analyses that permit basic and applied researchers, and practitioners, to predict and influence the behavior of individuals and groups.

The functional approach extends well beyond a brute form of empiricism, without collapsing into a collection of techniques for behavioral change, by holding fast to analyses with precision, scope, and depth as scientific goals (Hayes, Barnes-Holmes, & Roche, 2001; see also chapters 2 and 6). *Precision* requires that behavior analysis seeks to identify or generate a limited or parsimonious set of principles and theories of behavioral change. *Scope* requires that these principles and theories should apply across a wide range of behaviors or psychological events. And *depth* requires that such scientific analyses should not contradict or disagree with well-established scientific evidence and analyses in other scientific domains (e.g., a behavioral "fact" should be broadly consistent with facts established in neuroscience or anthropology).

A classic example of a functional-analytic concept is the three-term contingency (described in the previous chapter) that defines operant behavior (or the four-term contingency, if motivational factors are added). Nothing in the concept of an operant requires immediate contiguity—the focus is on the functional relation among classes of events.

# Stimulus Equivalence and Relational Frame Theory: A Functional-Analytic Approach to Human Language and Cognition

The concept of the operant has provided a core scientific unit of analysis in the development of relational frame theory (RFT; Hayes et al., 2001; see Hughes & Barnes-Holmes, 2016a, 2016b, for recent reviews), which is an account of human language and cognition. This theory emerged originally from a program of research devoted to the phenomenon of stimulus equivalence (see Sidman, 1994, for a book-length treatment). The basic effect is defined as the emergence of unreinforced or untrained matching responses based on a small set of trained responses. For example, when a person is trained to match two abstract stimuli to a third (e.g., select Paf in the presence of Zid, and select Vek in the presence of Zid), untrained matching responses frequently appear in the absence of additional learning (e.g., select Vek in the presence of Paf, and Paf in the presence of Vek). When such a pattern of unreinforced responses occurs, the stimuli are said to form an equivalence class or relation. Importantly, this behavioral effect, according to Sidman, appears to provide a functional-analytic approach to symbolic meaning or reference.

Initially, the stimulus equivalence effect appeared to challenge a functional explanation, based on operant contingencies, because whole sets of matching responses emerged in the absence of programmed reinforcers (e.g., selecting Paf in the presence of Vek without ever reinforcing this behavior). Indeed, the emergence of such untrained responses provides the critical defining property of the stimulus equivalence effect itself. However, RFT posits that stimulus equivalence is just one overarching or generalized operant class of arbitrarily applicable relational responding (AARR). According to this view, exposure to an extended history of relevant reinforced exemplars serves to establish particular patterns of overarching or generalized relational response classes, which are defined as relational frames (D. Barnes-Holmes & Barnes-Holmes, 2000).

For example, the verbal community would likely expose a young child to direct contingencies of reinforcement if, upon hearing the word "dog" or the specific dog's name (e.g., Rover), the child points to the family dog or emits other appropriate naming responses, such as saying "Rover" or "dog" when observing the family pet or saying "Rover" when asked, "What is the dog's name?" Across many such exemplars, involving other stimuli and contexts, eventually the operant class of coordinating stimuli would become abstracted in this way, such that the child would no longer require direct reinforcement for all the individual components of naming when encountering a novel stimulus. Imagine, for example, that the child is shown a picture of an aardvark and the written word and is told the animal's name. Subsequently, the child may say "That's an aardvark" when presented with a relevant picture or the word without any prompting or direct reinforcement for doing so. In this way, the generalized relational response of coordinating pictorial, spoken stimuli and written words is established, and by directly reinforcing a subset of the relating behaviors the complete set is "spontaneously" generated. More informally, as the result of many experiences of being rewarded for responding as if sets of stimuli are equivalent in certain ways, children acquire the capacity to respond as if other sets of stimuli are equivalent without being rewarded for doing so. Generalized relational responding thus refers to classes of responses that are applied to novel sets of stimuli.

Critically, once this pattern of relational responding has been established, it occurs in ways that are sensitive to specific contextual cues. A contextual cue can thus be seen as a type of discriminative stimulus for a particular pattern of relational responding. The cues acquire their functions through the types of histories described above. For example, the phrase "that is a," as in *That is a* dog," would be established across exemplars as a contextual cue for the complete pattern of relational responding (e.g., coordinating the word "dog" with actual dogs). Once the relational functions of such contextual cues are established in the behavioral repertoire of a young child, the number of stimuli that may enter into such relational response classes becomes almost infinite (Hayes & Hayes, 1989; Hayes et al., 2001).

The core analytic concept of the relational frame proposed by RFT provides a relatively precise technical definition of AARR. Specifically, a *relational frame* is defined as possessing three properties: mutual entailment (if A is related to B, then B is also related to A), combinatorial mutual entailment (if A is related to B, and B is related to C, then A is related to C, and C is related to A), and the transformation of functions (the functions of the related stimuli are changed or transformed based upon the types of relations into which those stimuli enter). Imagine, for example, that you are told that "Guff" is a really tasty new brand of beer, and that you will love it, but you are also told that another new brand, called "Geedy," is the complete opposite in terms of taste. It is likely that given a choice between the two beers, you will choose the former over the latter, in part because the two verbal stimuli—Guff and Geedy—have entered into a relational frame of opposition, and the functions of Geedy have been transformed based on its relationship to Guff (more informally, you respond as if you expect Geedy to have an unpleasant taste).

Much of the early research in RFT has been designed to test its basic assumptions and core ideas. Some of this work shows that relational framing as a process occurs in several distinct patterns. Numerous experimental studies (see Hughes &

Barnes-Holmes, 2016a, for a recent review) have demonstrated these patterns of responding, referred to as relational frames (e.g., coordination, opposition, distinction, comparison, spatial frames, temporal frames, deictic relations, and hierarchical relations), and some of the research has also reported reliable demonstrations of the property of transformation of functions (e.g., Dymond & Barnes, 1995). In addition, provided that key functional elements were present, research has shown that relational framing can be observed using a variety of procedures (e.g., Leader, Barnes, & Smeets, 1996), indicating that the phenomenon is not tied to a particular experimental preparation or mode of instruction. Studies have also shown that exposure to multiple exemplars during early language development is required to establish specific relational frames (e.g., Y. Barnes-Holmes, Barnes-Holmes, Smeets, Strand, & Friman, 2004; Lipkens, Hayes, & Hayes, 1993; Luciano, Gómez-Becerra, & Rodríguez-Valverde, 2007), which supports the idea that relational framing is a generalized operant (see D. Barnes-Holmes & Barnes-Holmes, 2000; Healy, Barnes-Holmes, & Smeets, 2000).

Relational framing provides a functional-analytic account of many of the specific domains within human language and cognition (Hayes et al., 2001; see Hughes & Barnes-Holmes, 2016b, for a recent review). For illustrative purposes, we will briefly consider three of them to show how cognitive phenomena can be addressed in purely functional-analytic terms without reference to a mental world of information processing.

**Rules as relational networks.** According to RFT, understanding and following verbal rules or instructions is a result of frames of coordination and temporal relations that contain contextual cues and transform specific behavioral functions. Consider this simple instruction: "If the light is green, then go." It involves frames of coordination among the words "light," "green," and "go" and the actual events to which they refer. In addition, the words "if" and "then" serve as contextual cues for establishing a temporal or contingency relation between the actual light and the act of actually going (i.e., first "light," then "go"). And the relational network as a whole involves a transformation of the functions of the light itself, such that it now controls the act of "going" whenever an individual who has been presented with the rule observes the light being switched on. Although the foregoing example is a relatively simple one, the basic concept may be elaborated to provide a functional-analytic treatment of increasingly complex rules and instructions (e.g., O'Hora, Barnes-Holmes, Roche, & Smeets, 2004; O'Hora, Barnes-Holmes, & Stewart, 2014).

**Analogical reasoning as relating relational frames.** Another example is *analogical reasoning* (e.g., Stewart, Barnes-Holmes, Hayes, & Lipkens, 2001), which is viewed as the act of relating relations themselves. Suppose participants are trained and tested for the formation of four separate frames of coordination (the actual stimuli may be graphical squiggles or anything else, but labeling using alpha-numerics helps keep the example clear: A1-B1-C1; A2-B2-C2; A3-B3-C3; A4-B4-C4). The critical test involves determining if participants will match pairs of stimuli to other pairs of stimuli in a manner that is consistent with the relations between the stimulus pairs. For example, if the stimulus pair B1-C1 is presented to participants with two choices, say B3-C3 and B3-C4, the correct choice would be B3-C3 because both stimulus pairs (B1-C1 and B3-C3) are in frames of coordination, whereas the B3-C4 pair is not (Barnes, Hegarty, & Smeets, 1997). This basic RFT model of analogical reasoning generated an entire program of research with adults and children (see Stewart & Barnes-Holmes, 2004, for a summary) that uncovered important facts concerning the development and use of analogy and metaphor.

**Implicit cognition and brief and immediate relational responding.** RFT researchers have developed ways to distinguish brief and immediate relational responses (BIRRs), which are emitted relatively quickly within a short window of time after the onset of some relevant stimuli, from extended and elaborated relational responses (EERRs), which occur over a longer period of time (D. Barnes-Holmes, Barnes-Holmes, Stewart, & Boles, 2010; Hughes, Barnes-Holmes, & Vahey, 2012). The relational elaboration and coherence (REC) model, which provides an initial RFT approach to implicit cognition (D. Barnes-Holmes et al., 2010; Hughes et al., 2012), has formalized the distinction between BIRRs and EERRs, and the Implicit Relational Assessment Procedure (IRAP) was developed (D. Barnes-Holmes et al., 2010) to assess this domain. The IRAP has proven to be a useful clinical tool, for example, in predicting individual failure in cocaine treatment programs (Carpenter, Martinez, Vadhan, Barnes-Holmes, & Nunes, 2012).

## Conclusion

At this point, it should be clear that it is indeed possible to conduct research in the broad domain of human language and cognition using either a mechanistic mental model or a functional model. Researchers interested in mentalistic models and theories will likely be dissatisfied with a functional-analytic explanation, and vice versa, due to the different sets of philosophical assumptions and scientific goals that characterize each approach to psychological science (see chapter 2). Nonetheless, in the next section we will briefly argue that one doesn't have to consider these two broad approaches as antagonistic or mutually exclusive.

# The Functional-Cognitive Framework

De Houwer (2011; see Hughes, De Houwer, & Perugini, 2016, for an update) argues that the functional and cognitive approaches in psychology can be situated at two separate levels of explanation. Whereas functional psychology focuses on explanations of behavior in terms of its dynamic interaction with the environment, cognitive psychology aims to explain environment-behavior relations in terms of mental mechanisms. Consider the example of a client who exhibits a fear of elevators (see also De Houwer, Barnes-Holmes, & Barnes-Holmes, 2016). At a functional level, one could argue that the fear originated from a panic attack that occurred in an elevator or in another context related to elevators via arbitrarily applicable relational responding. Fearful responding to elevators is thus explained as being a consequence of a particular environmental event. Cognitive psychologists, on the other hand, would want to know *how* such an event can lead to fear of elevators. They might argue that the event resulted in the person forming associations between representations in memory (e.g., between the representations for "elevator" and "panic") or propositional beliefs about elevators (e.g., "I will suffocate when I am in an elevator."), and that those associations or propositions then lead to a fear of elevators under certain conditions.

Importantly, because the explanations that are developed in functional and cognitive psychology are fundamentally different, there is no inherent conflict between the two approaches. The explanations offered by functional and cognitive psychologists address different types of questions, and as long as each approach remains firmly committed to its respective level of explanation, functional and cognitive psychologists can collaborate to their mutual benefit.

Cognitive psychology can benefit from the conceptual, theoretical, and empirical knowledge that functional psychologists have gathered about the ways the environment influences behavior (including the behavior of framing events relationally): the more we know about environment-behavior relations, the better able we are to constrain cognitive theories about the mental mechanisms by which the environment influences behavior. Likewise, knowledge generated by cognitive research can help functional researchers to identify environment-behavior relations.

Neither approach is necessarily superior to the other. Ultimately, choosing one of the two shows a preference for a particular type of explanation. Functional psychologists focus on functional (i.e., environment-behavior) explanations because this allows them to predict and influence behavior. Cognitive researchers, however, want to know the mental mechanisms that drive behavior and will therefore not be satisfied with "explanations" that specify only environment-behavior relations. There is little point in arguing about which type of explanation is superior because the answer depends on fundamental philosophical assumptions and aims. Rather than devoting energy to such unresolvable debates, we see more merit in accepting that different researchers can pursue different types of explanations while still learning from each other (see Hughes et al., 2016, for an overview of the strengths and challenges of this functional-cognitive framework for psychological research).

The functional-cognitive framework allows for a reconciliation of cognitive and functional perspectives on cognition—not by one collapsing into the other but by recognizing the different issues they address. From a functional-analytic perspective, cognition is behavior (also see Overskeid, 2008). Phenomena that are typically considered to be cognitive (e.g., reasoning, implicit cognition) are seen as patterns of responses that are the result of historical and situational events. From the perspective of cognitive psychology, cognition is a form of information processing that mediates such phenomena. For instance, from a cognitive perspective, the ability to reason arises because a multitude of learning events lead to mental representations and information-processing skills that allow one to act as if sets of stimuli are equivalent in certain ways. Likewise, the environment may be seen as shaping up mental representations and information-processing skills that allow one to relate relations (analogical reasoning) and display BIRRs (implicit cognition).

A synergy between functional and cognitive perspectives requires only that cognitive psychologists conceive of cognitive phenomena as (complex) environment-behavior relations that are mediated by (complex) information processing (see Liefooghe & De Houwer, 2016, for an example in the context of cognitive control phenomena). Once cognitive phenomena are approached from a functional-analytic level of explanation and clearly separated from the mental mechanisms that mediate them, a fruitful collaboration can be initiated between functional and cognitive approaches to cognition. On the one hand, functional researchers can then start benefiting from the enormous wealth of empirical findings and theoretical ideas about cognitive phenomena that have been and continue to be generated within cognitive psychology. On the other hand, cognitive psychologists can exploit the concepts, theories, and findings about cognitive phenomena that have accumulated in functional psychology. In the final section of this chapter, we discuss some implications of this functional-cognitive framework for clinical psychology.

# Implications for Clinical Psychology

Although clinical psychology, as both an applied and academic endeavor, places mental events at its very core, the concept of cognition is still somewhat controversial. This is likely due, as noted above, to lack of clarity and consensus about how best to operationally define this broad umbrella term. This lack of clarity and consensus is evident in the antipathy that sometimes arises among individuals or groups involved in behavior therapy and cognitive therapy/cognitive behavioral therapy (CBT). For decades, clinical psychology has embodied this polarization and, for the most part, seems unable to structure itself any other way (De Houwer et al., 2016).

What the functional-cognitive framework seems to offer psychologists is clarity about which level of analysis and through which therapeutic means they are operating. The framework does not suggest one of these over the other, nor does it attempt to integrate them. It simply asks the clinician to identify which concepts and which therapeutic means best serve her conceptual analyses and her therapeutic aims, and it appears to allow greater clarity in this endeavor than previously existed. Below, we provide several extended examples so the reader might better understand the approach we are suggesting.

Wells and Matthews (1994) offer a theoretical explanation for a typical client who presents with an anxiety disorder, suggesting that the client focuses too much attention on particular stimuli, such as social cues, including the facial expressions of others. Critically, they consider the concept of "attention" (or more precisely, in this context, attentional bias) to involve information processing in the traditional cognitive-psychological meaning of that term. Consequently, in therapy, the therapist instructs and encourages the client to focus some of his attentional (mental) resources on his attending, with a view to recognizing that it is excessive when he could be attending to more relevant stimuli.

If the same client was undergoing a more functionally oriented type of therapy, the therapist might ask him about the costs and/or benefits served by him attending to particular social cues, with a view to establishing a broader and more flexible behavioral repertoire in this regard. In this conceptualization, however, there is no appeal to attention as a mental event involving information processing. The language of "attending" is simply used to orient the client to how verbal rules and evaluations may be leading to patterns of broadening or narrowing stimulus control. In other words, the therapist encourages the client to engage in relational actions that transform the behavior-controlling properties of the facial stimuli of other people (e.g., "When other people look at me, I tend to think they're judging me, and this makes me uncomfortable, so I withdraw, but that leaves me isolated, and that is inconsistent with what I value").

Within the context of the functional-cognitive framework, the metacognitive therapy approach taken by Wells (2000) and a functional-analytic approach overlap in some important ways (e.g., the focus on the client's own attention to particular social cues). However, in the former case the theoretical analysis is driven heavily by an information-processing view of attention, whereas in the latter case attention is defined as involving particular functional-analytic classes of derived relational responding. In our view, these two approaches to understanding and changing the client's behavior are not necessarily in direct opposition, but rather they represent philosophically different ways of talking about broadly similar psychological events.

Let us consider a second classic example, taken from Padesky (1994), involving Beck's cognitive theory of depression. Cognitive therapists devote considerable attention to schemas, especially those pertaining to affective states and behavioral patterns, as core beliefs that play a strong role in psychological suffering. In line with an information-processing approach, Beck proposes that "a schema is a structure for screening, coding, and evaluating...stimuli" (see Harvey, Hunt, & Schroder, 1961, p. 283). Cognitive therapy focuses on simultaneously identifying and changing maladaptive core schemas and building alternative adaptive ones (Beck et al., 1990). Consider a female client who identifies the schema "The world is dangerous and violent," which the therapist deems maladaptive because fear and depression accompany it. In observing events that activate this schema, the client and therapist clarify that greater affect accompanies the schema "Kindness is meaningless in the face of pain and violence." Working with the alternative schema "Kindness is as strong as violence and pain" helps the client to cope with the violent and painful realities she faces and to sustain hope and effort.

Consider now the same client undertaking functionally oriented psychotherapy. The therapist and client would explore related thoughts and rules about the world as a violent place and about the futility of kindness as functionally related response classes that control avoidance and lead to further suffering. The therapist would contextualize the emergence of these patterns within the client's history (e.g., she tried hard to please her parents, but they were never suitably impressed). This would indicate how the role of history accounts for why these psychological events have such strong control over current behavior instead of values-controlling behavior. Work on the deictic (perspective-taking) relations, such as imagining what she would say to herself if she could talk to herself as small child, would also serve to support the client as the owner of this history and the mental events it generates, so that she can choose what to do with her own behavior when these events emerge in certain contexts.

Again, in our view, these two approaches to understanding and changing the client's behavior are not in opposition to one another but are simply philosophically different ways of talking about similar events. Once this is fully recognized, practitioners (and researchers) in both traditions can begin to have a meaningful and hopefully mutually beneficial dialogue about human cognition and how it may be changed. This very book is in part an example of such a dialogue.

## Concluding Remarks

In this chapter, we argue that cognition may be understood from a functional-analytical perspective, as involving complex environment-behavior relations, as well as in terms of information processing, which mediates those environment-behavior relations. Moreover, we posit that these two perspectives are not mutually exclusive. On the contrary, within a functional-cognitive framework, close interactions between functional and cognitive research could, in principle, lead to a better understanding of cognition in clinical psychology, whether it is defined in functional-analytical terms or in terms of information processing. This functional-cognitive framework thus provides a new perspective on the long-standing divide between functional and cognitive approaches in clinical psychology, and psychology more generally, and opens up avenues for future interactions between researchers and practitioners from both sides of the divide.

## References

Bargh, J. A. (2014). Our unconscious mind. *Scientific American, 30,* 30–37.

Barnes, D., Hegarty, N., & Smeets, P. (1997). Relating equivalence relations to equivalence relations: A relational framing model of complex human functioning. *Analysis of Verbal Behavior, 14,* 57–83.

Barnes-Holmes, D., & Barnes-Holmes, Y. (2000). Explaining complex behavior: Two perspectives on the concept of generalized operant classes. *Psychological Record, 50*(2), 251–265.

Barnes-Holmes, D., Barnes-Holmes, Y., Stewart, I., & Boles, S. (2010). A sketch of the implicit relational assessment procedure (IRAP) and the relational elaboration and coherence (REC) model. *Psychological Record, 60*(3), 527–542.

Barnes-Holmes, Y., Barnes-Holmes, D., Smeets, P. M., Strand, P., & Friman, P. (2004). Establishing relational responding in accordance with more-than and less-than as generalized operant behavior in young children. *International Journal of Psychology and Psychological Therapy, 4*(3), 531–558.

Barsalou, L. W. (2008). Grounded cognition. *Annual Review of Psychology, 59,* 617–645.

Bechtel, W. (2008). *Mental mechanisms: Philosophical perspectives on cognitive neuroscience.* New York: Routledge.

Beck, A.T., Freeman, A., Pretzer J., Davis, D. D., Fleming, B., Ottavani, R., et al. (1990). *Cognitive therapy of personality disorders.* New York: Guilford Press.

Brysbaert, M., & Rastle, K. (2013). *Historical and conceptual issues in psychology* (2nd ed.). Harlow, UK: Pearson Education.

Carpenter, K. M., Martinez, D., Vadhan, N. P., Barnes-Holmes, D., & Nunes, E. V. (2012). Measures of attentional bias and relational responding are associated with behavioral treatment outcome for cocaine dependence. *American Journal of Drug and Alcohol Abuse, 38*(2), 146–154.

Chaney, D. W. (2013). An overview of the first use of the terms cognition and behavior. *Behavioral Sciences (Basel), 3*(1), 143–153.

Chiesa, M. (1992). Radical behaviorism and scientific frameworks: From mechanistic to relational accounts. *American Psychologist, 47*(11), 1287–1299.

Chiesa, M. (1994). *Radical behaviorism: The philosophy and the science.* Boston: Authors Cooperative.

De Houwer, J. (2011). Why the cognitive approach in psychology would profit from a functional approach and vice versa. *Perspectives on Psychological Science, 6*(2), 202–209.

De Houwer, J., Barnes-Holmes, Y., & Barnes-Holmes, D. (2016). Riding the waves: A functional-cognitive perspective on the relations among behaviour therapy, cognitive behaviour therapy, and acceptance and commitment therapy. *International Journal of Psychology, 51*(1), 40–44.

De Houwer, J., Barnes-Holmes, D., & Moors, A. (2013). What is learning? On the nature and merits of a functional definition of learning. *Psychonomic Bulletin and Review, 20*(4), 631–642.

Dymond, S., & Barnes, D. (1995). A transformation of self-discrimination response functions in accordance with the arbitrarily applicable relations of sameness, more than, and less than. *Journal of the Experimental Analysis of Behavior, 64*(2), 163–184.

Gardner, H. (1987). *The mind's new science: A history of the cognitive revolution.* New York: Basic Books.

Harvey, O. J., Hunt, D. E., & Schroeder, H. M. (1961). *Conceptual systems and personality organization.* New York: Wiley.

Hayes, S. C., Barnes-Holmes, D., & Roche, B. (Eds.). (2001). *Relational frame theory: A post-Skinnerian account of human language and cognition.* New York: Kluwer Academic/Plenum Publishers.

Hayes, S. C., & Brownstein, A. J. (1986). Mentalism, behavior-behavior relations, and a behavior-analytic view of the purposes of science. *Behavior Analyst, 9*(2), 175–190.

Hayes, S. C., & Hayes, L. J. (1989). The verbal action of the listener as a basis for rule-governance. In S. C. Hayes (Ed.), *Rule-governed behavior: Cognition, contingencies, and instructional control* (pp. 153–190). New York: Plenum Press.

Healy, O., Barnes-Holmes, D., & Smeets, P. M. (2000). Derived relational responding as generalized operant behavior. *Journal of the Experimental Analysis of Behavior, 74*(2), 207–227.

Hughes, S., & Barnes-Holmes, D. (2016a). Relational frame theory: The basic account. In R. D. Zettle, S. C. Hayes, D. Barnes-Holmes, & A. Biglan (Eds.), *The Wiley handbook of contextual behavioral science* (pp. 129–178). West Sussex, UK: Wiley-Blackwell.

Hughes, S., & Barnes-Holmes, D. (2016b). Relational frame theory: Implications for the study of human language and cognition. In R. D. Zettle, S. C. Hayes, D. Barnes-Holmes, & A. Biglan (Eds.), *The Wiley handbook of contextual behavioral science* (pp. 179–226). West Sussex, UK: Wiley-Blackwell.

Hughes, S., Barnes-Holmes, D., & Vahey, N. (2012). Holding on to our functional roots when exploring new intellectual islands: A voyage through implicit cognition research. *Journal of Contextual Behavioral Science, 1*(1–2), 17–38.

Hughes, S., De Houwer, J., & Perugini, M. (2016). The functional-cognitive framework for psychological research: Controversies and resolutions. *International Journal of Psychology, 51*(1), 4–14.

Leader, G., Barnes, D., & Smeets, P. M. (1996). Establishing equivalence relations using a respondent-type training procedure. *Psychological Record, 46*(4), 685–706.

Liefooghe, B., & De Houwer, J. (2016). A functional approach for research on cognitive control: Analyzing cognitive control tasks and their effects in terms of operant conditioning. *International Journal of Psychology, 51*(1), 28–32.

Lipkens, R., Hayes, S. C., & Hayes, L. J. (1993). Longitudinal study of the development of derived relations in an infant. *Journal of Experimental Child Psychology, 56*(2), 201–239.

Luciano, C., Gómez-Becerra, I., & Rodríguez-Valverde, M. (2007). The role of multiple-exemplar training and naming in establishing derived equivalence in an infant. *Journal of Experimental Analysis of Behavior, 87*(3), 349–365.

McClelland, J. L., & Rumelhart, D. E. (1985). Distributed memory and the representation of general and specific information. *Journal of Experimental Psychology: General, 114*(2), 159–197.

Moors, A. (2007). Can cognitive methods be used to study the unique aspect of emotion: An appraisal theorist's answer. *Cognition and Emotion, 21*(6), 1238–1269.

Neisser, U. (1967). *Cognitive psychology.* New York: Appleton-Century-Crofts.

O'Hora, D., Barnes-Holmes, D., Roche, B., & Smeets, P. (2004). Derived relational networks and control by novel instructions: A possible model of generative verbal responding. *Psychological Record, 54*(3), 437–460.

O'Hora, D., Barnes-Holmes, D., & Stewart, I. (2014). Antecedent and consequential control of derived instruction-following. *Journal of the Experimental Analysis of Behavior, 102*(1), 66–85.

Overskeid, G. (2008). They should have thought about the consequences: The crisis of cognitivism and a second chance for behavior analysis. *Psychological Record, 58*(1), 131–151.

Padesky, C. A. (1994). Schema change processes in cognitive therapy. *Clinical Psychology and Psychotherapy, 1*(5), 267–278.

Sidman M. (1994). *Equivalence relations and behavior: A research story.* Boston: Authors Cooperative.

Skinner, B. F. (1974). *About behaviorism.* New York: Vintage Books.

Stewart, I., & Barnes-Holmes, D. (2004). Relational frame theory and analogical reasoning: Empirical investigations. *International Journal of Psychology and Psychological Therapy, 4*(2), 241–262.

Stewart, I., Barnes-Holmes, D., Hayes, S. C., & Lipkens, R. (2001). Relations among relations: Analogies, metaphors, and stories. In S. C. Hayes, D., Barnes-Holmes, & B. Roche (Eds.), *Relational frame theory: A post-Skinnerian account of human language and cognition* (pp. 73–86). New York: Kluwer Academic/Plenum Publishers.

Tolman, E. C., & Honzik, C. H. (1930). "Insight" in rats. *University of California Publications in Psychology, 4,* 215–232.

Wells, A. (2000). *Emotional disorders and metacognition: Innovative cognitive therapy.* London: Wiley.

Wells, A., & Matthews G. (1994). *Attention and emotion: A clinical perspective.* Hove, UK: Lawrence Erlbaum.

Wiener, N. (1961). *Cybernetics, or control and communication in animal and the machine* (2nd ed.). Cambridge, MA: MIT Press

Zettle, R. D., Hayes, S. C., Barnes-Holmes, D., & Biglan, A. (2016). *The Wiley handbook of contextual behavioral science.* West Sussex, UK: Wiley-Blackwell.

# CHAPTER 8

# Emotions and Emotion Regulation

Anthony Papa, PhD
Emerson M. Epstein, MA

*Department of Psychology, University of Nevada, Reno*

Emotional responding and dysregulation underlie or exacerbate most problems that are the focus of clinical intervention. In this chapter, we define what an emotion is, how it arises, how it becomes dysregulated, and the implications these understandings present for clinical practice.

The definitions of *emotion* vary. For some, emotions are constructions, culturally defined meanings ascribed to antecedent stimuli and imposed upon neurophysiological-based affective responses. From this perspective, simple valence and arousal dimensions characterize these affective responses, and when combined with a social-driven attributional process, they give rise to the perception of distinct emotions (Barrett, 2012). For others, emotions are discrete action tendencies representing naturally selected adaptations in mammals. These action tendencies provide a basic framework for fast responding to species-specific, historically recurring antecedents in order to promote individual evolutionary success (Keltner & Haidt, 1999; Tooby & Cosmides, 1990). Still others strike a balance between these perspectives and view emotions as distinct states, as in the basic evolutionary view, but appraisal processes elicited by specific species-typical situations mediate their emergence (Hofmann, 2016; Scherer, 2009).

## The Nature of Emotions

With respect to antecedent conditions, there is a general consensus across perspectives that emotions are responses to self-relevant stimuli (Frijda, 1986; Hofmann, 2016; Scherer, 1984). How a stimulus is recognized as being self-relevant in any given context appears to be driven by two distinct, but not incompatible, processes: top-down processing and bottom-up processing (e.g., Mohanty & Sussman, 2013; Pessoa, Oliveira, & Pereira, 2013). While both processes are accepted as a part of emotional responding, different theoretical perspectives of emotion debate the primacy of each process to the experience and regulation of emotion.

Bottom-up processing does not require higher-level cognitive processing or attribution. A pure evolutionary, bottom-up view would suggest that emotions are hardwired responses to common fitness-related stimuli in our evolutionary past (Tooby & Cosmides, 1990). Proponents of this view define "emotions" as the output that results from the interaction of a biologically based core emotional system and a control system that modulates core emotional responses to match the relevant contingencies in specific contexts in order to maximize the adaptiveness of the response (Campos, Frankel, & Camras, 2004; Cole, Martin, & Dennis, 2004; Levenson, 1999). From this perspective, emotions are recursive, synchronized responses that can recruit a broad array of resources. The elements recruited that make up an emotional response include the engagement of perceptual and attentional systems; the activation of associational memory and attributional sets; physiological, hormonal, and neural activation; and overt and covert behavioral responses, including overt expression and goal-relevant responding. The degree of recruitment of any of these constituent elements for any given emotional response is contingent on multiple factors related to the nature of the antecedent stimulus. This includes factors such as degree of self-relevance, in terms of facilitation or impedance of approach or avoidance goals in any given situation, and social display rules for responding (Izard, 2010).

An evolutionary view of emotion suggests that antecedent conditions are largely stereotyped and reflect evolutionarily recurrent situations/stimuli, such as threat to physical integrity or loss of resource-rich objects or statuses that would reduce individual fitness (Ekman & Friesen, 1982; Tooby & Cosmides, 1990). In this view, specific emotions evolved as adaptations to generalized antecedents defined by specific, distributed patterns of neural activation, physiological arousal, and behavioral display (Panksepp & Biven, 2012). Activation of these response tendencies, while largely biologically determined, is open to significant modification via learning and conditioning (e.g., Levenson, 1999). As stimuli are perceived, whether biologically driven or shaped by conditioning, associational neuronal activation gives rise to the patterned response associated with emotional reactions to specific classes of stimuli. Thus, evolutionary-based theories suggest an important part of the emotion-elicitation process is that there is a one-to-one correspondence between some classes of stimuli and some responses, whether this coupling is hardwired or modified by conditioning.

While there may be general similarities in antecedent stimuli and emotional responses as described by evolutionary theory, it is important to keep in mind that variability exists across cultures (e.g., Elfenbein & Ambady, 2002; Mesquita & Frijda, 1992). Experimental evidence of cultural variation in emotion situations and responses is evident even within the United States. In a series of studies, researchers found that members of the Southern US honor culture were more likely to show facial displays of anger and experience increased testosterone when they were insulted compared with those not from an honor culture (Cohen, Nisbett, Bowdle, & Schwarz, 1996). To understand this variability, we can define "culture" as a set of expectations for how to think, feel, and behave in a given context. In other words, it is a culturally defined set of rules defining the self-relevance of many situations and stimuli in a social environment given one's role in that culture. These expectations originally developed in response to different socioecological demands that different groups faced in their history and the meaning ascribed to them, highlighting the role for higher-order processing in the elicitation and subsequent elicitation of partially stereotyped emotion responses.

The top-down process for emotion generation is schema driven, in which learned appraisals and associations color the way people perceive and hence respond to conditions. They are in part learned during acculturation, and they are in part a product of an individual's unique learning history. In Scherer's Component Process Model of emotions (2009), people undergo a series of either unconscious or conscious appraisal steps to evaluate stimuli, including (1) relevance, such as the novelty of an event, relevance to goals, and intrinsic pleasantness; (2) implications, such as outcome probability, discrepancy from expectations, conduciveness to goals, and urgency to react; (3) coping potential; and (4) normative significance, such as compatibility with internal and external standards. Other appraisal theorists have discussed similar ideas (e.g., Ortony & Turner, 1990; Smith & Lazarus, 1993).

Some emotions, especially those described as "self-conscious" or "moral" emotions, such as pride, shame, and guilt, require some social evaluative process to engender them (Haidt, 2001; Tracy & Robins, 2004). These social evaluation processes involve the consideration of social status and hierarchy, the moral probity of one's behavior, and attributions about the mental states of others, among other processes. For example, pride can involve attributions that one has done something that increases social status, is socially valued, and evokes envy in others. Shame can involve attributions that one has decreased social status, is socially undesirable, and evokes disgust in others.

Those from an evolutionary perspective would say that these *hypercognitized* emotions are adjuncts or modifications of a basic evolutionary-derived subset of emotions (Levy, 1982). However, an alternative position states that it might be reasonable, given that all emotions can be linked to some specific attributional set, to conclude that all emotions are hypercognitized constructions of a basic core affective system that responds in terms of valence (positive/negative or approach/avoidance) and intensity or level of arousal. In this constructivist view, what differentiates emotions is the experience of different attributional sets and expressive behaviors and the associated differences in action readiness. The experience of the recruited elements of an emotional reaction is defined by cultural scripts associated with the antecedent conditions, and it is modified by individual learning histories (Mesquita & Boiger, 2014).

Support for this view comes from two main sources: emotion granularity research and research seeking to identify the biological underpinning of emotional reactions. Research on emotional granularity suggests that while emotional categories are common conceptualizations of how emotions exist, many people do not report differences between their emotions in their day-to-day emotional experience but instead report in "nongranular" terms related to the constructs underlying core affect (valence and arousal; e.g., Barrett, 2012). The general lack of consistent findings delineating a patterned response in physiological measures of emotional arousal unique to each emotional state, and the lack of consistent findings identifying dedicated neurophysiology or activation unique to each emotional state, support this observation (see Cameron, Lindquist, & Gray, 2015; but see Panksepp & Biven, 2012).

## Elements of Emotional Responding

One way to delineate an emotion from its antecedents and consequences is to consider it a state of the organism that creates a context that increases the likelihood of subsequent action. Most emotion theorists, regardless of theoretical orientation, would agree that emotions involve multidimensional, semicoupled response channels, including physiological, expressive, cognitive, and motivational changes (Levenson, 2014). However, many debate the extent to which it is necessary to define the coherence and specificity of these response channels (e.g., Gross & Barrett, 2011; Lench, Flores, & Bench, 2011).

**Physiological changes.** Emotion researchers have examined autonomic nervous system (ANS) and central nervous system (CNS) activation and deactivation as an indicator of emotion specificity. This line of thinking makes sense if neural circuits were adapted by natural selection to solve different adaptive problems (Tooby & Cosmides, 1990). In a meta-analysis, Cacioppo, Berntson, Larsen, Poehlmann, and Ito (2000) found that a number of claims regarding ANS discrimination among emotions hold up. For instance, anger, fear, and sadness were associated with greater heart rate activity than disgust, anger was associated with higher diastolic blood pressure than fear, and disgust was associated with greater increases in skin conductance than happiness. A recent meta-analysis of the neural correlates of emotional processing found some support for differentiation

(Vytal & Hamann, 2010). However, this meta-analysis also found that many neural structures overlap with different emotions.

Research examining not just neural structures but neural pathways has pinpointed a number of unique systems dedicated to processing specific types of emotional information. For instance, research has demonstrated that the behavioral activation system is related to the detection of reward (Coan & Allen, 2003), while Panksepp's PANIC system is related to the detection of loss, which is proposed to be neuroanatomically distinct from the substrates involved in PLAY (Panksepp & Biven, 2012). Researchers have investigated other emotional systems (e.g., Panksepp, 2007; see Barrett, 2012, for criticisms of neural specificity) as well as auxiliary systems, such as the neuroendocrine system, which is related to a general stress response (Buijs & van Eden, 2000). One caveat to all of this research, however, is that emotions unfold over time, and, as a result, it is likely that components of ANS activity vary with respect to time (Lang & Bradley, 2010). This suggests that to truly distinguish ANS patterning for different emotions, research must look at multiple components across time.

**Expressive changes.** In his 1872 book *The Expression of the Emotions in Man and Animals*, Darwin highlighted the commonalities of expressions across mammalian species. Today, functional theories of emotion hypothesize that expressions of emotion are adaptations to social environments. Although expressions initially evolved to promote individual survival (e.g., disgust and fear affect nasal inhalation volume and visual field size; Susskind et al., 2008), they also promote the survival of other members of the group because of the communicative benefit of recognizing expressions in others, thus improving the overall fitness of the group. From the functional perspective, facial expressions are ethologically defined as social signals, meaning they are behaviors that come under selection pressures because of the effect they have on the behavior or states of others, which are in turn subject to selection pressures (Mehu & Scherer, 2012). In other words, recognizing facial expressions was an evolutionary adaptation that promoted group fitness, thus placing expressions, recognition ability, and responses in the realm of natural selection. They were selected for because they facilitated interindividual communication and coordination both within and between species. Facial expressions of emotion have been shown to shape the responses of others by evoking corresponding emotional responses, thus reinforcing or discouraging behavioral expression in others (Keltner & Haidt, 1999).

However, it is abundantly evident in certain social conditions that facial expressions do not necessarily correspond to a felt emotion (e.g., power/status differentials; Hall, Coats, & LeBeau, 2005). In addition, the rate of correspondence goes up when a person is in the presence of others, leading to the hypothesis that facial expressions are learned, culturally defined behaviors for communicating social intent (e.g., Barrett, 2012). Research on whether facial expressions are universal across cultures is mixed, but on balance it suggests that people from different cultures around the world display and recognize similar facial expressions (Ekman et al., 1987; see Russell, 1995, for critique). What is clear from this research is that cultural variations and nuances in prototypical expressions exist (Marsh, Elfenbein, & Ambady, 2003), suggesting that different facial expressions of emotion more or less comprise both evolutionary-adapted signals *and* learned cultural sets (Barrett, 2012; Mehu & Scherer, 2012; Scherer, Mortillaro, & Mehu, 2013).

Interestingly, research examining facial feedback suggests that facial expressions associated with certain emotions can initiate and modulate emotion and ANS arousal (see McIntosh, 1996, for a review of this work) even when the contraction of muscles related to a specific facial expression is inadvertent (e.g., Soussignan, 2002). Work on embodiment suggests a similar feedback process. *Embodiment* is the idea that emotional concepts are meaningful because they are grounded in sensorimotor and interoceptive activities that can represent the content of emotional information and knowledge (Niedenthal, 2007). For instance, Strack, Martin, and Stepper (1988) found that participants who were made to smile while watching a cartoon were more likely to report that the cartoon was funny. Research has also shown that the suppression and enhancement of facial expressions hampers and facilitates the processing of emotional information, respectively (Neal & Chartrand, 2011).

**Changes in attention, memory, and appraisals.** Emotion has been shown to affect all stages of attention, including orientation toward, engagement with, shifting away from, and maintaining disengagement from a stimulus (Vuilleumier & Huang, 2009). Depending on the emotion in an emotional situation—that is, a situation of self-relevance—individuals can narrow their focus on central aspects of the situation or broaden it in a global way. In the case of negativity bias, research has shown that threat-related information is more readily attended to compared with other information (Koster, Crombez, Verschuere, & De Houwer, 2004). Attentional changes also occur when one is experiencing positive emotions. Using the global-local visual processing paradigm, Fredrickson and Branigan (2005) found that when participants are led to feel a positive emotion, they tend to focus on global features, whereas when led to feel a negative emotion, they tend to focus on local features.

Emotions can also influence the content of cognition by directing attention and by affecting memory. Bower's network theory of affect (1981) suggests that distributed, associational information processing, starting at the processing of perceptual information, facilitates the recall of affectively similar information, which explains phenomena such as mood-state-dependent recall (e.g., when you are sad, you're only able to recall ever being sad) and mood-congruent learning (recall is maximized when there is affective congruency between a learner's mood state and the type of material being presented). These factors lead to thought congruity (thoughts and associations congruent with mood state) that is heightened by the intensity of emotional arousal, with increases in intensity leading to greater activation of associational networks, which affect how information is processed. For example, Forgas and George's (2001) affect infusion model (AIM) is a dual-process model designed to explain how affective states influence cognition, such as judgments and decision making. In this model, situational demands, in terms of effort required and degree of openness of information-search processes, result in four information-processing approaches. These include top-down, reflective processing, such as (1) direct access processing (low effort, low openness) and (2) motivated processing (high effort, low openness); and bottom-up associational processing, such as (3) heuristic processing (low effort, high openness) and (4) substantive processing (high effort, high openness). In all cases, when a person uses open, more constructive information-search processes, emotion is more likely to affect cognition processing. When effort is low and sources of information are open and constructive, individuals use an affect-as-information heuristic in which their emotional state is a source of information about a situation, regardless of whether the situation elicited the emotion (Clore & Storbeck, 2006). This is consequential, as once emotion-related associations are activated, there is a tendency for people to appraise subsequent, temporally related and/or affectively related events similarly, regardless of the functionality of the appraisal (e.g., Lerner & Keltner, 2001; Small, Lerner, & Fischhoff, 2006). This could be problematic when anxiety from one source leads to attributions of high risk and uncontrollability across situations, independent of the risk inherent in a particular context. In situations demanding complex, effortful, constructive thinking (substantive processing), researchers have seen affect-priming effects on cognition, as the constructive process is more likely to incorporate information primed by associational memory recall.

## Do Emotions Have Functions?

An essential hypothesis of the evolutionary–basic emotion perspective is that emotions are states derived from conditions of evolutionary and cultural significance that have persisted across time, and thus they have important functions. The potential intrapersonal and interpersonal functions of emotions span different levels of analysis: dyadic, group, cultural, and individual (Hofmann, 2014; Keltner & Haidt, 1999). At the dyadic level, emotion informs others as to one's inner states, motivational tendencies, and intentions; evokes emotions in others;

and promotes social coordination by eliciting or deterring behavior in others. At the group level, the function of emotions has been thought to define in-group membership, roles, and status, thus facilitating the resolution of group conflict. Emotions at the cultural level are thought to promote acculturation, moral guidance, and social identity formation. At the individual level, emotions facilitate situated information processing and motivational changes (Scherer, 2005). This can be seen on the physiological level, where physiological changes in neuroendocrine and CNS activity create a biological context that supports some overt response. For example, early work by Levenson, Ekman, and Friesen (1990) demonstrated that when anger is elicited, blood flow shifts toward appendages. Information processing and motivational changes can also be seen in individuals when changes in cognition related to an emotion reorient the individual's attention to salient features of a situation. These action tendencies act as modal action patterns, in which the likelihood of a species-typical behavioral response pattern increases. For example, when an individual experiences fear, the action of fighting, fleeing, or freezing increases in probability. This concept is similar to the behavioral notion of an establishing operation. However, given that emotions are evolutionary-derived responses that a person's history of reinforcement can shape, it would be misleading to consider emotions as merely establishing operations without specifying any biological affordance.

However, even the question of whether emotions have any emergent properties other than the sum of the activated elements in any behavioral response to a stimulus is open for debate (Gross & Barrett, 2011). If the experience of emotion is the epiphenomenon of the conceptual act of imposing meaning to physiological responses to core affect, then the question regarding the function of emotions is mainly this: Does behavior that a social group recognizes as emotion have a symbolic function within the group (Barrett, 2011)? Thus, "functionalist" accounts of emotion comprise a loose range of perspectives that differentially emphasize the primacy of naturally selected adaptations to symbolic functions. In all cases, functionalist accounts of emotion are the flip sides of the ontological perspectives outlined above.

# Defining Emotion Regulation

All theorists would agree that current environmental conditions are more important to adaptive responding than ancestral conditions. Levenson's control theory of emotions (1999) takes this into consideration. Levenson postulates that there are two emotion systems: (1) a core system that is a hardwired emotion-response system that processes prototypical inputs and outputs stereotyped emotional responses, and (2) a control system that modulates or regulates these stereotyped responses through feedback loops affected by learning and immediate social context to maximize the adaptiveness of emotional responding. In Levenson's definition, the distinction between emotion generation and emotion regulation (ER) are blurred—the regulatory feedback processes of the control system are a critical component in emotion generation, linking the emotional response to the environmental context and maximizing the functional adaptiveness of the response. Moreover, the ongoing interactions between the core and regulatory processes that tune the behavioral manifestations of a person's interaction with his environment are transactional in nature, affecting both the ongoing experience and expression of an emotion, and also the nature of the situation itself.

Cognitive reappraisal affects the intensity and duration of a response by modifying the cognitions framing the situation and thus the experience. Scherer's Component Process model (2009; see above) and other cognitive theories of emotion outline aspects of attributions that might be changed. Similarly, response modulation affects the intensity and duration of an emotion by influencing the degree to which any elements of an emotional response (i.e., perceptual and attentional processes, attribution, memory, physiological, hormonal, neural activation, and behavioral responses) are activated. Gross (1998) proposes hat this response modulation could include trying to suppress thoughts and expressions related to the emotion, trying to relax, engaging in exercise, or using substances. Others have since proposed other forms of response modulation, including engaging in acceptance or mindfulness exercises (Hayes et al., 2004), deliberate attentional shift/redeployment (e.g., Huffziger & Kuehner, 2009), and positive reminiscence (e.g., Quoidbach, Berry, Hansenne, & Mikolajczak, 2010), among others. ER as a form of appraisal or cognitive process is consistent with the constructionist view that emotions are personal and have social meaning that informs the nature of emotional experience (Gross & Barrett, 2011).

From all perspectives, the cognitive processing of emotional stimuli may be conscious or nonconscious. Automatic, associational processing, which leads to nonconscious response modulation, can (1) engender nonconscious affect mimicry and embodiment, affecting an emotional state; (2) be influenced by automatic face perception and social judgment; (3) prime regulatory goals that are associated with enacting various response-focused and antecedent-focused ER strategies; and (4) activate implicit attitudes, preferences, and goals, which can affect the associated valence and reinforcement properties of environmental stimuli. All of these results have implications for how attentional, perceptual, and working memory resource allocation discriminate between emotional stimuli in any given context (Bargh, Schwader, Hailey, Dyer, & Boothby, 2012). At its extreme, automatic processing can result in selective attention being paid to stimuli related to prepotent depressogenic and anxiety-related schemas; biased attributions; congruent memories being overaccessible; and emotion dysregulation contributing to the development and maintenance of psychopathology (Hofmann, Sawyer, Fang, & Asnaani, 2012; Teachman, Joormann, Steinman, & Gotlib, 2012).

Emotion regulation can go beyond control system processes. Individuals can proactively modify if and how they interact with antecedent stimuli. Gross (1998) outlines the following antecedent-focused ER strategies (see also chapter 16): (1) situation selection (approaching or avoiding certain emotionally evocative stimuli), (2) situation modification (preemptive steps to change the environment), (3) attentional deployment (deliberately attending to certain or different aspects of a situation), and/or (4) cognitive change (preventively exploring new meanings ascribed to stimuli/situations). However, it should be noted that if the antecedent stimuli eliciting an emotion can be identified, one will find that emotional reactions are almost always tightly linked, preprogrammed, or culturally scripted responses that naturally follow antecedents. Emotions are functionally maladaptive when regulatory feedback insufficiently "tunes" the intensity of the response to the context in which the antecedent stimulus occurs, or when the emotion is in response to a nonrelevant antecedent in a given context, thus obviating the potential for preadapted fast-track responding. This suggests that in order to promote the functional adaption of responding in individuals, a therapist should encourage them to (1) discriminate between co-occurring antecedent stimuli; and/or (2) enhance the efficacy of control processes or the range of control processes they employ, or (3) better match the control processes to the response or situation (see Bonanno and Burton, 2013). Indeed, a growing body of research supports the idea that well-being is, in large part, influenced by the extent to which individuals engage in flexible, context-sensitive emotional responding and regulation (Kashdan & Rottenberg, 2010).

# Application for Clinical Science and Conclusions

Breakdowns in antecedent discrimination and/or the efficacy of control processes trigger or exacerbate most of the problems conceptualized as mental health difficulties, and they are the main targets of intervention for most psychotherapies. These breakdowns may be attributable, in part, to the effect of emotional arousal on selective attention to stimuli, to preattentive processing, to poor attentional control, and to interpretive bias for ambiguous stimuli that results in decontextualized emotional responding.

However, decontextualized emotional arousal and regulation may have its genesis in a number of different problems beyond those of poor in-the-moment antecedent discrimination and the breakdown of feedback in automatic control processes. In depression, cognitive vulnerabilities and latent depressogenic schemas from early adverse life events impair information acquisition, memory retrieval, and information processing, creating a reciprocal relationship in which bias toward negative stimuli—and subsequent negative emotional experience—reaffirms negative schemas (Disner, Beevers, Haigh, & Beck, 2011). These schematic biases that are engendered in attributional patterns of dichotomous thinking, negative filtering, and hopelessness are also associated with attentional bias toward negative self-referential information—not necessarily threat—and away from positive information in the environment (Peckham, McHugh, & Otto, 2010). Difficulty orienting away from negative information and the expedited neural processing of emotionally negative information both influence attentional bias; both also influence the encoding and retrieval of negatively valenced memory, further heightening depressed mood and the bottom-up activation of depressogenic schemas (Beevers, 2005; Disner et al., 2011; Joormann & Gotlib, 2010). The open-sourced, associative heuristic or reflexive processing delineated by Forgas and George's (2001) AIM model, outlined above, reflects this bottom-up processing. This bottom-up process becomes problematic, because individuals are not in contact with sources of information or stimuli that violate depressive expectancies and stimulate reflective, motivated processing to correct biases, thus maintaining a positive feedback loop for depressive symptoms (see Beevers, 2005). The closed nature of this process is demonstrated by a general insensitivity to emotion context, in which individuals demonstrate decreased emotional reactivity to positive and negative stimuli over time (Bylsma, Morris, & Rottenberg, 2008; see also Van de Leemput et al., 2014), resulting in noncontextual, inflexible emotional processing and regulation characterized by avoidance, suppression, and rumination (Aldao, Nolen-Hoeksema, & Schweizer, 2010).

Conceptualizing mental illness in terms of decontextualized emotional responding, and focusing on the elements of emotion and control processes that may be contributing to the dysfunction, has the potential to improve our understanding of psychopathology and how to treat it. However, the dominant, categorical approaches to understanding mental illness, which look at unique indicators of potential taxon and less at the common processes that drive these emotional disruptions, have hampered this concept's translation into clinical practice. Currently, there is a move to examine the elements of emotion and ER that contribute to the psychic dysregulation called "mental illness" as products of common processes in the emotion systems (e.g., Barlow, Allen, & Choate, 2004; Hayes et al., 2004; Kring & Sloan, 2010; Watkins, 2008). This chapter represents a brief introduction to the vast amount of basic research literature on emotion and the burgeoning translational literature.

# References

Aldao, A., Nolen-Hoeksema, S., & Schweizer, S. (2010). Emotion-regulation strategies across psychopathology: A meta-analytic review. *Clinical Psychology Review, 30*(2), 217–237.

Bargh, J. A., Schwader, K. L., Hailey, S. E., Dyer, R. L., & Boothby, E. J. (2012). Automaticity in social-cognitive processes. *Trends in Cognitive Sciences, 16*(12), 593–605.

Barlow, D. H., Allen, L. B., & Choate, M. L. (2004). Toward a unified treatment for emotional disorders. *Behavior Therapy, 35*(2), 205–230.

Barrett, L. F. (2011). Was Darwin wrong about emotional expressions? *Current Directions in Psychological Science, 20*(6), 400–406.

Barrett, L. F. (2012). Emotions are real. *Emotion, 12*(3), 413–429.

Beevers, C. G. (2005). Cognitive vulnerability to depression: A dual process model. *Clinical Psychology Review, 25*(7), 975–1002.

Bonanno, G. A., & Burton, C. L. (2013). Regulatory flexibility: An individual differences perspective on coping and emotion regulation. *Perspectives on Psychological Science, 8*(6), 591–612.

Bower, G. H. (1981). Mood and memory. *American Psychologist, 36*(2), 129–148.

Buijs, R. M., & van Eden, C. G. (2000). The integration of stress by the hypothalamus, amygdala and prefrontal cortex: Balance between the autonomic nervous system and the neuroendocrine system. *Progress in Brain Research, 126*, 117–132.

Bylsma, L. M., Morris, B. H., & Rottenberg, J. (2008). A meta-analysis of emotional reactivity in major depressive disorder. *Clinical Psychology Review, 28*(4), 676–691.

Cacioppo, J. T., Berntson, G. G., Larsen, J. T., Poehlmann, K. M., & Ito, T. A. (2000). The psychophysiology of emotion. In M. Lewis & J. M. Haviland-Jones (Eds.), *Handbook of emotions* (2nd ed., pp. 173–191). New York: Guilford Press.

Cameron, C. D., Lindquist, K. A., & Gray, K. (2015). A constructionist review of morality and emotions: No evidence for specific links between moral content and discrete emotions. *Personality and Social Psychology Review, 19*(4), 371–394.

Campos, J. J., Frankel, C. B., & Camras, L. (2004). On the nature of emotion regulation. *Child Development, 75*(2), 377–394.

Clore, G. L., & Storbeck, J. (2006). Affect as information about liking, efficacy, and importance. In J. P. Forgas (Ed.), *Affect in social thinking and behavior* (pp. 123–142). New York: Psychology Press.

Coan, J. A., & Allen, J. J. (2003). Frontal EEG asymmetry and the behavioral activation and inhibition systems. *Psychophysiology, 40*(1), 106–114.

Cohen, D., Nisbett, R. E., Bowdle, B. F., & Schwarz, N. (1996). Insult, aggression, and the Southern culture of honor: An "experimental ethnography." *Journal of Personality and Social Psychology, 70*(5), 945–959.

Cole, P. M., Martin, S. E., & Dennis, T. A. (2004). Emotion regulation as a scientific construct: Methodological challenges and directions for child development research. *Child Development, 75*(2), 317–333.

Darwin, C. (1872). *The expression of the emotions in man and animals.* London: John Murray.

Disner, S. G., Beevers, C. G., Haigh, E. A., & Beck, A. T. (2011). Neural mechanisms of the cognitive model of depression. *Nature Reviews Neuroscience, 12*(8), 467–477.

Ekman, P., & Friesen, W. V. (1982). Felt, false, and miserable smiles. *Journal of Nonverbal Behavior, 6*(4), 238–252.

Ekman, P., Friesen, W. V., O'Sullivan, M., Chan, A., Diacoyanni-Tarlatzis, I., Heider, K., et al. (1987). Universals and cultural differences in the judgments of facial expressions of emotion. *Journal of Personality and Social Psychology, 53*(4), 712–717.

Elfenbein, H. A., & Ambady, N. (2002). On the universality and cultural specificity of emotion recognition: A meta-analysis. *Psychological Bulletin, 128*(2), 203–235.

Forgas, J. P., & George, J. M. (2001). Affective influences on judgments and behavior in organizations: An information processing perspective. *Organizational Behavior and Human Decision Processes, 86*(1), 3–34.

Fredrickson, B. L., & Branigan, C. (2005). Positive emotions broaden the scope of attention and thought-action repertoires. *Cognition and Emotion, 19*(3), 313–332.

Frijda, N. H. (1986). *The emotions.* Cambridge, UK: Cambridge University Press.

Gross, J. J. (1998). Antecedent-and response-focused emotion regulation: Divergent consequences for experience, expression, and physiology. *Journal of Personality and Social Psychology, 74*(1), 224–237.

Gross, J. J., & Barrett, L. F. (2011). Emotion generation and emotion regulation: One or two depends on your point of view. *Emotion Review, 3*(1), 8–16.

Haidt, J. (2001). The emotional dog and its rational tail: A social intuitionist approach to moral judgment. *Psychological Review, 108*(4), 814–834.

Hall, J. A., Coats, E. J., & LeBeau, L. S. (2005). Nonverbal behavior and the vertical dimension of social relations: A meta-analysis. *Psychological Bulletin, 131*(6), 898–924.

Hayes, S. C., Strosahl, K. D., Wilson, K. G., Bissett, R. T., Pistorello, J., Toarmino, D., et al. (2004). Measuring experiential avoidance: A preliminary test of a working model. *Psychological Record, 54*(4), 553–578.

Hofmann, S. G. (2014). Interpersonal emotion regulation model of mood and anxiety disorders. *Cognitive Therapy and Research, 38*(5), 483–492.

Hofmann, S. G. (2016). *Emotion in therapy: From science to practice.* New York: Guilford Press.

Hofmann, S. G., Sawyer, A. T., Fang, A., & Asnaani, A. (2012). Emotion dysregulation model of mood and anxiety disorders. *Depression and Anxiety, 29*(5), 409–416.

Huffziger, S., & Kuehner, C. (2009). Rumination, distraction, and mindful self-focus in depressed patients. *Behaviour Research and Therapy, 47*(3), 224–230.

Izard, C. E. (2010). More meanings and more questions for the term "emotion." *Emotion Review, 2*(4), 383–385.

Joormann, J., & Gotlib, I. H. (2010). Emotion regulation in depression: Relation to cognitive inhibition. *Cognition and Emotion, 24*(2), 281–298.

Kashdan, T. B., & Rottenberg, J. (2010). Psychological flexibility as a fundamental aspect of health. *Clinical Psychology Review, 30*(7), 865–878.

Keltner, D., & Haidt, J. (1999). Social functions of emotions at four levels of analysis. *Cognition and Emotion, 13*(5), 505–521.

Koster, E. H., Crombez, G., Verschuere, B., & De Houwer, J. (2004). Selective attention to threat in the dot probe paradigm: Differentiating vigilance and difficulty to disengage. *Behaviour Research and Therapy, 42*(10), 1183–1192.

Kring, A. M., & Sloan, D. M. (2010). *Emotion regulation and psychopathology: A transdiagnostic approach to etiology and treatment.* New York: Guilford Press.

Lang, P. J., & Bradley, M. M. (2010). Emotion and the motivational brain. *Biological Psychology, 84*(3), 437–450.

Lench, H. C., Flores, S. A., & Bench, S. W. (2011). Discrete emotions predict changes in cognition, judgment, experience, behavior, and physiology: A meta-analysis of experimental emotion elicitations. *Psychological Bulletin, 137*(5), 834–855.

Lerner, J. S., & Keltner, D. (2001). Fear, anger, and risk. *Journal of Personality and Social Psychology, 81*(1), 146–159.

Levenson, R. W. (1999). The intrapersonal functions of emotion. *Cognition and Emotion, 13*(5), 481–504.

Levenson, R. W. (2014). The autonomic nervous system and emotion. *Emotion Review, 6*(2), 100–112.

Levenson, R. W., Ekman, P., & Friesen, W. V. (1990). Voluntary facial action generates emotion-specific autonomic nervous system activity. *Psychophysiology, 27*(4), 363–384.

Levy, R. I. (1982). On the nature and functions of the emotions: An anthropological perspective. *Social Science Information, 21*(4–5), 511–528.

Marsh, A. A., Elfenbein, H. A., & Ambady, N. (2003). Nonverbal "accents": Cultural differences in facial expressions of emotion. *Psychological Science, 14*(4), 373–376.

McIntosh, D. N. (1996). Facial feedback hypotheses: Evidence, implications, and directions. *Motivation and Emotion, 20*(2), 121–147.

Mehu, M., & Scherer, K. R. (2012). A psycho-ethological approach to social signal processing. *Cognitive Processing, 13*(2), 397–414.

Mesquita, B., & Boiger, M. (2014). Emotions in context: A sociodynamic model of emotions. *Emotion Review, 6*(4), 298–302.

Mesquita, B., & Frijda, N. H. (1992). Cultural variations in emotions: A review. *Psychological Bulletin, 112*(2), 179–204.

Mohanty, A., & Sussman, T. J. (2013). Top-down modulation of attention by emotion. *Frontiers in Human Neuroscience, 7*, 102.

Neal, D. T., & Chartrand, T. L. (2011). Embodied emotion perception amplifying and dampening facial feedback modulates emotion perception accuracy. *Social Psychological and Personality Science, 2*(6), 673–678.

Niedenthal, P. M. (2007). Embodying emotion. *Science, 316*(5827), 1002–1005.

Ortony, A., & Turner, T. J. (1990). What's basic about basic emotions? *Psychological Review, 97*(3), 315–331.

Panksepp, J. (2007). Criteria for basic emotions: Is DISGUST a primary "emotion"? *Cognition and Emotion, 21*(8), 1819–1828.

Panksepp, J., & Biven, L. (2012). *The archaeology of mind: Neuroevolutionary origins of human emotions.* New York: W. W. Norton.

Peckham, A. D., McHugh, R. K., & Otto, M. W. (2010). A meta-analysis of the magnitude of biased attention in depression. *Depression and Anxiety, 27*(12), 1135–1142.

Pessoa, L., Oliveira, L., & Pereira, M. (2013). Top-down attention and the processing of emotional stimuli. In J. Armony & P. Vuilleumier (Eds.), *The Cambridge Handbook of Human Affective Neuroscience* (pp. 357–374). Cambridge, UK: Cambridge University Press.

Quoidbach, J., Berry, E. V., Hansenne, M., & Mikolajczak, M. (2010). Positive emotion regulation and well-being: Comparing the impact of eight savoring and dampening strategies. *Personality and Individual Differences, 49*(5), 368–373.

Russell, J. A. (1995). Facial expressions of emotion: What lies beyond minimal universality? *Psychological Bulletin, 118*(3), 379–391.

Scherer, K. R. (1984). Emotion as a multicomponent process: A model and some cross-cultural data. *Review of Personality and Social Psychology, 5*, 37–63.

Scherer, K. R. (2005). What are emotions? And how can they be measured? *Social Science Information, 44*(4), 695–729.

Scherer, K. R. (2009). The dynamic architecture of emotion: Evidence for the component process model. *Cognition and Emotion, 23*(7), 1307–1351.

Scherer, K. R., Mortillaro, M., & Mehu, M. (2013). Understanding the mechanisms underlying the production of facial expression of emotion: A componential perspective. *Emotion Review, 5*(1), 47–53.

Small, D. A., Lerner, J. S., & Fischhoff, B. (2006). Emotion priming and attributions for terrorism: Americans' reactions in a national field experiment. *Political Psychology, 27*(2), 289–298.

Smith, C. A., & Lazarus, R. S. (1993). Appraisal components, core relational themes, and the emotions. *Cognition and Emotion, 7*(3–4), 233–269.

Soussignan, R. (2002). Duchenne smile, emotional experience, and autonomic reactivity: A test of the facial feedback hypothesis. *Emotion, 2*(1), 52–74.

Strack, F., Martin, L. L., & Stepper, S. (1988). Inhibiting and facilitating conditions of the human smile: A nonobtrusive test of the facial feedback hypothesis. *Journal of Personality and Social Psychology, 54*(5), 768–777.

Susskind, J. M., Lee, D. H., Cusi, A., Feiman, R., Grabski, W., & Anderson, A. K. (2008). Expressing fear enhances sensory acquisition. *Nature Neuroscience, 11*(7), 843–850.

Teachman, B. A., Joormann, J., Steinman, S. A., & Gotlib, I. H. (2012). Automaticity in anxiety disorders and major depressive disorder. *Clinical Psychology Review, 32*(6), 575–603.

Tooby, J., & Cosmides, L. (1990). The past explains the present: Emotional adaptations and the structure of ancestral environments. *Ethology and Sociobiology, 11*(4–5), 375–424.

Tracy, J. L., & Robins, R. W. (2004). Putting the self into self-conscious emotions: A theoretical model. *Psychological Inquiry, 15*(2), 103–125.

Van de Leemput, I. A., Wichers, M., Cramer, A. O., Borsboom, D., Tuerlinckx, F., Kuppens, P., et al. (2014). Critical slowing down as early warning for the onset and termination of depression. *Proceedings of the National Academy of Sciences, 111*(1), 87–92.

Vuilleumier, P., & Huang, Y.-M. (2009). Emotional attention: Uncovering the mechanisms of affective biases in perception. *Current Directions in Psychological Science, 18*(3), 148–152.

Vytal, K., & Hamann, S. (2010). Neuroimaging support for discrete neural correlates of basic emotions: A voxel-based meta-analysis. *Journal of Cognitive Neuroscience, 22*(12), 2864–2885.

Watkins, E. R. (2008). Constructive and unconstructive repetitive thought. *Psychological Bulletin, 134*(2), 163–206.

# CHAPTER 9

# Neuroscience Relevant to Core Processes in Psychotherapy

Greg J. Siegle, PhD

*Western Psychiatric Institute and Clinic,*
*University of Pittsburgh, Pittsburgh*

James Coan, PhD

*University of Virginia*

The goal of this chapter is to provide translational bridges from the common vocabulary of core processes in psychotherapy described throughout this book to neural mechanisms, which are increasingly the lingua franca of the rest of medical science. Success in this endeavor will ideally allow clinicians in the psychological sciences to speak with and make use of insights from the rest of medicine more effectively. In the short term this may also allow clinicians to put neuroscience behind their explanations of mechanisms of change for clients. In the longer term this type of thinking could lead to the adoption of neuroscience methods in predicting response to psychological treatments, and in designing treatments.

In this chapter, we focus specifically on qualitative associations of brain networks with key concepts. We have chosen this granularity as it is likely to have direct clinical applicability given the recent emphasis on brain networks in understanding change processes (Chein & Schneider, 2005; Lane, Ryan, Nadel, & Greenberg, 2014; Tryon, 2014). More quantitative associations, for example, what neural reactivity best predicts response to what treatments (e.g., Hofmann, 2013; Siegle et al., 2012), involve solving technical hurdles of generalizability and societal issues, such as expenses that insurance companies do not currently

Greg Siegle's work on this chapter was supported by the Netherlands Institute for Advanced Study.

reimburse. If clinicians understand basic units and principles of neural change, and the empirical associations of these units with clinical concepts, this knowledge may change how they explain interventions to clients and add to the skills they can capitalize on in current interventions, and eventually it may lead to the adoption of more neurally informed methods (prediction algorithms and treatments) as they become available. Our methodology for identifying clinically relevant networks utilizes whole-brain, meta-analytic (hence, quantitative) procedures so that our described intuitions are at least defensible and externally derivable.

# Brain Networks

Increasingly, the field of cognitive neuroscience is moving away from a focus on specific brain areas putatively associated with specific discrete functions to one of *networks* of linked brain regions that accomplish various behavioral or psychological functions by interacting with each other (Sporns, 2010). For example, neural circuits associated with attention may modulate activity in circuits associated with emotion such that the reactions to attended emotional stimuli are different than those to unattended emotional stimuli. In this way, clinicians and therapists can conceive of a disorder not only as the activity or inactivity of a discrete neural region or circuit, but also in terms of abnormalities of communication between brain neural regions or circuits (Cai, Chen, Szegletes, Supekar, & Menon, 2015).

## *Change in Brain Networks*

In this chapter we adopt the idea that change processes in psychotherapy are associated with neural change, generally described as "plasticity" or "learning" in the neuroscience literature. Neural change processes follow a few principles that are useful to highlight here. *Hebbian learning* (Choe, 2014) is the idea that when multiple brain mechanisms are active at the same time, the connection between them grows stronger. So, for example, the association of an event with an emotional quality could happen when neural representations of the memory for an event are coactive with neural representations of an emotion. Thus activity in brain systems associated with salience and emotion along with memory could be considered catalytic for emotional associative learning. Theoretically, change in psychotherapy could occur by systematically activating the memory without the emotional tone (extinction) when either of these associations is weakened. The idea of *plasticity* can seem redundant with *learning*, but the two terms are not conceptually identical. For example, the traditional belief that memories cannot change has largely been supplanted by the understanding that every time a memory is accessed, the neural representation of the memory itself becomes plastic and can change via reconsolidation (Axmacher & Rasch, 2017). With its emphasis on building new knowledge, lay notions of learning could be an imprecise description of memory reconsolidation. The practical outcome of this new understanding is that neurally informed therapies are increasingly working to intentionally optimize memory reconsolidation processes so as to maximize the potential for psychotherapeutic gains (Treanor, Brown, Rissman, & Craske, 2017), including the potential for integrating pharmacological and therapeutic mechanisms (Lonergan, Brunet, Olivera-Figueroa, & Pitman, 2013). In the remainder of this chapter, we concentrate on the potential effects of psychotherapeutic techniques in a handful of potential networks of interest and, in particular, the potential for change to how networks interact.

## Brain Networks of Particular Interest

In this chapter we concentrate on a few canonical brain networks that have been identified across many studies (e.g., Bressler & Menon, 2010; K. L. Ray et al., 2013; Smith et al., 2009). Though there are many such networks, we will highlight only those that appear repeatedly in analyses of processes associated with therapeutic change, as described in the following sections. Three networks, shown in figure 1, derived using methods described in this section and consistent with those found in more traditional analyses (such as Bressler & Menon, 2010), have been particularly well characterized across multiple imaging modalities. A *salience network* is associated with monitoring the salience of external and internal stimuli. It consists of the insula, which is particularly associated with interoceptive processing (Craig, 2009); the dorsal anterior cingulate cortex, which is associated with the interface of emotional and cognitive information processing (Bush, Luu, & Posner, 2000); and regions traditionally considered to process emotional information, such as the amygdala (Armony, 2013). A *central executive network* is associated with executive control and task planning and execution. It is anchored by the dorsolateral prefrontal cortex and posterior parietal cortices. A *default network* (sometimes *default mode*) is associated with the brain's resting state (Raichle et al., 2001); functional neuroimaging studies suggest that it activates, or becomes better synchronized, when there is no explicit task, and deactivates during explicit tasks. Its components are often detected in association with social information processing (Amodio & Frith, 2006), as well as self-referential processing (Davey, Pujol, & Harrison, 2016; Kim, 2012). It is anchored by the posterior cingulate cortex and the rostral anterior cingulate or more anterior medial structures in the orbitofrontal cortex. It also includes the hippocampus, which appears to be particularly involved in a subnetwork for learning and memory (Kim, 2012; Van Strien, Cappaert, & Witter, 2009).

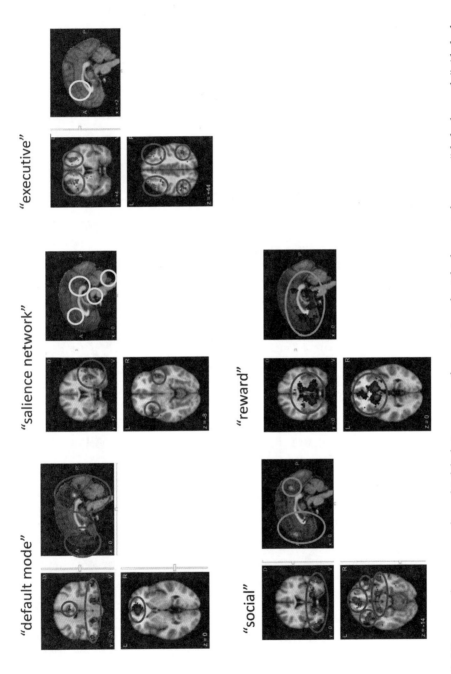

FIGURE 1. Neurosynth meta-analyses highlighting networks associated with the search terms "default mode" (default network; 516 studies), "salience network" (60 studies), and "executive" (executive network; 588 studies), as well as networks using the terms "social" (social information processing network; 1,000 studies) and "reward" (reward network; 671 studies)

Two other networks appear key to change in psychological interventions. Building on structures in the default network, researchers have observed that an expanded *social information processing network* (Burnett, Sebastian, Cohen Kadosh, & Blakemore, 2011) contains not only the rostral cingulate but structures such as the temporoparietal junction and superior temporal sulcus, suggesting they are involved in the perception of others' emotions and theory-of-mind. Often discussed in the literature is the *reward network*, which is really a set of networks that largely reflect the brain's responses to rewarding or positive stimuli. They are centered on the dopamine-producing ventral-tegmental area and reward-monitoring ventral striatum, or nucleus accumbens (Camara, Rodriguez-Fornells, Ye, & Münte, 2009).

By appealing to the putative function of these networks it is easy to speculate on how brain function may relate to specific therapeutic interventions. Interventions devoted to increasing reward responses might be expected to activate the reward network. Interventions devoted to decreasing self-focused processing might decrease activity in the default network. And interventions devoted to increasing social communication might activate the social information processing network. That said, these associations have not been rigorously tested, and brain reactions are often unintuitive. Thus, the forthcoming sections consist of empirical investigations of how these brain networks respond to the types of interventions discussed in this book.

# How Brain Networks Are Involved in Psychotherapeutic Change Processes

**Methods.** To describe brain networks involved in the concepts discussed in this book, we used the Neurosynth engine (http://neurosynth.org; Yarkoni, Poldrack, Nichols, van Essen, & Wager, 2011) to create meta-analytic images of associated concepts. We provide basic interpretations of the derived images with respect to the aforementioned brain networks. When other functional magnetic resonance imaging (fMRI) meta-analyses of similar concepts are available, we cite them as well and discuss similarities. Our searches used terms associated with each chapter in this book. When there were enough studies to create an interpretable map for a particular therapeutic or intervention technique, we included that map. That said, in general, neuroimaging studies of therapeutic techniques are sparse and in their infancy. Thus, we primarily report on studies of associated phenomena. So, for example, rather than reporting on studies of arousal reduction, we include neuroimaging meta-analytic maps for "arousal" and interpret what the associated networks might suggest about reducing arousal.

For the interested methodologist, in all cases maps are shown for reverse inference (chances that the term is used, given the presence of activation in the area), which is more conservative than typical fMRI strategies of forward inference (chances the area is observed, given the term that is used). We chose this strategy as many psychological terms tend to yield similar broad patterns of activation— reverse inference allows more specificity of network activity related to psychological constructs. We used a false discovery rate criterion of 0.01 as a threshold for the images.

The curious reader can directly access the neuroimaging meta-analyses reported in this chapter online. When primary Neurosynth terms were available, we used those. Otherwise, we did "custom" analyses based on Neurosynth's "studies" analyses; these can be accessed via the URLs listed in the appendix. The reader can thus regenerate any maps we describe. We generally show only a single representative axial, coronal, and sagittal image for each analysis; by directly regenerating the analyses, readers can see and interact with full brain maps slice by slice, as well as examine each associated study and its specific contributions to the meta-analysis. References for individual studies in the reported meta-analyses can be accessed by regenerating the associated searches.

**Contingency management and estimation.** *Contingency*, in the neuroimaging literature, has primarily been used to understand action contingencies—that is, what the consequences of some action or behavior will likely be. Neurosynth-nominated studies of "contingency" (figure 2; custom search URL in the appendix) were associated with increased activation in the reward network (throughout the striatum) and default network, including both ventromedial and posterior cingulate aspects. Indeed it has been increasingly understood that individuals with psychopathology estimate reward contingencies differently than healthy individuals (e.g., having decreased reactivity to temporally distant rewards in brain networks associated with reward perception; Vanyukov et al., 2016) or systematically estimate the probability of reward to be low (Olino et al., 2014). We found initial support for the idea that such associations can be exploited to yield psychological change; in the absence of other repetitive training, the ability to estimate high probabilities of reward is associated with not only decreased neural reactivity to negative information but decreased depressive symptomatology (Collier & Siegle, 2015). The described map may suggest the utility of not only explicitly managing reward contingencies but working with clients to associate reward contingencies with the types of calculations thought to be associated with the default network—which is to say, those involving self-related processing and impressions of the self with respect to others (Olino, McMakin, & Forbes, 2016). For example, one might help an individual to understand that a compliment is not just a positive outcome, but also a statement of deeper, ongoing personal (and interpersonal) relevance.

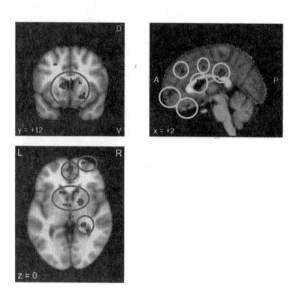

FIGURE 2. Neurosynth meta-analysis of "contingency" (eight studies)

**Stimulus control and shaping.** Generally, stimulus control and shaping techniques in psychotherapeutic processes occur in the context of manipulating associations to promote specific associative learning or to extinguish learned associations. Thus we examined neural features of associative learning, revealed by the term "associative." Neurosynth meta-analyses of both "associative" and "learning" (figure 3) primarily revealed activation of the bilateral hippocampus and parahippocampus, which is consistent with the hippocampus's frequently described role in indexing associative memories. To the extent that stimulus control is associated with manipulating hippocampal processes, we can see stimulus control through the lens of helping individuals to write new associative memories in place of dysfunctional associations, as well as other processes that promote clinically meaningful reconsolidation (Da Silva et al., 2007; Inaba, Kai, & Kida, 2016; Schmidt et al., 2017).

"associative"     "learning"

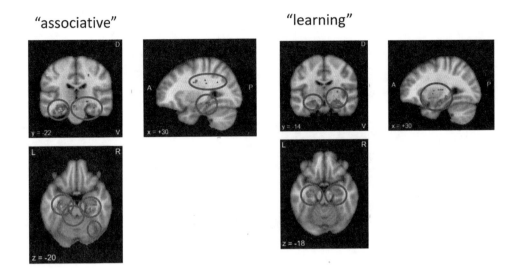

FIGURE 3. Neurosynth meta-analyses of "associative" (220 studies) and "learning" (876 studies)

**Self-management.** Self-management involves a wide collection of techniques unified by the idea of individuals taking responsibility for their behavior and well-being (e.g., by setting goals and managing priorities). In this sense, self-management can be seen as a combination of skills described in other sections of this chapter, such as contingency management, problem solving, and emotion regulation, with the constraint that these strategies are directed toward management of the self. Thus, we considered brain function to be specifically associated with self-processing. A Neurosynth meta-analysis of "self" (figure 4) revealed activity in the default network, which is strongly implicated, along with the superior temporal sulcus region of the social information processing network, in uncontrolled attention being paid to the self and one's self in relation to others. By "uncontrolled," we mean to suggest that default network processing is largely free of executive control, as measured by activity in the executive network. Indeed, default network processing is reliably inversely associated with outwardly directed attention and executive control (Uddin, Kelly, Biswal, Castellanos, & Milham, 2009). Together, these considerations suggest a fundamental tension between self (default network) and management (largely executive network) activities. Thus it may be intuitive why default network–mediated thinking about the self, particularly regarding distressing topics, can be "sticky"—that is, hard to get free of and manage. Increasing evidence suggests that default network processing is particularly competitive with executive network processing in psychopathology (Delaveau et al., 2017; Di & Biswal, 2014; Hamilton et al., 2011; Maresh, Allen, & Coan, 2014).

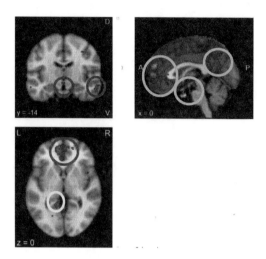

FIGURE 4. Neurosynth meta-analysis of "self" (903 studies)

**Arousal reduction.** A Neurosynth meta-analysis of "arousal" (figure 5) revealed increased activation throughout the salience network (e.g., amygdala, insula, and subgenual cingulate). Indeed, psychological disorders are often characterized by increased and sustained neural reactivity to negative information (Siegle et al., 2015), particularly in these regions. The literature suggests that reducing arousal likely involves decreasing the salience of emotional stimuli, an effect that should be reflected in diminished or inhibited salience network processing. The extensive literature showing mutual inhibition between the executive and salience networks could also speak to the potential for arousal reduction strategies to capitalize on the involvement of executive control (e.g., purposeful redirection of attention, as done in reframing; see "Values Choice and Clarification" below).

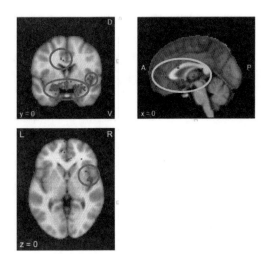

]FIGURE 5. Neurosynth meta-analysis of "arousal" (227 studies)

**Coping and emotion regulation.** A Neurosynth meta-analysis of "emotion regulation" (figure 6) yielded activation in the salience network (particularly the amygdala but also the posterior insula) as well as the executive network, including bilateral dorsolateral prefrontal and parietal regions, but no medial prefrontal regions. Indeed activity in these two networks has been specifically associated with response to emotion regulation therapy (Fresco et al., 2017). Associations with these networks may suggest that emotion regulation involves both effortful control and active emotional processing. This formulation may be more relevant to putatively "voluntary" or effortful forms of cognitive emotion regulation (Gross & Thompson, 2007), as opposed to more "automatic" manifestations (resulting from, for example, interventions such as exposure therapy), which are likely to be mediated through more medial prefrontal activity (R. D. Ray & Zald, 2012). The disruption of salience or threat signals by executive control could help individuals override prepotent responses that would otherwise trigger uncontrolled emotional reactions.

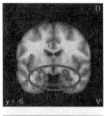
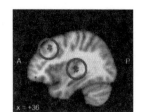
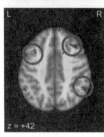

FIGURE 6. Neurosynth meta-analysis of "emotion regulation" (161 studies)

There were four Neurosynth-nominated studies of "coping," but we didn't report on them because they were not strongly related to therapeutic processes (e.g., two were on repressive coping style).

**Problem solving.** A Neurosynth meta-analysis of "problem solving" (figure 7; custom search URL in the appendix) revealed activations throughout aspects of the default network (posterior cingulate) and the rostrolateral prefrontal cortex (superior frontal gyrus)—a region strongly associated with relational integration and reasoning (Christoff et al., 2001; Davis, Goldwater, & Giron, 2017; Wendelken, Nakhabenko, Donohue, Carter, & Bunge, 2008), along with the caudate (part of the salience network), which, in combination with other regions, has also been associated with relational reasoning (Melrose, Poulin, & Stern, 2007). Taken together, these maps suggest that problem solving is likely a widely distributed activity requiring integration throughout multiple brain networks, consistent with the view that problem solving entails diverse cognitive operations, from conceptual encoding to the planning of contingencies and actions (Anderson & Fincham, 2014). Aspects of this wider network have been implicated in problem-solving failures, such as those observed in rumination in depression (Jones, Fournier, & Stone, 2017). Therapeutic interventions emphasizing problem solving may thus require the recruitment of systems associated with relating one domain to another, while preserving motivation for this type of activity.

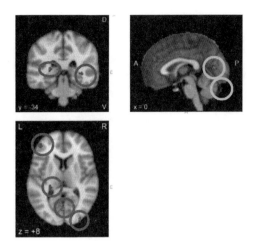

FIGURE 7. Neurosynth meta-analysis of "problem solving" (fifteen studies)

**Exposure strategies.** Exposure therapies generally rely on confronting individuals with situations or stimuli that they fear. While there are few neuroimaging studies of exposure per se (the Neurosynth engine has many references to "exposure" that are not relevant; e.g., drug cue exposure), the salience network was well represented in the Neurosynth meta-analysis of "fear" (figure 8), including the amygdala and dorsal anterior cingulate. It has been hypothesized that the salience network developed to prepare the brain for action in response to potential threat (Seeley et al., 2007); exposure therapies that signal a decreased need for action in response to threat likely reduce activity in this network. Contemporary investigations of pharmacological agents used to enhance exposure therapy, such as d-cycloserine (Hofmann, Mundy, & Curtiss, 2015), have shown that these drugs affect activity in the salience network (Wu et al., 2008), particularly during extinction (Portero-Tresserra, Martí-Nicolovius, Guillazo-Blanch, Boadas-Vaello, & Vale-Martínez, 2013; Wisłowska-Stanek, Lehner, Turzyńska, Sobolewska, & Płaźnik, 2010). A Neurosynth meta-analysis of "extinction" (figure 8) revealed activity in the ventromedial prefrontal cortex (vmPFC). This finding is consistent with work suggesting circuits of the vmPFC that inhibit activity in the salience network mediate the effects of exposure therapy (via extinction learning; Phelps, Delgado, Nearing, & LeDoux, 2004).

"fear"                 "extinction"

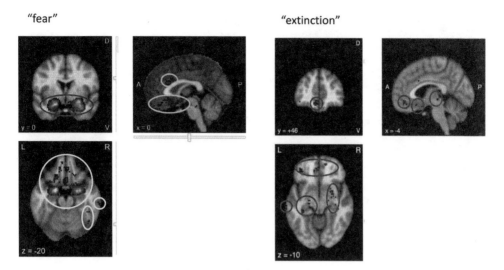

FIGURE 8. Neurosynth meta-analyses of "fear" (298 studies) and "extinction" (59 studies)

**Behavioral activation.** Behavioral activation involves using goal-directed activity and reward to increase appetitive behavior and pleasure responses. Key to the success of these interventions is increasing reward anticipation. A Neurosynth meta-analysis of "reward anticipation" (figure 9) revealed activity throughout the reward network, particularly within the striatum, along with activity in the hippocampus, potentially reflecting reward associations in memory. Indeed psychopathologies such as depression are characterized by disruptions in the reward network (Smoski, Rittenberg, & Dichter, 2011) and its connectivity to other networks (Sharma et al., 2017). The reward network has long been implicated in behavioral activation (Kalivas & Nakamura, 1999). Thus, it is possible that behavioral activation therapies work to restore connections between the reward network and networks more strongly associated with intentional action.

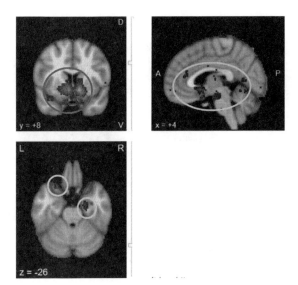

FIGURE 9. Neurosynth meta-analysis of "reward anticipation" (sixty-four studies)

**Interpersonal skills.** Access to quality social relationships is a major challenge in many psychological disorders. Indeed, difficulty reading and interpreting social cues, as well as responding appropriately to those cues, could be considered defining characteristics of many personality disorders. *Social cognition* is a broad term encompassing everything from distinguishing self from others to identifying action intentions to detecting and assigning agency to empathizing. A Neurosynth meta-analysis of "social cognition" (figure 10) revealed activation of the central executive network (dorsolateral and anterior portions of the PFC) and default network (dorsal posterior cingulate) as well the social information processing network (fusiform gyrus and temporoparietal junction), suggesting the potential for using executive processing to modulate otherwise more automatic aspects of social perception and interaction.

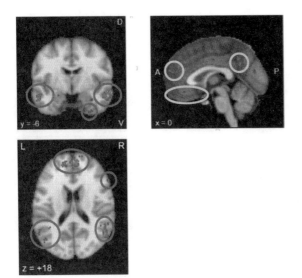

FIGURE 10. Neurosynth meta-analysis of "social cognition" (166 studies)

**Cognitive restructuring, challenging, or reframing.** Neuroimaging research has primarily studied cognitive restructuring and challenging using reappraisal designs in which participants are instructed to think differently about negative beliefs, images, or other stimuli. A Neurosynth meta-analysis of "reappraisal" (figure 11) revealed increased activation in aspects of the executive (e.g., dorsolateral prefrontal) and salience (e.g., amygdala, striatum) networks. These results largely match a recently published meta-analysis (Buhle et al., 2014; coordinates regenerated using Neurosynth), which also found deactivation in the salience network (insula, dorsal cingulate). These analyses could thus suggest that cognitive reframing/reappraisal represents an effortful but also emotional process, which appeals to voluntary cognitive, rather than body-based or more automatic, emotion regulation capabilities.

"reappraisal"                    meta-analysis by Buhle et al. (2014)

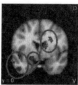
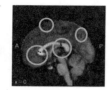
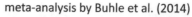
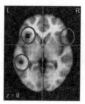
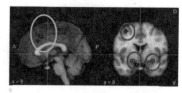
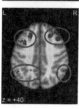

FIGURE 11. Neurosynth meta-analysis of "reappraisal" (sixty-four studies) and meta-analysis by Buhle and colleagues (2014)

**Modifying core beliefs.** From the reappraisal discussion above we can suggest that modifying core beliefs has elements of voluntary thought modification. The additional element of modifying core beliefs may involve other brain mechanisms. A Neurosynth meta-analysis of "belief" (figure 12) revealed activation in aspects of the default network associated with self-referential processing (BA10, posterior cingulate) and parietal aspects of the executive network. Thus, changing beliefs could be said to differ from more general thought challenging, as it involves activations and modifications of neural mechanisms of self-representation.

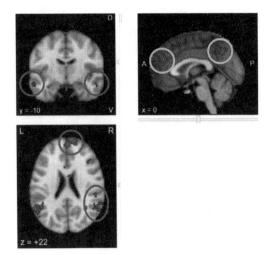

FIGURE 12. Neurosynth meta-analysis of "belief" (sixty-six studies)

**Defusion/distancing.** To date, we are aware of a single study that investigated distancing as an emotion regulation strategy (Koenigsberg et al., 2009, 2010; Neurosynth reconstruction in figure 13); it appears none have been done that nominally reference defusion. The study considered distancing to be a special case of reappraisal, and, indeed, the same networks of the brain were activated for both the distancing and reappraisal studies.

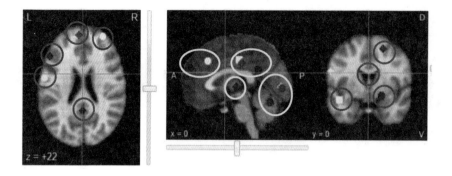

FIGURE 13. Neurosynth reconstruction of the map associated with "distancing" (Koenigsberg et al., 2010)

**Psychological acceptance.** The neuroimaging literature on psychological acceptance is sparse, with only two studies in the Neurosynth database through 2015 (Servaas et al., 2015; Smoski et al., 2015). Their aggregation (figure 14) revealed a variety of activations throughout the executive and salience networks. An additional study published after the Neurosynth database was completed (Ellard, Barlow, Whitfield-Gabrieli, Gabrieli, & Deckersbach, 2017) confirmed activations in the medial and ventrolateral frontal aspects of the executive network. To the extent that these findings are replicable, they may suggest that acceptance is an executive strategy that affects a wide range of cortical and subcortical functions, much like other executive regulatory strategies (e.g., reframing). The study by Ellard and colleagues (2017) specifically contrasted acceptance with other strategies, including suppression and worry, primarily finding that these other strategies required more prefrontal recruitment, possibly suggesting that acceptance can accomplish the same goals as these other regulatory strategies, but with less executive effort.

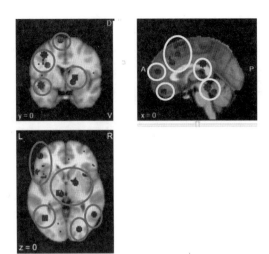

FIGURE 14. Neurosynth meta-analysis of "acceptance" (two studies)

**Values choice and clarification.** We consider values choice and clarification to involve iterative processes associated with specifying one's values and then reevaluating those specifications. There were 284 Neurosynth-nominated studies of "values" that primarily looked at unrelated concepts (e.g., "activation values") or reward valuation, which may or may not be involved in values choice and clarification. Of these studies, a Neurosynth meta-analysis of seventeen of them—which appeared to author Greg Siegle as being more clearly related to "subjective values" (figure 15; custom search URL in the appendix)—revealed activations primarily in default network regions associated with self-referential processing, such as the orbitofrontal cortex, rostral anterior cingulate, and hippocampus. Thus, we conclude that intervening on one's values may help individuals to evaluate self-relevant, if abstract, information.

The clarification of values involves an iterative process of belief refinement, which may be considered to reflect the large neuroscience literature on the adjustments of beliefs in response to errors in prediction (i.e., realizing that something you thought was incorrect and, thus, changing thinking). A Neurosynth meta-analysis of "prediction error" (figure 15) revealed reactivity almost exclusively in the basal ganglia, a key element of the reward network. Thus, we suggest that values clarification may involve the iterative refinement of what one views as rewarding or punishing, and how rewarding or punishing it is, with respect to the self.

"values"                              "prediction error"

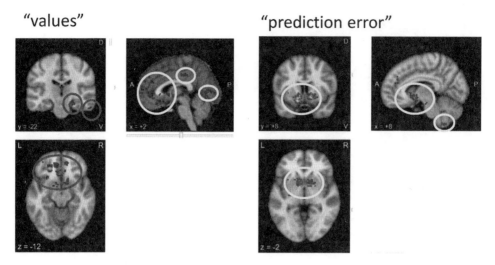

FIGURE 15. Neurosynth meta-analyses of (subjective) "values" (seventeen studies) and "prediction error" (sixty-six studies)

**Mindfulness.** A Neurosynth meta-analysis of "mindfulness" (figure 16; custom search URL in the appendix) revealed activations in the salience network (anterior insula) and frontal structures often implicated in attention (rostral cingulate). These results largely match a recent meta-analysis (Tomasino, Chiesa, & Fabbro, 2014) that also implicated a network of frontal structures associated with attention. Thus, mindfulness interventions appear to recruit brain networks consistent with often-described increases in attentional control and focus on internal body sensations.

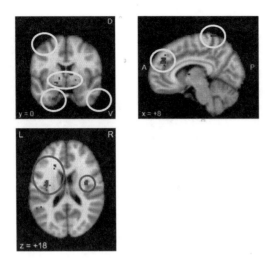

FIGURE 16. Neurosynth meta-analysis of "mindfulness" (fifteen studies)

**Motivational strategies.** Neurosynth meta-analyses of "motivation" and "motivational" (figure 17) revealed nearly identical maps. These data suggest that, much like the behavioral activation strategies discussed earlier, motivational features are associated with the activation of the reward network, particularly the basal ganglia (especially the striatum), subgenual anterior cingulate, and sublenticular extended amygdala, all of which have been associated with emotion/reward-based preparation for action, along with evaluation of the extent to which possible outcomes are estimated to be rewarding. Thus, the neural data could suggest that motivational strategies capitalize on the brain's ability to conceive of otherwise difficult actions as being rewarding.

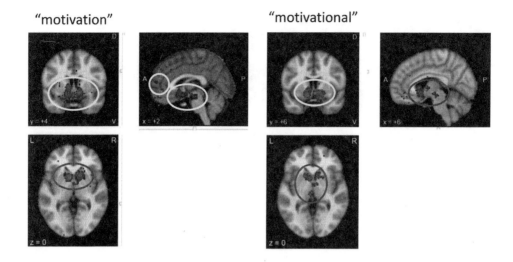

FIGURE 17. Neurosynth meta-analyses of "motivation" (135 studies) and "motivational" (149 studies)

## Conclusion

We highlighted brain networks that are associated with concepts addressed in therapeutic change generally and the contents of this book specifically. The similarities of maps and identified networks across the sections of this chapter suggest that different therapeutic techniques may share key elements and may have critical similarities despite their nominal differences. In particular, the evidence highlights increased executive control, increased reward, and the use of somatic processing as possible routes to emotional change. Taking advantage of inherent tensions between executive control and automatic processing of salient information, as well as the potential use of executive control to increase reward valuation, are common mechanisms across intervention techniques. Keeping such common principles in mind may help clinicians to unify and promote a translational appreciation of what they are doing in the therapy room.

## Appendix: Custom Neurosynth Meta-Analyses

These custom Neurosynth meta-analyses are not among Neurosynth's stored canonical meta-analyses. They represent searches of terms from article texts.

Acceptance: http://neurosynth.org/analyses/custom/69f0107f-ea71–437c

Alexithymia: http://neurosynth.org/analyses/custom/d6d48d7d-00ac-43a6

Contingency: http://neurosynth.org/analyses/custom/e7a9cb5c-e0f3-4fae

Dissociation: http://neurosynth.org/analyses/custom/ffaa34e4-d75e-4355

Mindfulness: http://neurosynth.org/analyses/custom/62bf31de-285b-4239

Problem solving: http://neurosynth.org/analyses/custom/9fbbed1a-9078-45e3

Subjective values: http://neurosynth.org/analyses/custom/ab283af2-32f0-49b6

# References

Amodio, D. M., & Frith, C. D. (2006). Meeting of minds: The medial frontal cortex and social cognition. *Nature Reviews Neuroscience, 7*(4), 268–277.

Anderson, J. R., & Fincham, J. M. (2014). Extending problem-solving procedures through reflection. *Cognitive Psychology, 74*, 1–34.

Armony, J. L. (2013). Current emotion research in behavioral neuroscience: The role(s) of the amygdala. *Emotion Review: Journal of the International Society for Research on Emotion, 5*(1), 104–115.

Axmacher, N., & Rasch, B. (2017). *Cognitive neuroscience of memory consolidation*. Charm, Switzerland: Springer.

Bressler, S. L., & Menon, V. (2010). Large-scale brain networks in cognition: Emerging methods and principles. *Trends in Cognitive Sciences, 14*(6), 277–290.

Buhle, J. T., Silvers, J. A., Wager, T. D., Lopez, R., Onyemekwu, C., Kober, H., et al. (2014). Cognitive reappraisal of emotion: A meta-analysis of human neuroimaging studies. *Cerebral Cortex, 24*(11), 2981–2990.

Burnett, S., Sebastian, C., Cohen Kadosh, K., & Blakemore, S.-J. (2011). The social brain in adolescence: Evidence from functional magnetic resonance imaging and behavioural studies. *Neuroscience and Biobehavioral Reviews, 35*(8), 1654–1664.

Bush, G., Luu, P., & Posner, M. I. (2000). Cognitive and emotional influences in anterior cingulate cortex. *Trends in Cognitive Sciences, 4*(6), 215–222.

Cai, W., Chen, T., Szegletes, L., Supekar, K., & Menon, V. (2015). Aberrant cross-brain network interaction in children with attention-deficit/hyperactivity disorder and its relation to attention deficits: A multisite and cross-site replication study. *Biological Psychiatry*. Retrieved from http://dx.doi.org/10.1016/j.biopsych.2015.10.017.

Camara, E., Rodriguez-Fornells, A., Ye, Z., & Münte, T. F. (2009). Reward networks in the brain as captured by connectivity measures. *Frontiers in Neuroscience, 3*(3), 350–362.

Chein, J. M., & Schneider, W. (2005). Neuroimaging studies of practice-related change: fMRI and meta-analytic evidence of a domain-general control network for learning. *Cognitive Brain Research, 25*(3), 607–623.

Choe, Y. (2014). Hebbian learning. In D. Jaeger & R. Jung (Eds.), *Encyclopedia of computational neuroscience* (pp. 1–5). New York: Springer Verlag.

Christoff, K., Prabhakaran, V., Dorfman, J., Zhao, Z., Kroger, J. K., Holyoak, K. J., et al. (2001). Rostrolateral prefrontal cortex involvement in relational integration during reasoning. *NeuroImage, 14*(5), 1136–1149.

Collier, A., & Siegle, G. J. (2015). Individual differences in response to prediction bias training. *Clinical Psychological Science, 3*(1), 79–90.

Craig, A. D. (2009). How do you feel—now? The anterior insula and human awareness. *Nature Reviews Neuroscience, 10*(1): 59–70.

Da Silva, W. C., Bonini, J. S., Bevilaqua, L. R. M., Medina, J. H., Izquierdo, I., & Cammarota, M. (2007). Inhibition of mRNA synthesis in the hippocampus impairs consolidation and reconsolidation of spatial memory. *Hippocampus, 18*(1), 29–39.

Davey, C. G., Pujol, J., & Harrison, B. J. (2016). Mapping the self in the brain's default mode network. *NeuroImage, 132,* 390–397.

Davis, T., Goldwater, M., & Giron, J. (2017). From concrete examples to abstract relations: The rostrolateral prefrontal cortex integrates novel examples into relational categories. *Cerebral Cortex, 27*(4), 2652–2670.

Delaveau, P., Arruda Sanchez, T., Steffen, R., Deschet, K., Jabourian, M., Perlbarg, V., et al. (2017). Default mode and task-positive networks connectivity during the N-Back task in remitted depressed patients with or without emotional residual symptoms. *Human Brain Mapping, 38*(7), 3491–3501. Retrieved from http://dx.doi.org/10.1002/hbm.23603.

Di, X., & Biswal, B. B. (2014). Modulatory interactions between the default mode network and task positive networks in resting-state. *PeerJ, 2,* e367.

Ellard, K. K., Barlow, D. H., Whitfield-Gabrieli, S., Gabrieli, J. D. E., & Deckersbach, T. (2017). Neural correlates of emotion acceptance versus worry or suppression in generalized anxiety disorder. *Social Cognitive and Affective Neuroscience, 12*(6), 1009–1021. Retrieved from http://dx.doi.org/10.1093/scan/nsx025.

Fresco, D. M., Roy, A. K., Adelsberg, S., Seeley, S., García-Lesy, E., Liston, C., et al. (2017). Distinct functional connectivities predict clinical response with emotion regulation therapy. *Frontiers in Human Neuroscience, 11,* 86.

Gross, J. J., & Thompson, R. A. (2007). Emotion regulation: Conceptual foundations. In J. J. Gross (Ed.), *Handbook of emotion regulation* (pp. 3–24). New York: Guilford Press.

Hamilton, J. P., Furman, D. J., Chang, C., Thomason, M. E., Dennis, E., & Gotlib, I. H. (2011). Default-mode and task-positive network activity in major depressive disorder: Implications for adaptive and maladaptive rumination. *Biological Psychiatry, 70*(4), 327–333.

Hofmann, S. G. (2013). Can fMRI be used to predict the course of treatment for social anxiety disorder? *Expert Review of Neurotherapeutics, 13*(2), 123–125.

Hofmann, S. G., Mundy, E. A., & Curtiss, J. (2015). Neuroenhancement of exposure therapy in anxiety disorders. *AIMS Neuroscience, 2*(3), 123–138.

Inaba, H., Kai, D., & Kida, S. (2016). N-glycosylation in the hippocampus is required for the consolidation and reconsolidation of contextual fear memory. *Neurobiology of Learning and Memory, 135,* 57–65.

Jones, N. P., Fournier, J. C., & Stone, L. B. (2017). Neural correlates of autobiographical problem-solving deficits associated with rumination in depression. *Journal of Affective Disorders, 218,* 210–216.

Kalivas, P. W., & Nakamura, M. (1999). Neural systems for behavioral activation and reward. *Current Opinion in Neurobiology, 9*(2), 223–227.

Kim, H. (2012). A dual-subsystem model of the brain's default network: Self-referential processing, memory retrieval processes, and autobiographical memory retrieval. *NeuroImage, 61*(4), 966–977.

Koenigsberg, H. W., Fan, J., Ochsner, K. N., Liu, X., Guise, K. G., Pizzarello, S., et al. (2009). Neural correlates of the use of psychological distancing to regulate responses to negative social cues: A study of patients with borderline personality disorder. *Biological Psychiatry, 66*(9), 854–863.

Koenigsberg, H. W., Fan, J., Ochsner, K. N., Liu, X., Guise, K., Pizzarello, S., et al. (2010). Neural correlates of using distancing to regulate emotional responses to social situations. *Neuropsychologia, 48*(6), 1813–1822.

Lane, R. D., Ryan, L., Nadel, L., & Greenberg, L. (2014). Memory reconsolidation, emotional arousal, and the process of change in psychotherapy: New insights from brain science. *Behavioral and Brain Sciences, 38*, e1. Retrieved from http://dx.doi.org/10.1017/s0140525x14000041.

Lonergan, M. H., Brunet, A., Olivera-Figueroa, L. A., & Pitman, R. K. (2013). Disrupting consolidation and reconsolidation of human emotional memory with propranolol: A meta-analysis11. In C. M. Alberni (Ed.), *Memory Reconsolidation* (pp. 249–272). Amsterdam: Elsevier.

Maresh, E. L., Allen, J. P., & Coan, J. A. (2014). Increased default mode network activity in socially anxious individuals during reward processing. *Biology of Mood and Anxiety Disorders, 4*, 7.

Melrose, R. J., Poulin, R. M., & Stern, C. E. (2007). An fMRI investigation of the role of the basal ganglia in reasoning. *Brain Research, 1142*, 146–158.

Olino, T. M., McMakin, D. L., & Forbes, E. E. (2016). Toward an empirical multidimensional structure of anhedonia, reward sensitivity, and positive emotionality: An exploratory factor analytic study. *Assessment*. Retrieved from http://dx.doi.org/10.1177/1073191116680291.

Olino, T. M., McMakin, D. L., Morgan, J. K., Silk, J. S., Birmaher, B., Axelson, D. A., et al. (2014). Reduced reward anticipation in youth at high-risk for unipolar depression: A preliminary study. *Developmental Cognitive Neuroscience, 8*, 55–64.

Phelps, E. A., Delgado, M. R., Nearing, K. I., & LeDoux, J. E. (2004). Extinction learning in humans: Role of the amygdala and vmPFC. *Neuron, 43*(6), 897–905.

Portero-Tresserra, M., Martí-Nicolovius, M., Guillazo-Blanch, G., Boadas-Vaello, P., & Vale-Martínez, A. (2013). D-cycloserine in the basolateral amygdala prevents extinction and enhances reconsolidation of odor-reward associative learning in rats. *Neurobiology of Learning and Memory, 100*, 1–11.

Raichle, M. E., MacLeod, A. M., Snyder, A. Z., Powers, W. J., Gusnard, D. A., & Shulman, G. L. (2001). A default mode of brain function. *Proceedings of the National Academy of Sciences of the United States of America, 98*(2), 676–682.

Ray, K. L., McKay, D. R., Fox, P. M., Riedel, M. C., Uecker, A. M., Beckmann, C. F., et al. (2013). ICA model order selection of task co-activation networks. *Frontiers in Neuroscience, 7*, 237.

Ray, R. D., & Zald, D. H. (2012). Anatomical insights into the interaction of emotion and cognition in the prefrontal cortex. *Neuroscience and Biobehavioral Reviews, 36*(1), 479–501.

Schmidt, S. D., Furini, C. R. G., Zinn, C. G., Cavalcante, L. E., Ferreira, F. F., Behling, J. A. K., et al. (2017). Modulation of the consolidation and reconsolidation of fear memory by three different serotonin receptors in hippocampus. *Neurobiology of Learning and Memory, 142*(Part A), 48–54.

Seeley, W. W., Menon, V., Schatzberg, A. F., Keller, J., Glover, G. H., Kenna, H., et al. (2007). Dissociable intrinsic connectivity networks for salience processing and executive control. *Journal of Neuroscience, 27*(9), 2349–2356.

Servaas, M. N., Aleman, A., Marsman, J.-B. C., Renken, R. J., Riese, H., & Ormel, J. (2015). Lower dorsal striatum activation in association with neuroticism during the acceptance of unfair offers. *Cognitive, Affective and Behavioral Neuroscience, 15*(3), 537–552.

Sharma, A., Wolf, D. H., Ciric, R., Kable, J. W., Moore, T. M., Vandekar, S. N., et al. (2017). Common dimensional reward deficits across mood and psychotic disorders: A connectome-wide association study. *American Journal of Psychiatry, 174*(7), 657–666.

Siegle, G. J., D'Andrea, W., Jones, N., Hallquist, M. N., Stepp, S. D., Fortunato, A., et al. (2015). Prolonged physiological reactivity and loss: Association of pupillary reactivity with negative thinking and feelings. *International Journal of Psychophysiology, 98*(2, Part 2), 310–320.

Siegle, G. J., Thompson, W. K., Collier, A., Berman, S. R., Feldmiller, J., Thase, M. E., et al. (2012). Toward clinically useful neuroimaging in depression treatment: Prognostic utility of subgenual cingulate activity for determining depression outcome in cognitive therapy across studies, scanners, and patient characteristics. *Archives of General Psychiatry, 69*(9), 913–924.

Smith, S. M., Laird, A. R., Glahn, D., Fox, P. M., Mackay, C. E., Filippini, N., et al. (2009). FMRI resting state networks match BrainMap activation networks. *NeuroImage, 47*, S147.

Smoski, M. J., Keng, S.-L., Ji, J. L., Moore, T., Minkel, J., & Dichter, G. S. (2015). Neural indicators of emotion regulation via acceptance vs. reappraisal in remitted major depressive disorder. *Social Cognitive and Affective Neuroscience, 10*(9), 1187–1194.

Smoski, M. J., Rittenberg, A., & Dichter, G. S. (2011). Major depressive disorder is characterized by greater reward network activation to monetary than pleasant image rewards. *Psychiatry Research: Neuroimaging, 194*(3), 263–270.

Sporns, O. (2010). *Networks of the brain.* Cambridge, MA: MIT Press.

Tomasino, B., Chiesa, A., & Fabbro, F. (2014). Disentangling the neural mechanisms involved in Hinduism- and Buddhism-related meditations. *Brain and Cognition, 90*, 32–40.

Treanor, M., Brown, L. A., Rissman, J., & Craske, M. G. (2017). Can memories of traumatic experiences or addiction be erased or modified? A critical review of research on the disruption of memory reconsolidation and its applications. *Perspectives on Psychological Science, 12*(2), 290–305.

Tryon, W. (2014). *Cognitive neuroscience and psychotherapy: Network principles for a unified theory.* Amsterdam: Elsevier.

Uddin, L. Q., Kelly, A. M., Biswal, B. B., Castellanos, F. X., & Milham, M. P. (2009). Functional connectivity of default mode network components: Correlation, anticorrelation, and causality. *Human Brain Mapping, 30*(2), 625–637.

Van Strien, N. M., Cappaert, N. L. M., & Witter, M. P. (2009). The anatomy of memory: An interactive overview of the parahippocampal–hippocampal network. *Nature Reviews Neuroscience, 10*(4), 272–282.

Vanyukov, P. M., Szanto, K., Hallquist, M. N., Siegle, G. J., Reynolds, C. F., III, Forman, S. D., et al. (2016). Paralimbic and lateral prefrontal encoding of reward value during intertemporal choice in attempted suicide. *Psychological Medicine, 46*(2), 381–391.

Wendelken, C., Nakhabenko, D., Donohue, S. E., Carter, C. S., & Bunge, S. A. (2008). "Brain is to thought as stomach is to ??": Investigating the role of rostrolateral prefrontal cortex in relational reasoning. *Journal of Cognitive Neuroscience, 20*(4), 682–693.

Wisłowska-Stanek, A., Lehner, M., Turzynska, D., Sobolewska, A., & Płaznik, A. (2010). The influence of D-cycloserine and midazolam on the release of glutamate and GABA in the basolateral amygdala of low and high anxiety rats during extinction of a conditioned fear. *Pharmacological Reports, 62*, 68–69.

Wu, S. L., Hsu, L. S., Tu, W. T., Wang, W. F., Huang, Y. T., Pawlak, C. R., et al. (2008). Effects of d-cycloserine on the behavior and ERK activity in the amygdala: Role of individual anxiety levels. *Behavioural Brain Research, 187*(2), 246–253.

Yarkoni, T., Poldrack, R. A., Nichols, T. E., van Essen, D. C., & Wager, T. D. (2011). Large-scale automated synthesis of human functional neuroimaging data. *Nature Methods, 8*(8), 665–670.

# CHAPTER 10

# Evolutionary Principles for Applied Psychology

Steven C. Hayes, PhD

*Department of Psychology, University of Nevada, Reno*

Jean-Louis Monestès, PhD

*Department of Psychology, LIP/PC2S Lab,*
*University Grenoble Alpes*

David Sloan Wilson, PhD

*Departments of Biology and Anthropology,*
*Binghamton University*

Evidence-based therapy (EBT) is *evidence based* in four distinct ways. First, it draws from and contributes to basic principles of behavior change. Second, it links these principles to applied models and theories. Third, it evaluates the technological extensions and methods in carefully controlled research. And fourth, it examines whether patterns of intervention results can be understood in terms of both basic principles and applied models or theories.

The cognitive and behavioral therapies have been especially clear about these empirical needs, or at least a portion of them. More than forty years ago, conformance to steps one and three above were said to be the defining features of early behavior therapy, in the form of "operationally defined learning theory and conformity to well established experimental paradigms" (Franks & Wilson, 1974, p. 7). The present volume, however, is organized around this full four-step vision. For example, chapters 6 through 9 focus on the basic principles of applied relevance, including those focused on behavior, cognition, emotion and emotional regulation, and neuroscience. All of these topics are perhaps expected in a book of this kind, but we are unaware of other such volumes including a foundational chapter on evolution science.

In some ways this is odd. After all, if neuroscientists are asked, "Why is the brain organized in this way?" they will soon run out of scientifically interesting things to say unless evolutionary explanations begin to appear. The same is true of those in behavioral, cognitive, or emotion science. In the modern era, Dobzhansky's (1973) famous title "Nothing in Biology Makes Sense Except in the Light of Evolution" needs to be extended to all of behavioral science, and with it, to cognitive behavioral therapy (CBT) and EBT.

The current chapter will show that evolution science provides useful guidance to research and practice in evidence-based psychological interventions. It will summarize contemporary evolution science in thumbnail form, focusing on a small set of processes that students of EBT can use to better understand psychopathology, or to develop and implement more efficient and effective therapeutic methods, regardless of the specific therapeutic model.

One reason evolution science is now better prepared to fulfill this role is that it also has changed, and changed rapidly. Evolution science is emerging from a period of isolation from the behavioral sciences. Until quite recently, modern evolution science was clearly gene-centric. Popular evolutionary authors, such as Richard Dawkins (1976), advanced the view that physical life-forms were merely part of the life cycle of genes as replicating units. Evolution was commonly defined straightforwardly as a "change in gene frequencies in a species due to selective survival" (Bridgeman, 2003, p. 325). The main application of this view in applied psychology was the idea that genes can cause behavior. There was the hope that once the human genome was fully mapped we would see that a good deal of psychopathology and human functioning was genetically determined, and that intervention could at least be targeted to high-risk groups, even if genetic causes could not be changed.

This view of the role of genetics in behavior has changed radically, especially as a result of the sequencing of the human genome, which was finally accomplished in 2003. The detailed knowledge from this scientific achievement shows conclusively that genes do not code for specific phenotypic attributes (Jablonka & Lamb, 2014), in psychopathology or anywhere else. Enormous studies have appeared, for example, with full genomic mapping of tens of thousands of participants who were or were not suffering from mental health problems (e.g., Cross-Disorder Group of the Psychiatric Genomics Consortium, 2013). Genetic risk factors were correlated with psychopathology only in broad, systemic, and very complex ways. This same pattern has been seen elsewhere. A recent genomic analysis of 250,000 participants (Wood et al., 2014) was able to explain only one-fifth of the differences in human height, and even that required nearly seven hundred genetic variations in over four hundred sites. The authors concluded that height was likely linked to thousands of genetic sites and variations.

The rise of knowledge about epigenetics has had a similarly profound effect. The term refers broadly to biological processes other than the sequence of DNA nucleotides that regulate gene activity, expression, transcription, and function. The greatest interest is in heritable epigenetic processes. For example, when a methyl group is chemically attached to the nucleotide cytosine, regions of DNA become difficult to transcribe and thus are unlikely to produce protein. Such methylation is heritable to a degree (Jablonka & Lamb, 2014), and along with other epigenetic processes it is itself regulated by environment and behavior. For example, the pups of mice exposed to aversive classical conditioning with olfactory stimuli show a startle response to the smell despite no previous history with it, apparently due to methylation of certain olfactory genes (Dias & Ressler, 2014).

Such effects are known to be relevant to psychological interventions. For example, eight weeks of mindfulness meditation reliably turns on or off about 6 percent of the genes in the human body (Dusek et al., 2008). Epigenetic processes impact the organization of the brain (Mitchell, Jiang, Peter, Goosens, & Akbarian, 2013), and experiences that are protective in mental health areas are known to have epigenetic effects (e.g., Uddin & Sipahi, 2013).

These data fundamentally change how environment and behavior are thought of in evolutionary terms. Evolution does not just mean that genes (or genes and cultural memes) impact behavior. The reverse is also true. It is increasingly plausible to think of physical organisms themselves as systems for turning environment and behavior into biology (Slavich & Cole, 2013). Learning is increasingly understood to be one of the major ladders of evolution (Bateson, 2013), as we will describe below. A more systemic and multidimensional version of evolutionary thinking that views fitness in a more inclusive way and considers genetic and nongenetic factors alike (Danchin et al., 2011) can now be used to organize behavioral interventions themselves (D. S. Wilson, Hayes, Biglan, & Embry, 2014).

# Evolutionary Principles: Six Key Concepts

Evolution science is a vast area of study comprising an equally vast literature, but in application the core of it can be distilled down to six key concepts. We will describe each of these concepts and give an example of its relevance to psychopathology or psychological intervention.

## *Variation*

Comedian Moms Mabley was right: "If you always do what you've always done, you'll always get what you've always got." Variation is the sine qua non of evolution.

Evolution originates in blind variation, and some evolutionary perspectives in the behavioral sciences have continued to emphasize this idea (e.g., Campbell, 1960), but taken on its own it can be a bit misleading, because evolution itself soon leads to targeted variation in response to environmental conditions. It is now known, for example, that when facing stressful environments, organisms from bacteria to human beings have an evolved capacity both to increase the rates of mutation and to decrease the precision of DNA repair (Galhardo, Hastings, & Rosenberg, 2007). Such observations have led some evolutionists to ask "whether the collection of species we have with us today is not only the product of the survival of the fittest, but also that of the survival of the most evolvable?" (Wagner & Draghi, 2010, p. 381). The evolution of evolvability is one of the main arguments in favor of an extended evolutionary synthesis (Pigliucci, 2007; Laland et al., 2015), which seeks to take evolution beyond a gene-centered approach to consider more organism- and ecology-centered approaches, which will be mentioned in this chapter, including multilevel selection, development, and epigenetics.

The evolution of evolvability is seen at the behavioral level as well, for instance, in the increase in response variation during extinction. For human beings, variation perhaps is at its apogee with the transformation of functions via language and higher cognition, a competency that permitted purposeful behaviors to emerge from nonteleological processes (Monestès, 2016; D. S. Wilson, 2016).

In psychopathology and psychological intervention, the evolutionary requirement for variability leads to the investigation of unhealthy cognitive, emotional, or behavioral rigidity on the one hand, and the promotion of healthy variation in these domains on the other. Consider such important transdiagnostic processes as rumination, worry, alexithymia, experiential avoidance, lack of self-control, social anhedonia, or lack of committed relationships: all of these processes can easily be defined as narrow and rigid repertoires in the cognitive, emotional, behavioral, or social domains. The specific forms of psychopathology also tend to include symptoms or features that undermine healthy variation or sensitivity to contextual change. For example, the social withdrawal seen in depression reduces the opportunity to learn new social behaviors; drug and alcohol consumption reduce the motivation to change; and so on. It is worth noting that clients entangled with such processes often describe themselves as "stuck," "in a rut," or "unable to change."

The development of psychopathology over time can be understood in part as having its roots in experiences that produce narrow and rigid forms of adjustment. For example, high and extended periods of unavoidable aversive control can often be found in the history of clients, whether it be in the form of trauma, abuse and neglect, lack of nurturance and social support, or pervasive environmental stressors such as poverty or racism. Aversive control of this kind leads to patterns of avoidance that limit healthy behavioral variation (Biglan, 2015).

Another source of pathological limitation for behavioral variation is the human capacity to respond to stimuli according to what they represent and not "simply" to what they are—that is, the capacity to derive functions between stimuli independently of their physical characteristics and in the absence of direct training (as was covered in chapter 7). Verbal rules based on this ability can dramatically improve behavioral variation (for example, one can use flowers to decorate the house, express love, or honor the dead), but this relational ability can also seriously limit behavioral variation, such as when someone avoids barbecues because meat evokes thoughts of dead animals and thus of the recent loss of her father.

Behavioral variation should not be thought of in merely topographical terms, however. The promotion of disorganized, impulsive, or chaotic behavior is hardly a goal of psychotherapy, and behavioral variability at a superficial level can readily be put into the service of maintaining existing nonadaptive functions, as when a person struggling with substance abuse shifts from one drug to another when supplies of her preferred substances of abuse are strained. Rather, what psychological intervention seeks to do is to target functionally more adaptive forms of living when existing forms are unsuccessful in achieving a healthy lifestyle. In short, for behavioral variation to be adaptive in the case of psychological issues, it has to be functionally different. New behaviors must give rise to different categories of consequences or a different organization of reinforcement. For example, if a person learns to open up to the emotions and sensations involved in stopping substance use so as to do a better job as a father, it is not just the change in drug use that is important. Other positive adaptations might include a shift from negative to positive reinforcement; or from being driven by urges to connecting with "values-based" forms of symbolic reinforcement; or from being directed more by long-term rather than short-term reinforcement. What is truly "new" is also functionally "new."

New and healthy forms of thinking, feeling, and doing also generally require a new and more supportive environment. That is exactly what psychotherapy is designed to create, by undermining repertoire-narrowing psychological processes and promoting psychosocial processes (trust, acceptance, respect, exploration, curiosity, and so on) that lead to successful variation. Clinically, psychotherapy can be thought of in part as the attempt to produce the healthy and functional emotional, cognitive, and behavioral flexibility needed to foster growth when encountering psychological dead ends (Hayes & Sanford, 2015). Psychotherapy constitutes a safe place for clients to experiment in the deployment of functionally different behaviors, and for psychotherapists to evoke behavioral variability by contributing to its selection.

## Selection

The second major evolutionary process is selection. In genetic evolution, *selection* includes anything that results in a difference in lifetime productive success, including survival, access to mates, and competitive ability. In the behavioral domain, within the lifetime of an individual, selection can easily be applied to operant learning: actions are selected by the consequences they produce. Skinner (1981) was especially forceful in noting this parallel.

Operant learning dramatically changes selection pressures by maintaining contact with environmental niches and by constructing these niches through behavior and its side effects. For example, a bird whose digging in river mud is reinforced by the acquisition of edible crustaceans may then be exposed, over generations, to a feeding environment in which adaptations of beak structure can be selected at the genetic level. New phenotypic forms can evolve fairly rapidly as a result. The flamingo's beak is a concrete example of exactly this process. Because eating crustaceans found in rivers was highly reinforcing, flamingoes spent a great deal of time digging through the mud. This led to the evolution of its very odd scoop-shaped beak that filters out food before expelling water as the bird eats with its head upside down—but the beginning of that physical evolutionary process was contingency learning that changed the selection pressure bearing on beak variations (Schneider, 2012). This effect—the rapid evolution of phenotypic forms in response to learning-based niche selection and construction—is one reason some evolutionists believe that the evolution of learning itself may have driven the explosion of life-forms during the so-called Cambrian explosion (Ginsburg & Jablonka, 2010). An analogous situation is the effect that nurturance has on positive social connections and the enjoyment of being with others (Biglan, 2015), which in turn establishes the conditions for the development of greater empathy, and greater social skills, in a self-amplifying developmental loop.

In the applied domain, selection may help us understand psychopathology and its treatment. Many forms of psychopathology can be thought of as evolutionary "adaptive peaks" (Hayes, Sanford, & Feeney, 2015). The metaphor of an adaptive peak refers to a situation in which phenotypic adjustments are made that promote progress "up a hill," but the "hill" runs out and no further progress is possible. For example, a predator may become more and more efficient in targeting certain prey via evolved physical (e.g., digging claws) or behavioral (e.g., hunting in teams) characteristics. This success may lead to an increase in the number of predators, but it may also lead to more dependence on the specific prey and to adaptations that eventually may not be used for anything else. If predation becomes so successful that the prey population collapses, the predator may even become extinct.

In much the same way, certain processes observed in psychopathology consist of patterns of behavior that are initially "adaptive" in the evolutionary sense of the word. The problem is that adaptations can occur to features of the environment (e.g., short-term contingencies, aversive control) that prevent positive development in less restrictive environments. "In other words, psychopathology is an evolutionary process gone awry in a specific way: it prevents further positive development via normal evolutionary processes" (Hayes et al., 2015, p. 224). For example, children raised in a chaotic, nonnurturing environment will tend to show more behavior that is controlled by short-term consequences (Biglan, 2015) because that behavior is adaptive: chaotic, nonnurturing environments are less predictable over longer time frames, and it only makes sense to enhance immediate gains. As an adult, the ability to control the environment may be much greater over longer time frames, but the "impulsive" behavior remains—and that very behavior makes it more difficult to contact the changes in the environment of the adult (who can act to avoid chaos or seek nurturance in healthy ways) as compared with that of the child.

The case of behavioral evolution within the lifetime raises special issues because differential selection is used to select behaviors. Since time and the number of behaviors that can be emitted are limited, each behavior is selected by its consequences in comparison with consequences of other behaviors (Herrnstein, 1961). Moreover, there is no such thing as death for behaviors, since unlearning is impossible. *Extinction* is inhibition, a decrease in the frequency of a behavior occurrence due to a diminution in reinforcement, but not "unlearning" per se. Previously reinforced behaviors may drown in competition with other response forms, but they don't totally disappear. Thus, in the case of behavior selection, criteria always need to be analyzed in competition with other behavioral alternatives. This suggests that therapists need to organize new and powerful sources of reinforcement for healthy behaviors that are competing with previous forms: to select against a given problem behavior, a superior alternative must be available in the repertoire. Thus psychotherapy is always a matter of building, not removing. Metaphorically, if you have too much salt in your soup, you won't be able to take it out. Your only solution is to add more soup. When dealing with unwanted behavior and behavioral excesses, the solution to pollution is dilution.

By examining and choosing values in therapy, the effectiveness of consequences can be altered through symbolic processes—the reinforcing effectiveness of existing behavioral consequences can be augmented, or new consequences for extinguished behaviors can be created. Religious commitments, or cultural practices in general, often appear to work in the same way: by creating new or augmented selection criteria for action. Just as we all have genotypes, once human language evolved we also had *symbotypes*, networks of cognitive relations that themselves evolve and impact other behavioral processes (D. S. Wilson et al., 2014).

## Retention

For selected variations to be useful to organisms or species, they have to be retained one way or another. At the species level, the genes transmitted from parents to offspring; their organization in DNA; and, to a certain degree, their expression through epigenetic processes ensure the retention of a selected trait. These reasons are why reproductive success stands as a central theme in evolutionary studies: the more offspring, the more that genes are transmitted to the next generation, and the better the retention of an advantageous characteristic across generations. Trade-offs between size and number of offspring observed in many species also prove that transmission success matters across generations (Rollinson & Hutchings, 2013). Considering only parental fitness, to maximize the number of copies of advantageous characteristics, the better strategy would be to breed as many offspring as possible. However, if the retention of selected traits across generations also matters, survival of the offspring is important too. Many species give birth to fewer descendants than possible and concentrate effort on their survival.

At the behavioral level, retention includes both a within-individual component, corresponding to the modification of the repertoire of the organism via repetition and contingent consequences, and a between-individual component, corresponding to social learning and cultural transmission. Without retention, learning would be meaningless as a behavioral process, and imitation or culture would be meaningless as a social process. For example, the fact that reinforcement changes the probability of forthcoming behavior is itself a kind of retention. However, we need to be sure not to think of retention and heritability as necessarily matters of "storage." A gene is composed of tangible matter, and it is indeed stored and transmitted from one generation to the next on the chromosomes of gametes, but behavioral retention is more like what happens when one folds a sheet of paper. If you roll a sheet of paper, it will easily take its initial state back when released. When folded several times on the same crease, the sheet will stay in this creased state. The actions of rolling or folding are not "stored" in a literal sense: the paper has simply changed. In the case of behavior within a lifetime, retention is consequently more a matter of practice than transmission.

It is a fascinating challenge for psychotherapists to change behavioral repertoires durably while meeting with clients for a tiny fraction of time. A number of the chapters in section 3 of this volume can be understood as efforts to help clients retain behavior through the provision of portable cues or prompts that set the opportunity for actions outside therapy (see chapter 12 on stimulus control), to develop environments that support and reinforce behavioral patterns (see chapter 14 on self-management), to augment motivation to help clients obtain existing consequences (see chapter 27 on motivational interviewing, or chapter 25 on values selection). In a slightly different vein, evolution favors the retention of overt behaviors associated with emotions (see chapter 8), which may explain why greater emotional openness in session can aid in the retention of clinical material (see chapter 24).

Variation and selective retention are at the core of evolutionary perspectives, but particularly when evolutionary principles are being used intentionally, three more concepts are needed: a focus on context and multilevel and multidimensional approaches.

## Context

Evolution is inherently context sensitive. All organisms experience many different contexts during the course of their lives, each potentially requiring adaptive responses. Context determines which variations are selected. All species capable of contingency learning can select environments by their behavior (we described an instance of such niche selection in the example of the flamingo's beak earlier). Many species are also capable of creating particular physical and social contexts by their actions that alter the selection pressures impacting issues of production and reproduction—what is termed *niche construction*. Learning may help form these larger functional patterns, which can then become more efficient by cultural and genetic adaptations. That is part of why learning can be thought of as a ladder of evolution (Bateson, 2013).

If applied psychologists are in essence engaged in a process of applied evolution, it does little good to foster behavioral changes that will not be supported in the context in which they occur. When evolving on purpose, either a context needs to be selected that will retain desired behavioral innovation, or the current context needs to be modified so that it does so. Understanding the natural place of behavioral innovation requires mindful and open attention to the current environment within and without. The chapters on mindfulness (chapter 26) and acceptance (chapter 24) can be seen in this light.

To some degree, an understanding of the context of psychological actions can itself change the conditions under which such actions are selected. For example, values work (chapter 25) might link seemingly unimportant, everyday behaviors to larger qualities of being and doing. Shaving in the morning may seem boring and trivial, but showing respect for others could be both important and linked to that very act.

## Multilevel Selection

Selection operates simultaneously at different levels of organization: not just genes, but gene systems; not just behaviors, but behavioral classes and repertoires; not just thoughts, but cognitive themes and schemas. Selection at different levels can go in the same or in different directions. There can be interlevel cooperation or conflict (Okasha, 2006).

Consider the body as a multicellular system. The body of a normal human adult is composed of thirty to thirty-seven trillion cells (Bianconi et al., 2013). Millions of them die every second, but what looks like enormous carnage at the level of individual cells is what sustains robust living at the level of that group of cells called "you." The major evolutionary advance of multicellular organisms happened the same way cooperation at any given level happens: when selection occurs based on between-group competition, greater success on average at the group level is augmented by adaptations that restrict selfishness at lower levels of organization. For example, on average cells do better and live longer when they cooperate together to be "you" than they would alone—even if millions die every minute. Competition between multicellular bodies is how that came to be. If some of your cells begin to replicate regardless of their usefulness to you, that is called cancer. If left unchecked it would soon cause your death, and with it, the death of your individual cells. To prevent that, there are evolved systems in your body to repair DNA, to detect anomalous and precancerous cells, or even to kill those cancerous rebels that do appear.

This example contains some of the core ideas in multilevel selection theory (D. S. Wilson, 2015), which has experienced a major resurgence in the last several years (e.g., Nowak, Tarnita, & Wilson, 2010). There is a continuous balancing act between levels of selection. The one-two punch of selection at the higher level of organization—due to small group competition—and the suppression of selfishness at a lower level is what sometimes tilts the balance toward cooperation and becomes an engine of major evolutionary transitions, such as the development of multicellular organisms; eukaryotic cells (which are an ancient cooperative partnership with another life-form, mitochondria); and eusocial species, such as termites, bees, and arguably humans, which have evolved forms of social cooperation that have been extremely successful in evolutionary terms.

Multilevel selection theory suggests that human beings are extremely cooperative as compared with other primates because we evolved in competition between small groups and bands, and various adaptations evolved (likely in part cultural and symbolic) that restricted selfishness (e.g., moral dictates against stealing). However, as the example of cancer shows, in the far more ancient system of multicellular organisms, the selfish interests of the individual never fully disappear.

As an applied matter, the concept of multilevel selection reminds applied psychologists to constantly consider the balance of helpful cooperation at the group level and the restriction of selfishness at lower levels. For example, therapists working on the psychological issues of an individual still need to be concerned with fostering social connection, attachment, and intimacy and not letting these human needs be undermined by psychological selfishness. It is not by accident that social support and nurturance are among the most powerful known contributors to psychological health, while social isolation and disconnection are among the largest known contributors to psychopathology (Biglan, 2015). Humans are social primates. Intergroup competition designed us to function in small groups for the simple reason that cooperative groups function better than groups in conflict.

The balance between the group and the individual applies to every topic in applied psychology because the levels of selection are present no matter how fine grained the focus. We began with an example of a single human body, in part, for that reason: the body is the very definition of the "individual," and yet it is actually an enormous cooperating group of trillions of cells. In the same way, the psychological "individual" contains multiple selves, behaviors, emotions, thoughts, and so on—and a key applied issue is how these can become cooperative.

Consider some of the common topics in psychopathology that appear in this volume. Part of the problem with, say, rumination, worry, unhelpful core beliefs (see chapter 22), or avoidant emotional regulation processes (see chapter 16) is that these specific psychological issues can come to demand more of our client's time and resources than is their fair due. It is not that anxiety or worry has no role in healthy living—rather, its specific role can become out of balance relative to the interest of the psychological (and not just cellular) group called "your client." Psychotherapy attempts to right that balance and to promote personality integration. For example, an emphasis on mindfulness and acceptance in therapy can be thought of, in part, as an attempt to establish peace at the level of the psychological whole by fostering success at that level (e.g., through values work) and by confronting the selfish interests of specific thoughts, feelings, and actions that demand more time and attention than is beneficial.

## Multidimensional Selection

At any level of analysis, researchers and practitioners generally abstract a number of relevant domains to study. The emphasis at the psychological level in EBT, for example, is usually on domains such as behavior, emotion, and cognition. Some will remind evidence-based therapists of the centrality of the social level and its various domains (family, relationships, attachment, social learning, culture, and so on), while others emphasize the biological level and its domains (the brain, the nervous system, genes, the limbic system, and so on).

An evolutionary perspective provides the opportunity for real consilience (E. O. Wilson, 1998) between these many domains by linking them to those that can be thought of as inheritance streams within the lifetime of the individual or the species. These dimensions of evolution are of a more limited set. The genetic level is clearly such a dimension, but so too are epigenetics, behavior, and symbolic communication (Jablonka & Lamb, 2014).

For example, in this chapter we have already mentioned the opportunities and costs in terms of healthy and unhealthy behavioral variation that symbolic processes present. Symbolic processes are clearly a distinct inheritance stream. The writing you are now reading, for example, could easily influence the actions of readers long after the authors are dead and buried.

Symbolic processes seem far removed from the genetics of psychopathology, but empirically that is not the case. Consider the gene that controls the serotonin transporter protein (*SERT* or *5HTT*). An initial and highly influential study found that two short alleles of the *SERT* gene were associated with higher levels of depression when combined with life stress (Caspi et al., 2003). The effect weakened or disappeared in later studies across various cultural groups and individuals (for a meta-analysis, see Risch et al., 2009). Recent evidence, however, suggests that the inconsistent effect may have been, in part, the result of a genetic feature functionally interacting with experiential avoidance (Gloster et al., 2015), a process that in turn is largely driven by symbolic thought (Hayes, Wilson, Gifford, Follette, & Strosahl, 1996), which varies across groups and individuals. In other words, for the system to be understood, the impact of the genetic polymorphism may require knowledge at the psychological level. Multidimensional systems that sustain common problematic functions are often more resistant to change than problems in a single evolutionary dimension.

The reverse is also true. It is clinically helpful to target keystone functions that operate across evolutionary dimensions, such as those that undermine rigidity and promote context-sensitive selective retention. Mindfulness training, which is now known to produce not just increased psychological flexibility but also the epigenetic down-regulation of stress-promoting genes, is a good example (Dusek et al., 2008). As a positive practice of health promotion, psychotherapy is a process of helping people learn to respond adaptively to contextual conditions so as to foster actions linked to chosen selection criteria across dimensions and levels.

# Using Evolutionary Principles in Psychotherapy

We can turn the six dimensions we have covered into a kind of prescription for evidence-based interventions at the metalevel. Therapists foster healthy functional variation and undermine needless rigidity so as to retain variations that meet desired selection criteria (values, goals, needs, and so on) and can be sustained in the current context, across appropriate levels and dimensions. The broad scope and applicability of these evolutionary ideas means that even when EBT systems are not explicitly linked to evolutionary concepts, these systems tend to contain concepts that focus on the detection and change of unhealthy rigidity, or the promotion of greater context sensitivity, which allows deliberate variation to be linked to chosen selection criteria. And these systems all tend to foster retention by practice and the creation of sustaining contextual features.

This description of key features is not meant to minimize any therapeutic tradition but rather to point out that empirically successful methods operate knowingly or unknowingly in broad accord with basic principles of behavior change. We are used to that insight in the area of behavioral principles, but there is every reason to apply it to other sets of principles, including those drawn from emotion science, cognitive science, neuroscience, and, perhaps above all others, evolution science. Indeed, one of the most important implications of evolution science is that it allows principles from different theories and models to be used without incoherence if they are consistent with evolutionary principles.

Process-based therapy is an old idea in CBT and EBT generally. As the chapters in section 2 of this book show, there is a wide variety of principles to guide clinical practice. These principles ultimately all stand together, and the umbrella provided by evolution science is the broadest of all. Behavioral principles evolved— and indeed they are most powerful when they are cast as an example of evolutionary thinking. The same is true of functional-cognitive principles and symbotypes, or of emotional and neurobiological development. Modern multidimensional and multilevel evolution science provides an extended evolutionary synthesis that increasingly allows evidence-based psychopathologists and psychotherapists to view themselves as applied evolution scientists.

# References

Bateson, P. (2013). Evolution, epigenetics and cooperation. *Journal of Biosciences, 38,* 1–10.

Bianconi, E., Piovesan, A., Facchin, F., Beraudi, A., Casadei, R., Frabetti, F., et al. (2013). An estimation of the number of cells in the human body. *Annals of Human Biology, 40*(6), 463–471.

Biglan, A. (2015). *The nurture effect: How the science of human behavior can improve our lives and our world.* Oakland, CA: New Harbinger Publications.

Bridgeman, B. (2003). *Psychology and evolution: The origins of mind.* Thousand Oaks, CA: Sage Publications.

Campbell, D. T. (1960) Blind variation and selective retention in creative thought as in other knowledge processes. *Psychological Review, 67,* 380–400.

Caspi, A., Sugden, K., Moffitt, T. E., Taylor, A., Craig, I. W., Harrington, H., et al. (2003). Influence of life stress on depression: Moderation by a polymorphism in the 5-HTT gene. *Science, 301*(5631), 386–389.

Cross-Disorder Group of the Psychiatric Genomics Consortium. (2013). Identification of risk loci with shared effects on five major psychiatric disorders: A genome-wide analysis. *Lancet, 381*(9875), 1371–1379.

Danchin, E., Charmantier, A., Champagne, F. A., Mesoudi, F., Pujol, B., & Blanchet, S. (2011). Beyond DNA: Integrating inclusive inheritance into an extended theory of evolution. *Nature Reviews: Genetics, 12*(7), 475–486.

Dawkins, R. (1976). *The selfish gene.* Oxford: Oxford University Press.

Dias, B. G., & Ressler, K. J. (2014). Parental olfactory experience influences behavior and neural structure in subsequent generations. *Nature Neuroscience, 17*(1), 89–96.

Dobzhansky, T. (1973). Nothing in biology makes sense except in the light of evolution. *American Biology Teacher, 35*(3), 125–129.

Dusek, J. A., Otu, H. H., Wohlhueter, A. L., Bhasin M., Zerbini L. F., Joseph, M. G., et al. (2008). Genomic counter-stress changes induced by the relaxation response. *PLoS One, 3*(7), e2576.

Franks, C. M., & Wilson, G. T. (1974). *Annual review of behavior therapy: Theory and practice.* New York: Brunner/Mazel.

Galhardo, R. S., Hastings, P. J., & Rosenberg, S. M. (2007). Mutation as a stress response and the regulation of evolvability. *Critical Reviews in Biochemistry and Molecular Biology, 42*(5), 399–435.

Ginsburg, S., and Jablonka, E. (2010). The evolution of associative learning: A factor in the Cambrian explosion. *Journal of Theoretical Biology, 266*(1), 11–20.

Gloster, A. T., Gerlach, A. L., Hamm, A., Höfler, M., Alpers, G. W., Kircher, T., et al. (2015). 5HTT is associated with the phenotype psychological flexibility: Results from a randomized clinical trial. *European Archives of Psychiatry and Clinical Neuroscience, 265*(5), 399–406.

Hayes, S. C., & Sanford, B. T. (2015). Modern psychotherapy as a multidimensional multilevel evolutionary process. *Current Opinion in Psychology, 2,* 16–20.

Hayes, S. C., Sanford, B. T., & Feeney, T. K. (2015). Using the functional and contextual approach of modern evolution science to direct thinking about psychopathology. *Behavior Therapist, 38*(7), 222–227.

Hayes, S. C., Wilson, K. G., Gifford, E. V., Follette, V. M., & Strosahl, K. (1996). Experiential avoidance and behavioral disorders: A functional dimensional approach to diagnosis and treatment. *Journal of Consulting and Clinical Psychology, 64*(6), 1152–1168.

Herrnstein, R. J. (1961). Relative and absolute strength of response as a function of frequency of reinforcement. *Journal of the Experimental Analysis of Behavior, 4*(3), 267–272.

Jablonka, E., & Lamb, M. J. (2014). *Evolution in four dimensions* (2nd rev. ed.). Cambridge, MA: MIT Press.

Laland, K. N., Uller, T., Feldman, M. W., Sterelny, K., Müller G. B., Moczek, A., et al. (2015). The extended evolutionary synthesis: Its structure, assumptions and predictions. *Proceedings of the Royal Society B: Biological Sciences, 282*(1813), 1–14.

Mitchell, A. C., Jiang, Y., Peter, C. J., Goosens, K., & Akbarian, S. (2013). The brain and its epigenome. In D. S. Charney, P. Sklar, J. D. Buxbaum, & E. J. Nestler (Eds.), *Neurobiology of mental illness* (4th ed., pp. 172–182). Oxford: Oxford University Press.

Monestès, J. L. (2016). A functional place for language in evolution: Contextual behavior science contribution to the study of human evolution. In R. D. Zettle, S. C. Hayes, D. Barnes-Holmes, & A. Biglan (Eds.), *The Wiley handbook of contextual behavior science* (pp. 100–114). West Sussex, UK: Wiley-Blackwell.

Nowak, M. A., Tarnita, C. E., & Wilson, E. O. (2010). The evolution of eusociality. *Nature, 466,* 1057–1062

Okasha, S. (2006). The levels of selection debate: Philosophical issues. *Philosophy Compass, 1*(1), 74–85.

Pigliucci, M. (2007). Do we need an extended evolutionary synthesis? *Evolution, 61*(12), 2743–2749.

Risch, N., Herrell, R., Lehner, T., Liang, K. Y., Eaves, L., Hoh, J., et al. (2009). Interaction between the serotonin transporter gene (*5-HTTLPR*), stressful life events, and risk of depression: A meta-analysis. *JAMA, 301*(23), 2462–2471.

Rollinson, N., & Hutchings, J. A. (2013). The relationship between offspring size and fitness: Integrating theory and empiricism. *Ecology, 94*(2), 315–324.

Schneider, S. M. (2012). *The science of consequences: How they affect genes, change the brain, and impact our world.* Amherst, NY: Prometheus Books.

Skinner, B. F. (1981). Selection by consequences. *Science, 213*(4507), 501–504.

Slavich, G. M., & Cole, S. W. (2013). The emerging field of human social genomics. *Clinical Psychological Science, 1*(3), 331–348.

Uddin, M., & Sipahi, L. (2013). Epigenetic influence on mental illnesses over the life course. In K. C. Koenen, S. Rudenstine, E. S. Susser, & S. Galea (Eds.), *A life course approach to mental disorders* (pp. 240–248). Oxford: Oxford University Press.

Wagner, G. P., & Draghi, J. (2010). Evolution of evolvability. In M. Pigliucci & G. B. Müller (Eds.), *Evolution: The extended synthesis* (pp. 379–399). Cambridge, MA: MIT Press.

Wilson, D. S. (2015). *Does altruism exist? Culture, genes, and the welfare of others.* New Haven, CT: Yale University Press.

Wilson, D. S. (2016). Intentional cultural change. *Current Opinion in Psychology, 8,* 190–193.

Wilson, D. S., Hayes, S. C., Biglan, A., & Embry, D. D. (2014). Evolving the future: Toward a science of intentional change. *Behavioral and Brain Sciences, 34*(4), 395–416.

Wilson, E. O. (1998). *Consilience: The unity of knowledge.* New York: Vintage Books.

Wood, A. R., Esko, T., Yang, J., Vedantam, S., Pers, T. H., Gustafsson, S., et al. (2014). Defining the role of common variation in the genomic and biological architecture of adult human height. *Nature Genetics, 46*(11), 1173–1186.

PART 3

# CHAPTER 11

# Contingency Management

Stephen T. Higgins, PhD

*Vermont Center on Behavior and Health; Departments of Psychiatry and Psychological Science, University of Vermont*

Allison N. Kurti, PhD

*Vermont Center on Behavior and Health; Department of Psychiatry, University of Vermont*

Diana R. Keith, PhD

*Vermont Center on Behavior and Health; Department of Psychiatry, University of Vermont*

## Definitions and Background

*Contingency management* (CM) involves the systematic delivery of reinforcement contingent on achieving predetermined clinical targets or goals (e.g., abstinence from drug use) and withholding reinforcement or providing punitive consequences when those goals are unmet. This approach is based on the principles of operant conditioning, an area of psychology that focuses on the effects of environmental consequences on the probability of future behavior. *Reinforcement* refers to the behavioral process whereby an environmental consequence increases the

This research was supported by research grants R01HD075669 and R01HD078332 from the National Institute of Child Health and Human Development and award P20GM103644 of the National Institute of General Medical Sciences, Centers of Biomedical Research Excellence. Other than financial support, the funding sources had no other role in this project.

future probability of a response, and *punishment* refers to the process whereby a consequence decreases the future probability of a response (see chapter 6). CM extends back to the 1960s and the advent of applied behavior analysis, behavior modification, and behavior therapy. More recently, the approach has come to be aligned with behavioral economics, although often under the heading of "financial incentives" rather than CM per se (S. T. Higgins, Silverman, Sigmon, & Naito, 2012). CM is typically used in combination with another psychosocial or pharmacological intervention rather than as a stand-alone intervention.

Beginning in the 1960s, case studies suggested that CM could be used as an applied intervention. Controlled studies in the areas of substance abuse (e.g., Stitzer, Bigelow, & Liebson, 1980), weight loss (Jeffery, Thompson, & Wing, 1978), and other applied areas soon provided proof-of-concept evidence that CM was a powerful therapeutic process. Nevertheless, CM garnered only relatively modest attention in the larger area of applied psychosocial approaches.

The growing use of cocaine fostered a striking rekindling of interest and research on CM (S. T. Higgins, Heil, & Lussier, 2004) for two major reasons. First, while virtually every other type of pharmacological and psychosocial intervention with cocaine-dependent outpatients was failing miserably, controlled clinical trials showed that CM reliably kept cocaine-dependent outpatients in treatment and substantially increased cocaine abstinence levels (S. T. Higgins et al., 1994). Second, researchers developed a monetary-based incentive program (i.e., vouchers exchangeable for retail items) to use with cocaine-dependent outpatients that was readily adaptable to a wide range of other clinical problems, unlike earlier programs that were often specific to a particular population (e.g., medication take-home privileges among methadone-maintained opioid-dependent outpatients).

A programmatic series of literature reviews on the use of vouchers and related financial incentives with substance-use disorders provides a continuous record of efficacy, from the seminal reports on treating cocaine dependence through the present (Lussier, Heil, Mongeon, Badger, & Higgins, 2006; S. T. Higgins, Sigmon, & Heil, 2011; Davis, Kurti, Redner, White, & Higgins, 2015). Between 1991 and 2015, 177 controlled studies reported in peer-reviewed journals examined the efficacy of systematically delivered financial incentives for reducing drug use (the vast majority of studies) or increasing adherence with other treatment regimens, such as clinic attendance or medication adherence. Eighty-eight percent (156/177) of those studies supported the efficacy of the CM intervention.

Researchers are now turning their attention in this area to reach into and dissemination in routine care; for example, studies are looking at interventions that integrate various technologies in order to increase their reach to populations living in remote areas, and interventions that integrate the treatment approach into routine care (Kurti et al., 2016). Two examples of the latter dissemination effort are CM becoming part of routine care in intensive substance-abuse treatment centers in the US Veterans Health Administration hospital system (Petry, DePhilippis, Rash, Drapkin, & McKay, 2014) and the use of CM to promote smoking cessation among pregnant women in economically disadvantaged communities in the United Kingdom (Ballard & Radley, 2009).

The use of CM has grown, reaching well beyond substance-use disorders to include exercise (e.g., Finkelstein, Brown, Brown, & Buchner, 2008), medication adherence (e.g., Henderson et al., 2015), and the use of shared physician and patient financial incentives to reduce biomarkers for cardiovascular disease (Asch et al., 2015). Because incentives are highly effective at promoting initial behavior change, researchers are now shifting attention to strategies to sustain treatment effects after the incentive programs have been discontinued (John, Loewenstein, & Volpp, 2012; Leahey et al., 2015).

The largest-scale interventions involving CM are in the area of global health (Ranganathan & Legarde, 2012). Conditional cash-transfer programs involve many millions of families throughout Latin America, Africa, and Asia. In Latin America impoverished mothers of young children can earn additional public assistance contingent on having their children immunized, participating in routine medical preventive care, and enrolling their children in school. In Africa, similar large-scale CM interventions have curtailed the AIDS epidemic by reducing sexually transmitted diseases, increasing rates of HIV testing, and promoting adult male circumcision, among other outcomes. These are complex efforts for which thorough and complete evaluations are not yet available, but reviews of this emerging literature offer many reasons for optimism regarding the effectiveness of large-scale incentive programs to promote health-related behavior change (Ranganathan & Legarde, 2012).

The institutional and cultural support for CM appears to be increasing. In the United States, financial incentives were thoroughly integrated into the landmark 2009 Patient Protection and Affordable Care Act (ACA). The ACA established the groundwork for US employers to use incentives as part of employee wellness programs, and the majority of major US employers are now doing so (Mattke et al., 2013). The ACA also requires the US Center for Medicare and Medicaid Services to allocate funds (roughly $85 million annually) to examine the use of financial incentives to promote health-related behavior change in such areas as smoking cessation, weight loss, medication adherence, and the like to prevent chronic disease among economically disadvantaged individuals (Centers for Medicare and Medicaid Services, 2017).

# Basic Components

Simply offering financial incentives for behavior change does not qualify as CM. CM is dependent on basic design features that have been developed from CM research, and the principle of reinforcement, which is the core process of this treatment approach (S. T. Higgins, Silverman, & Washio, 2011). Below we outline ten features of CM interventions that are important to their efficacy:

1. Explain the details of the intervention carefully prior to treatment and provide a written description when possible.

2. Define objectively the response (e.g., drug-negative urine toxicology results) being targeted by the CM intervention (e.g., drug abstinence).

3. Identify in advance the methods to be used for verifying that the target response has occurred (e.g., urine toxicology testing).

4. Outline clearly the schedule for monitoring progress.

5. Monitor progress frequently to provide opportunities for patients to experience the programmed consequences.

6. Stipulate clearly in advance the duration of the intervention.

7. Pinpoint a single rather than multiple behavioral targets when possible.

8. Make clear the consequences of success and failure in meeting targeted goals.

9. Keep delays as short as practical when delivering earned incentives since treatment effect size varies inversely with delay.

10. Be mindful that treatment effect size varies inversely with the monetary value of the incentive provided.

# Case Study

To outline the CM treatment approach in greater detail, we will use an example of smoking cessation among pregnant women. Cigarette smoking during pregnancy continues to represent a serious public health problem that increases risk for catastrophic pregnancy complications, adverse effects on fetal development, and disease throughout the life span. While the prevalence of smoking during pregnancy has decreased over time, economically disadvantaged pregnant women continue to smoke at much higher rates than more-affluent women. Meta-analyses of more than seventy-seven controlled trials and twenty-nine thousand women show that CM produces the largest effect sizes by several orders of magnitude as compared with pharmacological or other psychosocial interventions (Lumley et al., 2009; Chamberlain et al., 2013). Across eight controlled trials of CM (see figure 1), the odds of late-pregnancy abstinence were 3.79 (95% confidence intervals, or CIs: 2.74–5.25) times greater than with control interventions (Cahill, Hartmann-Boyce, & Perera, 2015).

**University of Vermont model.** The CM model developed at the University of Vermont is the most thoroughly researched for this population (S. T. Higgins, Washio et al., 2012). In this body of work, women who enter prenatal care and report that they continue to smoke are recruited from community ob-gyn providers. After entering the study, they are encouraged to begin their cessation effort on either of the following two Mondays. For the initial five consecutive days (Monday through Friday) of the quit attempt, they report to the clinic daily to have their smoking status monitored. During those initial visits, "abstinence" is defined as having a breath carbon monoxide (CO) level of less than or equal to six parts per million. Because of the relatively long half-life of cotinine (the principal metabolite of nicotine), it cannot be used to verify abstinence in the initial days of the quit attempt. Starting on Monday of the second week of the quit attempt, biochemical verification transitions from breath CO to urine cotinine testing ($\leq$ 80 ng/ml). At that point, the frequency of clinic contact to monitor smoking status decreases to twice weekly, where it remains for the next seven weeks, at which point it decreases to once weekly for four weeks, and then to every other week until delivery. During the postpartum period, abstinence monitoring increases again to once weekly for four weeks, and then decreases to every other week through twelve weeks postpartum. Follow-up assessments are conducted at twenty-four weeks and, more recently, fifty weeks postpartum.

The voucher-based incentive program is in place from the start of the quit attempt through twelve weeks postpartum. Voucher value begins at $6.25 and escalates by $1.25 for each consecutive negative specimen, reaching a maximum of $45.00, where it remains through the remainder of the intervention. However, a positive test result, failure to provide a scheduled specimen, or a missed visit resets the value of vouchers back to their initial low value, and two consecutive negative tests restore voucher value to the pre-reset level. A woman who is continuously abstinent throughout the duration of treatment typically can earn around $1,180, depending on how many weeks pregnant she is when she starts treatment. In a clinical trial to improve treatment response that is currently under way, women who smoke ten or more cigarettes per day at study intake are eligible

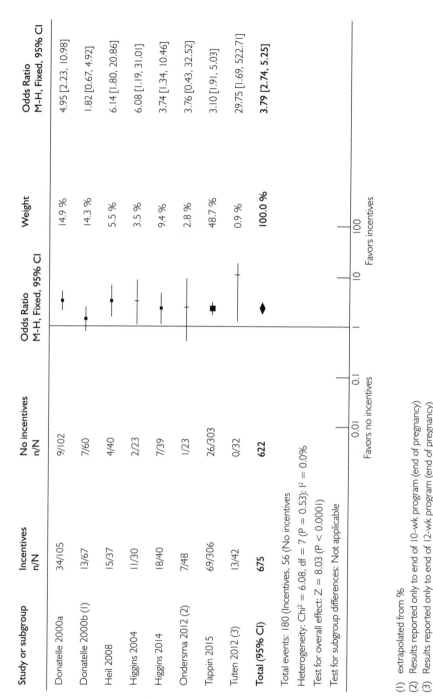

FIGURE 1. Odds ratios and 95 percent CIs for late-pregnancy point-prevalence abstinence among women treated with financial incentives versus control treatments. Results are shown separately for individual randomized controlled trials and with total results collapsed across trials. Reprinted with permission from Cahill et al. (2015).

202

to receive vouchers according to the same schedule described above, but at double the incentive value.

Figure 2 compares the combined results from the initial three trials conducted with the intervention using the $1,180 maximal-earnings model to a control condition wherein vouchers of the same values were delivered independent of smoking status. Late-pregnancy abstinence levels were almost fivefold greater among women treated with abstinence-contingent versus noncontingent vouchers (34% versus 7%). Abstinence rates in both treatment conditions decreased during the postpartum period, but abstinence-contingent incentives continued to show an advantage even twelve weeks after the discontinuation of the incentives.

Table 1 shows birth outcomes among women from those trials. Mean birth weight was significantly greater, and the percentage of infants born with especially low birth weight (< 2,500 g) was significantly lower, among infants born to mothers treated with abstinence-contingent vouchers compared to noncontingent vouchers.

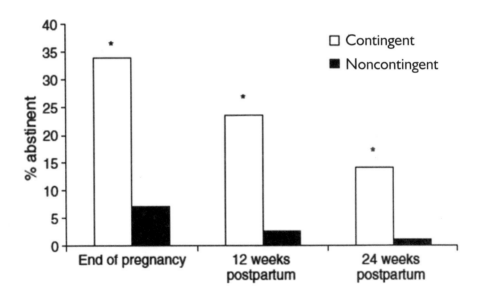

FIGURE 2. Assessments of seven-day point-prevalence abstinence at the end of pregnancy and at twelve and twenty-four weeks postpartum in contingent (n = 85) and noncontingent (n = 81) voucher-treatment conditions. The asterisk (*) indicates a significant difference between conditions ($p \leq .003$ across the three assessments).

203

# Table 1. Infant outcomes at delivery

| Measure | Contingent (n = 85) | Noncontingent (n = 81) | p values |
|---|---|---|---|
| Birth weight (grams) | 3,295.6 ± 63.8 | 3,093.6 ± 67.0 | .03 |
| % Low birth weight | 5.9 | 18.5 | .02 |
| Gestational age (weeks) | 39.1 ± 0.2 | 38.5 ± 0.3 | .06 |
| % Preterm births | 5.9 | 13.6 | .09 |
| % NICU admissions | 4.7 | 13.8 | .06 |

Values represent mean ± standard error, unless specified otherwire. NICU: neonatal intensive care unit.

Although the incentives of these programs may sound expensive, a recent formal analysis of the largest trial yet reported of this treatment approach for pregnant smokers (Tappin et al., 2015) demonstrates that it is highly cost-effective (Boyd, Briggs, Bauld, Sinclair, & Tappin, 2016). Furthermore, research shows that CM can be moved into a community setting without losing efficacy. A recent study implemented CM using regular obstetrical staff and community smoking-cessation personnel in a large urban hospital (Ierfino et al., 2015) and found that 20 percent of women achieved abstinence as compared with 0 percent among historical controls.

To convey a sense of the use of this incentives intervention at the level of an individual participant, we share the experience of Jamie, an unemployed twenty-one-year-old who was living in low-income housing when she learned that she was pregnant with her second child. She had smoked throughout her first pregnancy, and although her daughter from that pregnancy had been born within the normal range of birth weight, Jamie did not want to risk smoking through a second pregnancy.

Age when initiating smoking and the number of prior quit attempts are important predictors of success, and both indicated that quitting was going to be difficult for Jamie: she had started smoking at age fourteen and had made only two quit attempts in the preceding seven years, with her longest attempt lasting a mere two days. Even after learning of her second pregnancy, when entering pre-natal care Jamie was still smoking ten cigarettes per day, and she smoked her first cigarette of the day within thirty minutes of waking (an empirically based indica-tor of nicotine dependence). Ten cigarettes per day is considered relatively heavy smoking in the pregnant population, as most women reduce the daily number of cigarettes they smoke by approximately half before entering prenatal care (Heil et al., 2014). Despite having numerous characteristics associated with a poor progno-sis for successful cessation, Jamie expressed strong determination to quit.

Jamie was enrolled in the CM intervention when she was approximately seven weeks pregnant. Her cotinine level on the day of enrollment was 729 ng/ml, quite a bit higher than the 80 ng/ml cut point needed to earn vouchers during the intervention. However, in her eagerness to quit, Jamie selected the earliest possi-ble Monday as her quit date—a mere six days away.

Other than the two puffs that Jamie took on her first day of treatment, she reported abstaining from smoking entirely during her first week, earning a total $87.50, which she opted to redeem in the form of a gift card to the nearest grocery store. After a successful first week, Jamie recognized the importance of remaining abstinent over the weekend. The following Monday was her "transition day," when urine cotinine replaced breath CO levels for bioverification of abstinence. Breath CO has a much shorter half-life than cotinine and thus is less sensitive to low-level or intermittent smoking (S. T. Higgins et al., 2006). Even one puff could have shown up in her urine cotinine test, thereby resetting her voucher earnings to the initial value of $12.50.

Despite living with a smoker and having a substantial number of friends who smoked, Jamie managed to avoid smoking over the weekend, and her urine coti-nine levels were well below the cut point for abstinence. This transition day is a robust predictor of late-pregnancy abstinence (S. T. Higgins et al., 2007), and consistent with this pattern Jamie remained abstinent throughout the remainder of her pregnancy and through 1 year postpartum—9 months after the discontinu-ation of the incentive program. Jamie used her voucher earnings to pay for practi-cal economic demands (e.g., groceries, gas, phone bills) and items for her soon-to-arrive second daughter.

Importantly, Jamie gave birth to a healthy baby girl and had a normal vaginal delivery without complications. Emily was born at a gestational age of 39.1 weeks and a birth weight of 3,221 grams. These outcomes align well with those achieved by women who received this intervention in our prior trials, in which mean gesta-tional age was 39.1 weeks and birth weight was 3,295 grams (see table 1; also see S. T. Higgins et al., 2010). Mean gestational age and birth weight among women in the control conditions in those prior trials were 38.5 weeks and 3,093 grams, respectively. Moreover, had Jamie not been successful in quitting smoking, her baby may have been among the 14 percent of infants of the control condition who were born preterm (< 37 weeks), or the 18.5 percent who met the medical cut point for low birth weight (< 2,500 g), or the 14 percent who were admitted to the NICU. Instead, Emily was admitted to the newborn nursery on December 23 and discharged the following day. Jamie's abstinence through the postpartum period leading to the one-year follow-up was a strong indication that Jamie was well on her way to life as a nonsmoker. It also suggested that Emily will be protected from the serious adverse health effects of secondhand smoke exposure from Mom's smoking. Jamie breast-fed exclusively for approximately one month and then breast-fed and formula-fed for 10.75 months, which far exceeds the pattern of early weaning typical of maternal smokers. This pattern is associated with important short- and longer-term maternal and child health benefits (T. M. Higgins et al., 2010).

## Future Directions

Although practitioners are using CM treatments to treat substance abuse and other problem areas, CM is potentially relevant to a much wider range of clinical problems. As just one example, cardiac rehabilitation is an efficacious and cost-effective program for improving the health outcomes and reducing the rehospitalization rates of individuals with cardiovascular disease. Unfortunately, economically disadvantaged patients use this service far less frequently than more affluent patients, despite their medical insurance covering the costs and, on average, having greater medical need for the care (Ades & Gaalema, 2012). Initial research is showing that CM is effective at increasing participation in cardiac rehabilitation and improving health outcomes among economically disadvantaged patients (Gaalema et al., 2016).

CM interventions do not represent a silver bullet. For example, even in studies in which CM is efficacious, half or more of the treated individuals fail to benefit. Nonresponders typically are individuals who have more severe problems and may need a more intensive intervention. Significantly increasing incentives has been shown to reach many nonresponders (Silverman, Chutuape, Bigelow, & Stitzer, 1999), and other treatment combinations may be possible. For example, at least one study has associated CM nonresponse among cocaine users with avoidance and behavioral inflexibility in the presence of cocaine-related thoughts (Stotts et al., 2015). Perhaps combining CM with treatments that have efficacy in that domain, or emotion regulation skills more generally, could be helpful (Bickel, Moody, & Higgins, 2016; Hayes, Luoma, Bond, Masuda, & Lillis, 2006).

It is also important for CM developers to attend to how behavior change can be sustained once incentives are discontinued. For example, developers could pay more attention to how more-natural incentives already available in the physical and electronic community could be leveraged to support treatment gains once formal treatment is discontinued (people treated with incentives to increase physical activity or weight loss could join community walking or running groups following treatment, or CM could be integrated with online support groups that continue beyond the incentive period).

It's also going to be important to examine the cost-effectiveness of long-term CM interventions. CM is being used to assist in the management of chronic conditions. Just as chronic medications are often necessary to effectively manage these chronic conditions, chronic behavior-change interventions may be necessary as well. It is relatively easy to think through the logistics of providing long-term incentives for healthy behavior change with employee wellness programs. While the logistics may be less straightforward in the public sector, the efficacy and cost-effectiveness of longer-term CM interventions should be carefully examined. Cost-effectiveness will be an important guidepost in all such efforts.

We used the long-standing problem of smoking cessation among pregnant women to illustrate the potential power of this treatment approach. The growing body of evidence on the efficacy of CM, and its close alignment to fundamental principles of behavioral science, should give psychology and psychotherapy practitioners confidence that this approach has the potential to substantially help reduce the adverse individual and societal impacts of behavior and health problems. The tremendous growth in the use of CM in the public and private sectors in the past two decades suggests that CM has a home in mental and behavioral health care across the board.

# References

Ades, P. A., & Gaalema, D. E. (2012). Coronary heart disease as a case study in prevention: Potential role of incentives. *Preventive Medicine, 55*(Supplement 1), S75–S79.

Asch, D. A., Troxel, A. B., Stewart, W. F., Sequist, T. D., Jones, J. B., Hirsch, A. G., et al. (2015). Effect of financial incentives to physicians, patients, or both on lipid levels: A randomized clinical trial. *JAMA, 314*(18), 1926–1935.

Ballard, P., & Radley, A. (2009). Give it up for baby: A smoking cessation intervention for pregnant women in Scotland. *Cases in Public Health Communication and Marketing, 3*, 147–160.

Bickel, W. K., Moody, L., & Higgins, S. T. (2016). Some current dimensions of the behavioral economics of health-related behavior change. *Preventive Medicine, 92*, 16–23.

Boyd, K. A., Briggs, A. H., Bauld, L., Sinclair, L., & Tappin, D. (2016). Are financial incentives cost-effective to support smoking cessation during pregnancy? *Addiction, 111*(2), 360–370.

Cahill, K., Hartmann-Boyce, J., & Perera, R. (2015). Incentives for smoking cessation. *Cochrane Database of Systematic Reviews, 5*(CD004307).

Centers for Medicare and Medicaid Services. (Updated Feb. 13, 2017). Medicaid incentives for the prevention of chronic diseases model. https://innovation.cms.gov/initiatives/MIPCD/index.html.

Chamberlain, C., O'Mara-Eves, A., Oliver S., Caird, J. R., Perlen, S. M., Eades, S. J., et al. (2013). Psychosocial interventions for supporting women to stop smoking in pregnancy. *Cochrane Database of Systematic Reviews, 10*(CD001055).

Davis, D. R., Kurti, A. N., Redner, R., White, T. J., & Higgins, S. T. (2015, June). *Contingency management in the treatment of substances use disorders: Trends in the literature*. Poster presented at the meeting of the College on Problems of Drug Dependence, Phoenix, AZ.

Finkelstein, E. A., Brown, D. S., Brown, D. R., & Buchner, D. M. (2008). A randomized study of financial incentives to increase physical activity among sedentary older adults. *Preventive Medicine, 47*(2), 182–187.

Gaalema, D. E., Savage, P. D., Rengo, J. L., Cutler, A. Y., Higgins, S. T., & Ades, P. A., (2016). Financial incentives to promote cardiac rehabilitation participation and adherence among Medicaid patients. *Preventive Medicine, 92*, 47–50.

Hayes, S. C., Luoma, J. B., Bond, F. W., Masuda, A., & Lillis, J. (2006). Acceptance and commitment therapy: Model, processes, and outcomes. *Behaviour Research and Therapy, 44*(1), 1–25.

Heil, S. H., Herrmann, E. S., Badger, G. J., Solomon, L. J., Bernstein, I. M., & Higgins, S. T. (2014). Examining the timing of changes in cigarette smoking upon learning of pregnancy. *Preventive Medicine, 68*, 58–61.

Henderson, C., Knapp, M., Yeeles, K., Bremner, S., Eldridge, S., David, A. S., et al. (2015). Cost-effectiveness of financial incentives to promote adherence to depot antipsychotic medication: Economic evaluation of a cluster-randomised controlled trial. *PLoS One, 10*(10), e0138816.

Higgins, S. T., Bernstein, I. M., Washio, Y., Heil, S. H., Badger, G. J., Skelly, J. M., et al. (2010). Effects of smoking cessation with voucher-based contingency management on birth outcomes. *Addiction, 105*(11), 2023–2030.

Higgins, S. T., Budney, A. J., Bickel, W. K., Foerg, F. E., Donham, R., & Badger, G. J. (1994). Incentives improve outcome in outpatient behavioral treatment of cocaine dependence. *Archives of General Psychiatry, 51*(7), 568–576.

Higgins, S. T., Heil, S. H., Badger, G. J., Mongeon, J. A., Solomon, L. J., McHale, L., et al. (2007). Biochemical verification of smoking status in pregnant and recently postpartum women. *Experimental and Clinical Psychopharmacology, 15*(1), 58–66.

Higgins, S. T., Heil, S. H., Dumeer, A. M., Thomas, C. S., Solomon, L. J., & Bernstein, I. M. (2006). Smoking status in the initial weeks of quitting as a predictor of smoking-cessation outcomes in pregnant women. *Drug and Alcohol Dependence, 85*(2), 138–141.

Higgins, S. T., Heil, S. H., & Lussier, J. P. (2004). Clinical implications of reinforcement as a determinant of substance use disorders. *Annual Review of Psychology, 55*, 431–461.

Higgins, S. T., Sigmon, S. C., & Heil, S. H. (2011). Contingency management in the treatment of substance use disorders: Trends in the literature. In P. Ruiz & E. C. Strain (Eds.), *Lowinson and Ruiz's substance abuse: A comprehensive textbook* (5th ed., 603–621). Philadelphia: Lippincott, Williams & Wilkins.

Higgins, S. T., Silverman, K., Sigmon, S. C., Naito, N. A. (2012). Incentives and health: An introduction. *Preventive Medicine, 55*, S2–S6.

Higgins, S. T., Silverman, K., & Washio, Y. (2011). Contingency management. In M. Galanter & H. D. Kleber (Eds.), *Psychotherapy for the treatment of substance abuse* (pp. 193–218). Washington, DC: American Psychiatric Publishing.

Higgins, S. T., Washio, Y., Heil, S. H., Solomon, L. J., Gaalema, D. E., Higgins, T. M., et al. (2012). Financial incentives for smoking cessation among pregnant and newly postpartum women. *Preventive Medicine, 55*(Supplement 1), S33–S40.

Higgins, T. M., Higgins, S. T., Heil, S. H., Badger, G. J., Skelly, J. M., Bernstein, I. M., et al. (2010). Effects of cigarette smoking cessation on breastfeeding duration. *Nicotine and Tobacco Research, 12*(5), 483–488.

Ierfino, D., Mantzari, E., Hirst, J., Jones, T., Aveyard, P., & Marteau, T. M. (2015). Financial incentives for smoking cessation in pregnancy: A single-arm intervention study assessing cessation and gaming. *Addiction, 110*(4), 680–688.

Jeffery, R. W., Thompson, P. D., & Wing, R. R. (1978). Effects on weight reduction of strong monetary contracts for calorie restriction or weight loss. *Behaviour Research and Therapy, 16*(5), 363–369.

John, L. K., Loewenstein, G., & Volpp, K. G. (2012). Empirical observations on longer-term use of incentives for weight loss. *Preventive Medicine, 55*(Supplement 1), S68–S74.

Kurti, A. N., Davis, D. R., Redner, R., Jarvis, B. P., Zvorsky, I., Keith, D. R., et al. (2016). A review of the literature on remote monitoring technology in incentive-based interventions for health-related behavior change. *Translational Issues in Psychological Science, 2*(2), 128–152.

Leahey, T. M., Subak, L. L., Fava, J., Schembri, M., Thomas, G., Xu, X., et al. (2015). Benefits of adding small financial incentives or optional group meetings to a web-based statewide obesity initiative. *Obesity (Silver Spring), 23*(1), 70–76.

Lumley, J., Chamberlain, C., Dowswell, T., Oliver, S., Oakley, L., & Watson, L. (2009). Interventions for promoting smoking cessation during pregnancy. *Cochrane Database of Systematic Reviews, 3*(CD001055).

Lussier, J. P., Heil, S. H., Mongeon, J. A., Badger, G. J., & Higgins, S. T. (2006). A meta-analysis of voucher-based reinforcement therapy for substance use disorders. *Addiction, 101*(2), 192–203.

Mattke, S., Hangsheng, L., Caloyeras, J. P., Huang, C. Y., van Busum, K. R., Khodyakov, D., et al. (2013). *Workplace wellness programs study.* Santa Monica, CA: RAND Corporation. Retrieved from http://aspe.hhs.gov/hsp/13/WorkplaceWellness/rpt_wellness.pdf.

Patient Protection and Affordable Care Act of 2009, H.R. 3590, 111th Cong. (2009–2010). Retrieved from https://www.congress.gov/bill/111th-congress/house-bill/3590/.

Petry, N. M., DePhilippis, D., Rash, C. J., Drapkin, M., & McKay, J. R. (2014). Nationwide dissemination of contingency management: The Veterans Administration initiative. *American Journal of Addictions, 23*(3), 205–210.

Ranganathan, M., & Lagarde, M. (2012). Promoting healthy behaviours and improving health outcomes in low and middle income countries: A review of the impact of conditional cash transfer programmes. *Preventive Medicine, 55*(Supplement 1), S95–S105.

Silverman, K., Chutuape, M. A., Bigelow, G. E., & Stitzer, M. L. (1999). Voucher-based reinforcement of cocaine abstinence in treatment-resistant methadone patients: Effects of reinforcement magnitude. *Psychopharmacology, 146*(2), 128–138.

Stitzer, M. L., Bigelow, G. E., & Liebson, I. (1980). Reducing drug use among methadone maintenance clients: Contingent reinforcement of morphine-free urines. *Addictive Behaviors, 5*(4), 333–340.

Stotts, A. L., Vujanovic, A., Heads, A., Suchting, R., Green, C. E., & Schmitz, J. M. (2015). The role of avoidance and inflexibility in characterizing response to contingency management for cocaine use disorders: A secondary profile analysis. *Psychology of Addictive Behaviors, 29*(2), 408–413.

Tappin, D., Bauld, L., Purves, D., Boyd, K., Sinclair, L., MacAskill, S., et al. (2015). Financial incentives for smoking cessation in pregnancy: Randomised controlled trial. *BMJ.* Jan 27; 350: h134.

# CHAPTER 12

# Stimulus Control

William J. McIlvane, PhD
*University of Massachusetts Medical School*

## Definitions and Background

Like many terms in the clinical and behavioral sciences, different people use *stimulus control* for different purposes relating to their interests, activities, needs, and verbal conventions. For example, some clinicians may recognize *stimulus control* as a name for specific kinds of behavior therapy or therapeutic procedure (e.g., for compulsive gambling; Hodgins, 2001). By contrast, behavioral scientists often use the term when describing one component of a three-term contingency relation used in analyzing the environmental control of behavior (stimulus, response, consequence; see Skinner, 1935). Still others use this term as a name for an entire subfield of scientific inquiry (stimulus control research) that encompasses analytic studies of behavior—attention, memory, executive functions, concept formation, and symbolic classification (e.g., Sidman, 2008). All of these uses are relevant for the purposes of this chapter.

A *stimulus* is a measurable environmental event that has a measurable effect on behavior. While a tree falling in a forest may be an event that could be measured, the falling tree is not a stimulus unless someone observes it and that observation results in reactions that would not have occurred otherwise (e.g., yelling "Watch out!"). Even if someone is present to observe the tree fall, it is not a stimulus unless a behavior occurs with respect to it. If a birdwatcher's full visual

I gratefully acknowledge the long-term support of the National Institute of Child Health and Human Development (grant numbers HD25995 and HD04147) and the Commonwealth Medicine Division of the University of Massachusetts Medical School. I also thank Charles Hamad, David Smelson, and Beth Epstein for helpful input in the formulation of this chapter.

attention was captured by a rare species, for example, an observer might judge that the birdwatcher didn't seem to notice the tree fall (i.e., it would not be a stimulus for the latter from the perspective of the former). However, if the sound of the tree falling caused a change in the birdwatcher's blood pressure, it would be a potentially measurable event that had a potentially measurable effect on the birdwatcher. If the effect *was* measured via remote sensors that detected both the sound and the change in blood pressure, the tree falling could be classified as a stimulus, by my definition, even though the on-site observer detected no behavior change.

From a more functional perspective, stimuli cannot be defined independently of behavior, and behavior cannot be defined independently of stimuli. Stimuli are defined in relation to their effects on behavior as measured directly or indicated by strong inferential processes. The two events constitute a functional unit of analysis that also includes a third term—the positive or negative *consequence*—when defining a reinforcement contingency (see Sidman, 2008).

# Stimulus Classes

Early on, Skinner (1935) defined stimuli (and responses) generically in terms of their function, much as I have done here. This emphasis on function led to the idea of further defining stimuli in terms of functional classes. If the functions of stimulus events X, Y, and Z can be shown to relate to behavior and its effects in a similar manner, then these events may constitute a *functional stimulus class*. There are two basic types of functional stimulus classes: those defined by shared physical features or in purely functional terms.

## *Feature/Perceptual Stimulus Classes*

Functional classes defined by shared physical features have been termed "feature classes" (McIlvane, Dube, Green, & Serna, 1993) or "perceptual classes" (Fields et al., 2002). To exemplify such classes, consider a simple sorting task that is used often in behavior therapy for children with autism spectrum disorders. One might teach the child to sort both coins and plastic washers from a pool containing these items and noncircular distractors to attempt to have the feature of circularity come to control behavior. Accurate sorting alone of the items does not necessarily demonstrate that a feature/perceptual class defined by *circularity* has been established, because the child might merely have attended to specific features of each of the items sorted (i.e., this could be a case of rote learning and nothing more). To assess whether the child was responding on the basis of the abstract property of circularity, however, one could add new circular items (e.g., buttons) and new noncircular distractors to the pool. If buttons are also immediately sorted along with the coins and washers, one has evidence that a functional feature or perceptual class (in this case, one defined by circularity) has been established.

To assess whether the circular stimuli relate in a similar manner to environmental operations, one might change the sorting task such that buttons but not coins or washers are available in the pool, and some other noncircular items (e.g., dominoes) are instead defined as correct choices. After the child masters the new task—now avoiding the buttons but selecting the dominoes—one might add back in the coins and washers. If the child now does *not* select those previously correct items, then it has been shown that changing the function of one class member (buttons) spontaneously changed the functions of the coins and washers, thus providing strong evidence that a functional class has been established.

Humans and nonhumans share this ability to develop such functional classes. For example, Herrnstein (1979) showed that even pigeons can (1) be taught certain generalized concepts, such as tree versus nontree or water versus nonwater, and (2) pass tests similar to those just described. The teaching method most commonly used has been termed *multiple exemplar training* (MET), in which several—sometimes many—examples sharing defining physical properties are contrasted with other examples lacking those properties. For example, Herrnstein's MET required pigeons to discriminate forty scenes containing trees from forty scenes without trees to establish the concept targeted. Normally, capable humans are quite adept at such tasks and may abstract concepts such as these from only a few examples.

Feature/perceptual classes show *primary stimulus generalization*, in which the behavioral effects of the stimulus class apparently extend beyond the original situation in which control was observed. This is what occurred in the earlier example: the ability of buttons to control behavior after the child was trained with coins and washers was an instance of primary stimulus generalization that verified the control by circularity. To specify a feature/perceptual class, one assumes that the individual *does* attend to the stimulus features specified and further assumes that the individual will respond similarly when other stimuli containing that feature are presented.

As a practical application of this feature/perceptual class analysis, consider a case of phobia: A client reports that he was severely frightened by the sudden appearance of a large rat in his bedroom. After that experience, he reports not only a phobic reaction to rats and mice, but also substantial discomfort with physically similar animals (e.g. squirrels, chipmunks, rabbits). Assuming that a feature/perceptual class exists, a therapist might first teach the client to relax and/or behave more flexibly in the presence of animals that aren't rats; she might assume also that this MET procedure will make it easier for the client to learn to relax and/or behave flexibly in the presence of rats, the animal that caused the original fright (see chapter 18). If the procedure proves successful, it is evidence that the therapist's feature/perceptual class analysis was correct. If not, the result suggests that the stimulus class was incorrectly or incompletely specified (e.g., a furless tail not shared by the other animals was a particularly frightening component of the rat's overall appearance).

## Contingency/Arbitrary Stimulus Classes

A functional stimulus class may also include physically *dissimilar* stimuli. These classes may be termed *contingency (only) classes* or *arbitrary stimulus classes* to emphasize that class membership is defined by similarity of function rather than physical similarity (see Goldiamond, 1966). To understand an arbitrary stimulus class, consider a red traffic light, a STOP sign, and a policeman's upraised hand; all set the stage for one to step on the car's brakes. Skinner (1935) implicitly and Goldiamond (1966) explicitly defined a functional stimulus class as having two properties: (1) stimuli must exhibit the same function(s) in the control of behavior, and (2) operations that influence the function of one member of the stimulus class must influence the function of the others. Using the traffic example, motorists fleeing an imminent disaster who observe others ignoring a policeman's directions without apparent negative consequences are more likely to also ignore other traffic-control measures. In technical terms, a transfer or transformation of functions occurs to all members of the class, although the procedure that changes the function is applied only to a subset of its members (see chapters 6 and 7).

It is an active point of discussion in behavior theory whether arbitrary stimulus classes can be extended to account for the kinds of stimulus control commonly noted in human language and cognition (e.g., Hayes, Barnes-Holmes, & Roche, 2001; Sidman, 2000). Notably, however, cognitive neuroscience methods (e.g., functional MRI, evoked cortical potentials) are increasingly showing that procedures used in basic stimulus control research have the same or similar effects on neural activities as the language and cognitive stimulus events they are intended to model (e.g., Bortoloti, Pimentel, & de Rose, 2014).

## Stimulus Control Defined

In summary, a given stimulus or stimulus class exhibits control when any measured behavior or class of behaviors is more probable in the presence of that stimulus/stimulus class than in its absence. Whether in research or clinical applications, one should not make assumptions about the specific elements and/or properties of controlling relations. It will be most useful to specify what these are by using direct measurements or inferences based on strong empirical evidence. In addition, the concept of "more probable in the presence of a stimulus/stimulus class than in its absence" is critical to understanding stimulus control. For example, suppose that behavior X occurs with a 10 percent frequency when stimulus X is present and with only a 5 percent frequency when stimulus X is absent. If one can reliably demonstrate a frequency difference using quantitative analysis techniques (see McIlvane, Hunt, Kledaras, & Deutsch, 2016), then one can say that stimulus control has been exhibited despite the low frequency of occurrence overall. As I'll discuss below, the frequency of occurrence of a given stimulus control relation need not indicate anything about its probable persistence or other similar concerns that a clinician might have.

# Clinical and Educational Practice

Feature/perceptual classes and arbitrary classes constitute a central component to the scientific analysis of complex behavior, human and otherwise. When combined with procedures exemplified in the next section, one has a strongly evidence-based conceptual, analytical, and methodological framework within which to understand critical components of therapeutic and educational procedures broadly.

At a practical level, the clinician or educator can benefit from stimulus control/stimulus class analyses, using them to promote client success or, when confronted with the failure of applied procedures that seem well designed, to understand and perhaps ameliorate puzzling treatment failures—as one illustration from my own research program shows. We conducted a long-term program aimed at developing methods for reducing so-called impulsive responding in individuals with autism spectrum and other neurodevelopmental disorders (i.e., responding too rapidly on tasks that required participants to carefully inspect stimuli in order to discriminate them). Stimuli were presented in locations defined by square borders on a computer display, thus emulating well-established procedures from much prior stimulus control research and its applications. Our procedures were able to eliminate impulsive responding in most individuals. Nevertheless, such responding persisted in a few people despite our best efforts to eliminate it. A breakthrough occurred, however, when a member of our team suggested eliminating the borders that defined stimulus locations to further simplify the display. Although we thought these borders were irrelevant constant features of the display, eliminating them instantaneously eliminated impulsive responding.

The preceding example illustrates a more general consideration in stimulus control analysis: the controlling properties of stimuli that the researcher, teacher, or therapist deems relevant may be strongly influenced by the broader context in which those stimuli are presented. We have found stimulus class analysis particularly useful in thinking about contextual stimuli and stimulus classes that relate to the critical issue of treatment generalization, and especially the failure thereof (see McIlvane & Dube, 2003). One reason that behavior therapists may prefer to provide therapy in everyday environments in which problem behavior occurs is to minimize the likelihood that they may miss critical contextual determinants of the stimulus control of behavior. Sometimes, however, therapy must be conducted outside such contexts (e.g., when the problem behavior is dangerous or socially repugnant). In such cases, the therapist may want to design the treatment contexts to include stimuli from feature/perceptual and/or arbitrary stimulus classes that simulate natural counterparts to maximize the potential for the treatment effects to be generalized.

## Implementation

**Simple differential reinforcement.** To establish control using two formerly neutral stimuli (A versus B), one can provide positive reinforcing consequences when a targeted behavior occurs in the presence of A and deliver no such consequences when B is present. Soon, one may find the target behavior occurring more frequently in the presence of A than of B. As I noted earlier, even a small difference in differential responding indicates some measure of stimulus control. After the continued application of these contingencies, however, one might find that the individual virtually always responds to A and virtually never to B.

The first sustained efforts of applying differential reinforcement procedures in clinical and educational settings began more than sixty years ago. For example, Skinner's *The Technology of Teaching* (1968) was intended for broad application in both regular and special education. His goal was to translate procedures and findings of basic research with nonhumans to such applications. Work in this tradition included the extensive development of instructional technology for normally capable populations, ranging from young children to advanced professional trainees. Other efforts to develop this technology were directed at finding effective therapeutic procedures for special populations (e.g., people with neurodevelopmental and neuropsychiatric problems; Ferster & DeMyer, 1961). In the decades since *Technology of Teaching*, a voluminous literature has developed, reporting many thousands of studies of reinforcement procedures for a vast range of beneficial clinical and educational applications. These studies have addressed a range of populations, including normally capable children and adults as well as individuals with a broad range of neurodevelopmental, neuropsychiatric, and other neurobehavioral deficits and disorders.

There are emerging issues in differential reinforcement–based methods for establishing stimulus control. Applied behavioral research has highlighted individual differences in response to reinforcement procedures in clinical populations. For example, it may be difficult to identify and/or maintain the potency of reinforcers for some children with autism spectrum and related neurodevelopmental disorders (see Higbee, 2009). Even if seemingly effective reinforcers have been identified, however, research tells us there is another critical consideration to the design of effective therapy: the degree to which the client's behavior is sensitive to disparities between reinforcement schedules.

As noted, if one reinforces behaviors within a given class and extinguishes behaviors in other classes, the former will come to predominate. In everyday experience, however, one rarely (if ever) encounters situations in which desirable behaviors can be consistently reinforced, nor ones in which undesirable behaviors can be consistently extinguished. Most often, one merely hopes that (1) desirable behavior will be reinforced often (rich schedules of reinforcement) and undesirable behavior only rarely (lean schedules), and that (2) client behavior will prove sensitive to the disparity between these schedules.

My stimulus control research group has long been interested in why some individuals with neurodevelopmental disorders show good sensitivity to rich-versus-lean schedule disparities, whereas others seem almost indifferent to these schedules—even in cases in which traditional reinforcer function tests show strong evidence of reinforce potency (e.g., tests contrasting continuous reinforcement versus extinction schedules, reinforcer preference tests). We are especially interested in cases in which indifference to a rich-versus-lean schedule persists despite programmed training aimed at making the schedule disparities easy to detect (McIlvane & Kledaras, 2012).

Schedule insensitivity/indifference may be a hidden variable when children with autism spectrum disorders do not respond well to applied behavior analysis therapies (see Sallows & Graupner, 2005). An increasing number of studies reference individuals with other neurodevelopmental and neuropsychiatric disorders exhibiting deviant responses to reinforcement procedures. For example, findings from clinical neuroscience research suggest that individuals with ADHD exhibit altered reinforcement sensitivity (e.g., Luman, Tripp, & Scheres, 2010).

**Shaping.** Much research has shown that some individuals do not respond well to differential reinforcement methods aimed at establishing stimulus control (due perhaps to unrecognized insensitivity to reinforcement schedules). Moreover, the unreinforced behaviors that result seem to interfere with learning. Put simply, such individuals do not seem to learn from their mistakes. In an effort to ameliorate this situation, researchers have pursued studies of procedures that could potentially establish stimulus control while minimizing unreinforced responding (so-called errorless learning procedures; e.g., Terrace, 1963). A typical procedure uses highly salient, easy-to-discriminate stimuli that capture attention readily and promote rapid, even virtually instantaneous, learning (e.g., a task that requires one merely to discriminate dissimilar colors). Thereafter, the color differences can be used as added prompts to direct attention to more subtle differences between potentially controlling stimuli. Many studies document the superiority of such errorless methods for promoting stimulus control in special populations (Snell, 2009). One can also minimize unreinforced behavior without using prompt procedures; programmed instructional procedures establish behavioral prerequisites with each new, learned behavior, making it likely that subsequent learning will proceed with a minimum of unreinforced behavior (McIlvane, Gerard, Kledaras, Mackay, & Lionello-DeNolf, 2016).

**Verbal instructions.** For people with adequately developed language skills, verbal instructions that describe environmental contingencies may suffice to establish stimulus control, though the exact processes by which this occurs is still a point of discussion (see chapter 7). In stimulus control therapy for insomnia, for example, verbal cognitive behavioral therapy has proven to be very helpful (Jacob, 1998). In this approach, insomnia is attributed, in part, to maladaptive habits that may develop when sleep does not occur in the typical manner and renders falling asleep even more difficult than it should be (e.g., watching the clock, worrying about the time remaining before one must start his or her day). Cognitive behavioral therapy for insomnia (CBT-I) aims to break down the stimulus control of such behaviors by, for example, instructing clients to remove the clock from the bedroom, to limit time in bed when one is not asleep, to establish standard bedtimes and wake times, and so on. Like all rule-governed behavior, however, the effectiveness of CBT-I and other verbal stimulus control therapies depends critically on whether the control established in this way yields the desired outcomes.

**Persistence.** In general, behavior therapists are concerned with making positive behaviors persist and weakening negative behaviors. Nevin's (1992) behavioral momentum analysis makes analogies between the relationships described in the physics of motion and the environmental determinants of behavioral persistence. He suggests that reinforcement variables associated with controlling stimuli determine the persistence of stimulus control. If a given stimulus predicts rich reinforcement, behavior is likely to persist. If reinforcement is reduced, he argues that behavior becomes less persistent. On its face, the momentum analysis might seem in conflict with the well-known partial reinforcement extinction (PRE) effect, wherein behavior tends to extinguish more slowly with intermittent versus continuous reinforcement. As Nevin (1992) pointed out, however, the resistance-to-extinction test introduces other variables that confound the analysis.

Nevin's studies, and direct and systematic replications by others, have lent substantial empirical support for the momentum analysis. For example, Dube and McIlvane (2002) showed that the momentum analysis can inform procedures aimed at increasing behavioral flexibility in children with autism spectrum disorders. The target task was to reverse a previously established discrimination (a basic requirement for learning educationally relevant tasks, such as matching to sample). In cases where children experienced relatively lean reinforcement schedules in learning A+ versus B– during training, they learned B+ versus A– discrimination faster than in cases where children experienced relatively richer A+ versus B– training schedules. Viewing the literature as a whole, behavioral momentum analyses of stimulus control are a promising development that will increasingly have a beneficial impact on behavior therapy.

**Altering.** When it comes to altering established maladaptive stimulus control in ways that benefit the client, there are many challenges for practicing clinicians and behavior therapists. Superficially, the obvious approach would be to use extinction (i.e., whatever consequence maintains the behavior is eliminated) to break the contingency relationship between stimuli and the behavior(s) controlled. In the world outside the laboratory, however, one often does not control consequences to a level adequate to impose extinction conditions. Moreover, even under laboratory conditions, extinction may merely reduce the probability of undesired stimulus control—and not actually destroy the "bond" between stimuli and the behavior(s) of interest. This outcome can be clearly shown in animal behavior models (e.g., Podlesnik & Kelley, 2014), which may inform analyses of people who relapse after finishing successful behavior therapy for reward system–related clinical disorders (RSRCDs), such as substance abuse, compulsive gambling, obesity, and so on.

In this context, there is clearly a downside to the potentially beneficial relationship described previously in the discussion of stimulus control therapies. Suppressing the control of stimuli associated with RSRCDs may merely reduce their frequency temporarily. Any challenge that causes the resurgence and strengthening of stimulus control by any member of an RSRCD class may increase the probability that other class members will exert stimulus control, even in situations that do not present such challenges.

The potential for resurgence may help account for the unimpressive results of cue exposure therapy (CET) for the treatment of addictive behavior (see Martin, LaRowe, & Malcolm, 2010). In CET, addicts are exposed to a series of drug-related stimuli (e.g., MET with various exemplars of drug paraphernalia) in a setting in which the resulting cravings cannot lead to drug use. The rationale is that the extinction of these cravings should at first lead to withdrawal symptoms and ultimately to the extinction of the drug-seeking/taking behavior. There are two problems with the CET approach. First, any subsequent exposure to even a small subset of stimuli associated with the addictive behavior that leads to relapse (e.g., meeting an old friend who was involved in past drug taking) may reestablish high-probability control by other members of the stimulus class, thus defeating the intent of the CET. Second, contextual stimuli (i.e., those in familiar drug-use settings) may be an unappreciated component of the stimulus control of addictive behavior. If that is the case, CET will fail if those stimulus control variables are not addressed in therapy.

## Conclusions

These days, one cannot open the many compendiums such as this one without seeing many citations to and discussions of evidence-based practice. For both practical and ethical reasons, clinicians and educators want to apply therapeutic and/or educational procedures that are supported by scientific evidence. In my experience, most practicing clinicians and educators tend to think in terms of broad classes of procedures (e.g., applied behavior analysis versus sensory integration/occupational therapy for autism). In this chapter, I illustrate a less commonly discussed approach to defining evidence-based practice—that is, relating therapeutic/educational procedures to scientific principles, which must undergird whatever approach one chooses. By doing so, I think one can promote behavioral development, health, and wellness, and have a secure evidential foundation on which to base one's practice and potentially improve its effectiveness, without being captured by fads and fancies that may temporarily dominate fields.

## References

Bortoloti, R., Pimentel, N. S., & de Rose, J. C. (2014). Electrophysiological investigation of the functional overlap between semantic and equivalence relations. *Psychology and Neuroscience, 7*(2), 183–191.

Dube, W. V., & McIlvane, W. J. (2002). Reinforcer rate and stimulus control in discrimination reversal learning. *Psychological Record, 52*(4), 405–416.

Ferster, C. B., & DeMyer, M. K. (1961). The development of performances in autistic children in an automatically controlled environment. *Journal of Chronic Diseases, 13*(4), 312–345.

Fields, L., Matneja, P., Varelas, A., Belanich, J., Fitzer, A., Shamoun, K. (2002). The formation of linked perceptual classes. *Journal of the Experimental Analysis of Behavior, 78*(3), 271–290.

Goldiamond, I. (1966). Perception, language and conceptualization rules. In B. Kleinmuntz (Ed.), *Problem solving: Research, method and theory* (pp. 183–224). New York: Wiley.

Hayes, S. C., Barnes-Holmes, D., & Roche, B. (Eds.). (2001). *Relational frame theory: A post-Skinnerian account of human language and cognition.* New York: Kluwer Academic/Plenum Publishers.

Herrnstein, R. J. (1979). Acquisition, generalization, and discrimination reversal of a natural concept. *Journal of Experimental Psychology: Animal Behavior Processes, 5*(2), 116–129.

Higbee, T. S. (2009). Reinforcer identification strategies and teaching learner readiness skills. In R. A. Rehfeldt & Y. Barnes-Holmes (Eds.), *Derived relational responding: Applications for learners with autism and other developmental disabilities.* Oakland, CA: New Harbinger Publications.

Hodgins, D. C. (2001). Processes of changing gambling behavior. *Addictive Behaviors, 26*(1), 121–128.

Jacob, G. D. (1998). *Say good night to insomnia.* New York: Henry Holt.

Luman, M., Tripp, G., & Scheres, A. (2010). Identifying the neurobiology of altered reinforcement sensitivity in ADHD: A review and research agenda. *Neuroscience and Biobehavioral Reviews, 34*(5), 744–754.

Martin, T., LaRowe, S. D., & Malcolm R. (2010). Progress in cue extinction therapy for the treatment of addictive disorders: A review update. *Open Addiction Journal, 3*, 92–101.

McIlvane, W. J., & Dube, W. V. (2003). Stimulus control topography coherence theory: Foundations and extensions. *Behavior Analyst, 26*(2), 195–213.

McIlvane, W. J., Dube, W. V., Green, G., & Serna, R. W. (1993). Programming conceptual and communication skill development: A methodological stimulus class analysis. In A. P. Kaiser & D. B. Gray (Eds.), *Enhancing children's language: Research foundations for intervention* (pp. 242–285). Baltimore, MD: Paul H. Brookes Publishing.

McIlvane, W. J., Gerard, C. J., Kledaras, J. B., Mackay, H. A., & Lionello-DeNolf, K. M. (2016). Teaching stimulus-stimulus relations to nonverbal individuals: Reflections on technology and future directions. *European Journal of Behavior Analysis, 17*(1), 49–68.

McIlvane, W. J., Hunt, A., Kledaras, J. K., & Deutsch, C. K. (2016). Behavioral heterogeneity among people with severe intellectual disabilities: Integrating single-case and group designs to develop effective interventions. In R. Sevcik & M. A. Romski (Eds.), *Communication interventions for individuals with severe disabilities: Exploring research challenges and opportunities* (pp. 189–207). Baltimore, MD: Paul H. Brookes Publishing.

McIlvane, W. J., & Kledaras, J. B. (2012). Some things we learned from Sidman and some things we did not (we think). *European Journal of Behavior Analysis, 13*(1), 97–109.

Nevin, J. A. (1992). An integrative model for the study of behavioral momentum. *Journal of the Experimental Analysis of Behavior, 57*(3), 301–316.

Podlesnik, C. A., & Kelley, M. E. (2014). Resurgence: Response competition, stimulus control, and reinforcer control. *Journal of the Experimental Analysis of Behavior, 102*(2), 231–240.

Sallows, G. O., & Graupner, T. D. (2005). Intensive behavioral treatment for children with autism: Four-year outcome and predictors. *American Journal on Mental Retardation, 110*(6), 417–438.

Sidman, M. (2000). Equivalence relations and the reinforcement contingency. *Journal of the Experimental Analysis of Behavior, 74*(1), 127–146.

Sidman, M. (2008). Reflections on stimulus control. *Behavior Analysis, 31*(2), 127–135.

Skinner, B. F. (1935). The generic nature of the concepts of stimulus and response. *Journal of General Psychology, 12*(1), 40–65.

Skinner, B. F. (1968). *The technology of teaching.* New York: Appleton-Century-Crofts.

Snell, M. E. (2009). Advances in instruction. In S. L. Odom, R. H. Horner, M. E. Snell, & J. Blacher (Eds.), *Handbook of developmental disabilities* (pp. 249–268). New York: Guilford Press.

Terrace, H. S. (1963). Discrimination learning with and without "errors." *Journal of the Experimental Analysis of Behavior, 6*(1), 1–27.

# CHAPTER 13

# Shaping

Raymond G. Miltenberger, PhD
Bryon G. Miller, MS
Heather H. Zerger, MS
Marissa A. Novotny, MS

*Department of Child and Family Studies,
University of South Florida*

## Definitions and Background

*Shaping* is the differential reinforcement of successive approximations of a target behavior. That definition relies on a handful of basic behavioral principles. *Reinforcement* refers to an increase in the future probability of a given class of behavior under similar conditions due to the relatively immediate occurrence of a consequence. Reinforcement, used for the acquisition and maintenance of a behavior, is a component of most applied behavior analysis procedures. The behavioral principle of *extinction* is the reduction and eventual near elimination of a behavior; extinction has occurred when a behavior no longer produces a reinforcing consequence. The combination of reinforcement and extinction is referred to as *differential reinforcement*, defined as the reinforcement of a specific response, while other response forms are placed on extinction (i.e., reinforcement is withheld). The outcome of differential reinforcement is the increased probability of the reinforced response and a reduction in all other nonreinforced responses. *Successive approximations* are the steps in response forms that lead incrementally to the target behavior. When successive approximations are differentially reinforced, response forms probabilistically change in the direction of the target. Shaping is a training procedure that can be used to generate novel behavior, to reinstate a previously exhibited behavior, or to change a dimension of an existing behavior; these applications are discussed in detail below.

# Examples

Shaping can be conceptualized as both an explicit training procedure and a behavioral phenomenon that can occur naturally or unintentionally. As a training procedure, a simple yet illustrative example of shaping is teaching a pigeon to make a complete clockwise turn (Chance, 2014). At first, any turn in either direction (i.e., the starting behavior) results in reinforcement (i.e., typically a conditioned reinforcer, such as an auditory stimulus, paired periodically with an unconditioned reinforcer, such as grain). After this response occurs reliably, only turns in a clockwise direction are reinforced, whereas counterclockwise turns are placed on extinction. The next several steps involve reinforcing closer and closer approximations of a complete clockwise turn (e.g., quarter-, half-, and three-quarter-clockwise turns), with all previous approximations placed on extinction. In this example, the pigeon is specifically trained to engage in a selected target behavior. However, shaping often occurs naturally or unintentionally as a result of the prevailing contingencies of reinforcement (both social and nonsocial) and extinction.

The intensity of problem behavior such as tantrums or self-injury can be shaped unintentionally, where new and often disruptive or dangerous topographies of behavior emerge (e.g., Rasey & Iversen, 1993; Schaefer, 1970). For example, parents may reinforce a child's tantrum by removing their demands, such that engaging in tantrums typically results in the child not having to comply with the parents' instructions. Initially, the problem behavior consists of the child stating an emphatic "No!" when instructed to complete a task, which results in the parents removing the demand (i.e., giving in). In an attempt to increase compliance, the child's parents begin to follow through with their instructions by not removing the demand when the child protests (i.e., extinction). In this context, extinction is often associated with an extinction burst, which can consist of a temporary increase in the severity of the problem behavior, the occurrence of novel behavior, or emotional responding. When faced with an extinction burst consisting of more-severe problem behavior (e.g., vocal protest and yelling at the parents), the parents might give in again, thus reinforcing a successive approximation to what will ultimately emerge as tantrum behavior. This process is then repeated as the parents begin to inadvertently reinforce more and more severe topographies of their child's tantrums. This can result in the problem behavior being shaped, from a low-severity vocal protest to a severe tantrum, such as yelling, crying, throwing objects, and engaging in aggressive behavior.

It's important for therapists to understand the inadvertent use of shaping so they can make sure that caregivers do not succumb to this practice. However, the rest of this chapter discusses shaping as a training procedure and reviews the steps involved in using shaping consistently and correctly. It presents illustrative examples of shaping from the literature and discusses them in further detail.

# Implementation

To implement shaping, the starting behavior is reinforced until the individual consistently engages in that response. Once this occurs, the next approximation is reinforced and the previous approximation is not reinforced (extinction). Once the individual consistently exhibits the second approximation, it is placed on extinction as the third approximation is now reinforced. The first and second approximations should stop occurring, as reinforcement is provided only for the subsequent approximation. This use of differential reinforcement is implemented for each successive approximation until the individual consistently engages in the target behavior. Although the number of approximations within a specific application of shaping might vary due to an individual's ability or the complexity of the target response, in general, the following steps should ensure that shaping is implemented correctly (Miltenberger, 2016).

**1. Identify the target behavior.** The target behavior must be identified and clearly defined to determine when the shaping procedure has successfully produced the target behavior.

**2. Determine whether shaping is the best procedure for getting the target behavior to occur.** The purpose of shaping is to generate a behavior or a dimension of the behavior that does not already occur. With shaping, the target behavior (or desired level of the target behavior) is achieved in a stepwise fashion. If the individual is already engaging in the target behavior, at least occasionally, then shaping is not necessary. Differential reinforcement can be used to strengthen the behavior. Additionally, if more efficient teaching strategies, such as prompting and fading, behavioral skills training, and behavioral chaining, can be used to promote the behavior, then shaping is not necessary.

**3. Identify the first approximation to be reinforced.** Before the shaping process begins, the first approximation, or starting behavior, must be identified. The starting behavior should be a response—relevant to the target behavior—that the individual already exhibits.

**4. Determine the remaining approximations of the target behavior.** The remaining approximations should also be determined before the shaping process begins. This is important, because the individual must master each step before proceeding to the next one. Once the starting behavior (and each subsequent approximation) has been reinforced and then placed on extinction, an extinction burst will generate novel behaviors, one of which will be reinforced as a closer approximation of the target behavior. Shaping steps should not be too big, such that the individual cannot easily go from one step to the next. The steps also should not be too small, such that the shaping process is slow. Steps should be set such that there is a reasonable expectation that the learner can advance from one to the next. Although shaping steps should be determined ahead of time, it is not uncommon for steps to be consolidated, or for additional steps to be added, during training (see step 7).

**5. Identify the reinforcer that will be delivered for each approximation.** The reinforcer to be used during the shaping process should be one that can be delivered immediately upon the occurrence of the appropriate response. Furthermore, the reinforcer must be an established reinforcer for the learner. Additionally, the reinforcer should be an item that, when presented repeatedly, will be unlikely to produce satiation. For example, although food is a reinforcer for most learners, it is likely to lose its reinforcing value as the learner continues to receive the food. Conditioned reinforcers (e.g., tokens or praise) are often used to avoid satiation.

**6. Provide differential reinforcement for each successive approximation.** To begin the shaping process, provide the reinforcer for the occurrence of the starting behavior. Once this step occurs consistently, it is placed on extinction, and the next approximation is reinforced. Once the second approximation occurs consistently, it is placed on extinction and the next approximation is reinforced. This process continues until the target behavior is reached.

**7. Determine the pace at which you will move through the shaping process.** Each approximation is a stepping-stone for the next approximation. Therefore, once the learner consistently exhibits the starting behavior, the trainer can place that response on extinction and move to the next approximation to be reinforced. It is important to progress through the shaping steps at a proper pace. If one approximation is reinforced too many times, it may be difficult to move to the next step. If progression is not successful, the trainer may cue or prompt the individual to engage in the next approximation. If the trainer finds that the shaping steps were originally set too large for the learner to accomplish, the successive approximations can be broken down into smaller steps.

# Applications

Shaping is used to get an individual to engage in a target behavior that he or she is not already exhibiting. In the sections that follow we describe the three applications of shaping: (1) generating novel behavior (i.e., behavior that is not in the learner's repertoire), (2) reinstating a previously exhibited behavior, and (3) changing some dimension of an existing behavior.

## Generating Novel Behavior

Shaping can be used to promote the acquisition of a behavior that an individual has never exhibited (Miltenberger, 2016). For example, Ferguson and Rosales-Ruiz (2001) used eight shaping steps and a clicker (and occasional food) as a reinforcer to get five horses to walk into a transport trailer. Previously, aversive procedures (whips and ropes) were used to get the horses loaded into the trailer.

In a human example of developing a novel behavior, Shimizu, Yoon, and McDonough (2010) used shaping to teach preschool-aged children diagnosed with intellectual disabilities to point and click with a computer mouse. The first shaping step was moving the mouse around the computer screen. The reinforcer consisted of visual and auditory stimulation (rectangles on the screen disappeared or changed color and a bubbling sound occurred). The second shaping step was pointing the cursor to a single rectangle to produce the reinforcer. In the final shaping step, the subject was required to move the mouse, point it to a single rectangle, and press and release the mouse for the reinforcer to be delivered.

Mathews, Hodson, Crist, and LaRouche (1992) used shaping to increase children's compliance with the use of contact lenses. Four children under the age of five who had previously demonstrated noncompliance with physician instructions during routine eye exams were chosen to participate in the study. Eight shaping steps, or variations of these steps, were used to teach contact lens wear. The shaping steps included touching the child's face, pulling open an eyelid, having the child pull open an eyelid, placing drops in eyes, approaching the child's eye with a finger, touching the child's eye with a finger, touching a soft lens to the corner of the child's eye, and touching a hard lens to the corner of the child's eye. Compliance with each shaping step was reinforced with praise, stars, bubbles, food, or access to toys. This use of shaping increased contact lens use with three of the four children. It should be noted that this example is a variation of shaping; it did not involve successive approximations of the target behavior but rather successive changes in stimulation, to which the participants were exposed while holding an eyelid open and remaining compliant.

## Reinstating a Previously Exhibited Behavior

Shaping can be used to teach an individual to engage in a previously exhibited behavior that no longer occurs. In some cases the individual may no longer exhibit the behavior because he or she lost the ability to do so (e.g., teaching someone to talk after traumatic brain injury) or refuses to do so.

Meyer, Hagopian, and Paclawskyj (1999) used shaping to increase the number of steps a student with intellectual disability correctly performed each day. Previously, he had engaged in severe aggressive behavior when asked to get ready for school. The shaping procedure included ten steps, from brushing teeth to remaining in school each day. The reinforcers they delivered were contingent on a specific number of steps being completed each day, and the number of steps required was systematically increased. Results of the study suggest that shaping can be used successfully to increase compliance with morning hygiene skills and to increase attendance at school.

Taub and colleagues (1994) used shaping and verbal feedback/praise as a reinforcer to increase the motor movements of stroke victims who had lost movement in one of their limbs. The authors restricted the movement of the unaffected limb and used shaping to promote the use of the affected limb with a variety of tasks, including turning a Rolodex file, pushing a disc in a shuffleboard game, and rolling a ball. The researchers showed that shaping increased the number of turns of a Rolodex file and the distance a subject pushed the shuffleboard disc. Additionally, the time it took individuals to move a ball from side to side decreased. This study shows that shaping can facilitate behavioral rehabilitation in individuals who suffered neurological damage due to a stroke. Shaping has since been shown to lead to greater cortical recovery as well (Liepert, Bauder, Miltner, Taub, & Weiller, 2000).

O'Neill and Gardner (1983) used a shaping procedure to reinstate independent walking with a walker in an older adult who was noncompliant with physical therapy (PT) after hip replacement surgery. To start the shaping procedure, the therapist reinforced going to the PT room (i.e., the starting behavior). Once the subject was consistently going to the PT room, the therapist reinforced standing between two parallel bars for an increasing number of seconds, and going to the PT room was placed on extinction. This process continued through a list of successive approximations, including walking between the parallel bars for an increasing number of steps and walking the full length of the bars, until the subject walked independently with a walker.

When using shaping to reinstate a previously exhibited behavior, it is essential to first determine the reason the individual is not engaging in the behavior. For example, the presence of an aversive condition associated with the behavior might decrease an individual's motivation to engage in the behavior, and in that case manipulating the environment in a way that removes this aversive condition might be enough to promote responding without the use of shaping. Before initiating shaping, however, it is essential to identify a powerful reinforcer to strengthen each approximation in the shaping process. The use of motivational strategies to augment the impact of reinforcers (see chapter 27) can also increase the effectiveness of shaping.

## Changing Some Dimension of an Existing Behavior

Shaping can be used to increase or decrease some dimension of a behavior (frequency, intensity, duration, or latency of a target response) that is not present at a satisfactory level. In this application of shaping, the target is a change in the behavioral dimension, such as an increase in speaking volume or a decrease in the number of cigarettes smoked per day.

Hagopian and Thompson (1999) used shaping with an eight-year-old boy with cystic fibrosis and an intellectual disability to increase his compliance with respiratory treatments. The target behavior was having the boy keep a mask on his face that released a medication mist. Initially they required the boy to keep the mask on his face for five seconds, after which he received praise and access to preferred items. The time he had to keep the mask on his face was systematically increased in five-second increments, until a goal of forty seconds was reached. Results of the study show that the duration of compliance increased from a mean of thirteen seconds to a mean of thirty-seven seconds, and the results were maintained at a fourteen-week follow-up.

In another example, Jackson and Wallace (1974) shaped behavior along the intensity dimension by reinforcing successively louder speech in a young girl diagnosed with a mild intellectual disability. In this study a reinforcer was delivered when she spoke at successively higher levels, as measured by a decibel meter.

Hall, Maynes, and Reiss (2009) used shaping to increase the duration of eye contact for two out of three individuals with fragile X syndrome. Participants received edible reinforcers and praise if they engaged in eye contact for a specified period of time. The time they had to make eye contact increased after each trial using percentile schedules of reinforcement.

Dallery, Meredith, and Glenn (2008) used shaping to decrease the number of cigarettes eight adults smoked. Following baseline, the researchers calculated a criterion that specified the number of cigarettes participants could smoke, which they determined from measured carbon monoxide (CO) levels. If participants' CO levels were at or below the set criterion level, they received a monetary voucher. CO levels for five of the participants had decreased to levels of abstinence by the conclusion of the study.

In a novel example of shaping, Scott, Scott, and Goldwater (1997) enhanced the performance of a track-and-field athlete. The target behavior was for a pole-vaulter to raise the pole as high above his head as possible just before planting the pole to launch himself over the bar. Scott and colleagues used auditory feedback as a reinforcer for reaching a certain height with the pole. The height that was required for reinforcement was raised in five-centimeter increments over seven shaping steps until the athlete achieved his maximum arm extension.

O'Neill and Gardner (1983) describe a situation in which a woman diagnosed with multiple sclerosis interrupted her therapy program more than once per hour for bathroom visits. Ultimately, the therapist wanted the subject to wait two hours between each bathroom visit. The starting behavior, waiting one hour between bathroom visits, was reinforced until she consistently waited this amount of time. The next approximation was to wait seventy minutes. At this point, waiting one hour was placed on extinction, whereas waiting seventy minutes was reinforced with praise and approval from the therapist. This process of reinforcing increasing latencies between bathroom visits continued until the subject consistently waited two hours between bathroom visits.

## Opportunities for Using Shaping in Psychotherapy

Although behavior analysts have most commonly been the ones to use shaping, the opportunities for applied psychologists to use it are all around. For example, a clinician conducting psychotherapy who is interested in shaping self-disclosure, or emotional openness, or attention to the present moment can target and change this behavior in session. Potential reinforcers, such as attention, leaning forward, adopting a posture that mirrors the client's posture, making clinical comments, clinician self-disclosure, or praise, can be explored in session, and if they function as reinforcers the clinician can systematically use them to draw out clients or help them to venture into new areas in terms of their relationships with others. Indeed, this idea is commonly used in clinical behavior analysis and contextual forms of cognitive behavioral therapy, such as functional analytic psychotherapy, which has been shown empirically to work in part through shaping in the psychotherapy session itself (Busch et al., 2009).

# Summary

Shaping is a training procedure used to develop behavior that an individual is currently not exhibiting. More specifically, shaping is used to generate novel behavior, to reinstate a previously exhibited behavior, and to change the dimension of an existing behavior. A goal of most applied behavior analysis procedures is to promote the occurrence of desirable behavior that improves the quality of life of the individual engaging in that behavior. However, reinforcement cannot be used to strengthen desirable behavior if it does not already occur at least occasionally. Shaping provides a way for individuals to acquire desirable behavior in a stepwise fashion and for it to be strengthened through the application of several basic principles of behavior. Although shaping is used as a training procedure, it can also occur accidentally (e.g., the inadvertent shaping of problem behavior). The prevailing contingencies of reinforcement can occur in such a way that a variety of target behaviors can be acquired and shaped inadvertently.

Although shaping is a valuable training tool, it is not always the best-suited or most efficient method of teaching. Again, shaping is typically used to help an individual acquire behavior that is currently not strong or has never been established as part of the individual's behavioral repertoire. A trainer can use differential reinforcement to increase behavior that does occur only occasionally. In addition, a trainer can deliver prompts or manipulate antecedent events to increase motivation so that the behavior is more likely to occur and contact reinforcement. Additionally, shaping is not ideal for training complex chains of behavior involving multiple topographies of behavior to be performed in sequence. To train these behaviors it is more appropriate to create a task analysis, which breaks a chain of behaviors down into individual stimulus-response components. The trainer can then use behavioral-chaining strategies that use prompting and fading to teach each stimulus-response component of the behavioral chain.

# References

Busch, A. M., Kanter, J. W., Callaghan, G. M., Baruch, D. E., Weeks, C. E., & Berlin, K. S. (2009). A micro-process analysis of functional analytic psychotherapy's mechanism of change. *Behavior Therapy, 40*(3), 280–290.

Chance, P. (2014). *Learning and behavior.* Belmont, CA: Wadsworth Publishing.

Dallery, J., Meredith, S., & Glenn, I. M. (2008). A deposit contract method to deliver abstinence reinforcement for cigarette smoking. *Journal of Applied Behavior Analysis, 41*(4), 609–615.

Ferguson, D. L., & Rosales-Ruiz, J. (2001). Loading the problem loader: The effects of target training and shaping on trailer-loading behavior of horses. *Journal of Applied Behavior Analysis, 34*(4), 409–424.

Hagopian, L. P., & Thompson, R. H. (1999). Reinforcement of compliance with respiratory treatment in a child with cystic fibrosis. *Journal of Applied Behavior Analysis, 32*(2), 233–236.

Hall, S. S., Maynes, N. P., & Reiss, A. L. (2009). Using percentile schedules to increase eye contact in children with fragile X syndrome. *Journal of Applied Behavior Analysis, 42*(1), 171–176.

Jackson, D. A., & Wallace, R. F. (1974). The modification and generalization of voice loudness in a fifteen-year-old retarded girl. *Journal of Applied Behavior Analysis, 7*(3), 461–471.

Liepert, J., Bauder, H., Miltner, W. H. R., Taub, E., & Weiller, C. (2000). Treatment-induced cortical reorganization after stroke in humans. *Stroke, 31*(6), 1210–1216.

Matthews, J. R., Hodson, G. D., Crist, W. B., & LaRouche, G. R. (1992). Teaching young children to use contact lenses. *Journal of Applied Behavior Analysis, 25*(1), 229–235.

Meyer, E. A., Hagopian, L. P., & Paclawskyj, T. R. (1999). A function-based treatment for school refusal behavior using shaping and fading. *Research in Developmental Disabilities, 20*(6), 401–410.

Miltenberger, R. G. (2016). *Behavior modification: Principles and procedures* (6th ed.). Boston: Cengage Learning.

O'Neill, G. W., & Gardner, R. (1983). *Behavioral principles in medical rehabilitation: A practical guide.* Springfield, IL: Charles C. Thomas.

Rasey, H. W., & Iversen, I. H. (1993). An experimental acquisition of maladaptive behavior by shaping. *Journal of Behavior Therapy and Experimental Psychiatry, 24*(1), 37–43.

Schaefer, H. H. (1970). Self-injurious behavior: Shaping "head banging" in monkeys. *Journal of Applied Behavior Analysis, 3*(2), 111–116.

Scott, D., Scott, L. M., & Goldwater, B. (1997). A performance improvement program for an international-level track and field athlete. *Journal of Applied Behavior Analysis, 30*(3), 573–575.

Shimizu, H., Yoon, S., & McDonough, C. S. (2010). Teaching skills to use a computer mouse in preschoolers with developmental disabilities: Shaping moving a mouse and eye-hand coordination. *Research in Developmental Disabilities, 31*(6), 1448–1461.

Taub, E., Crago, J. E., Burgio, L. D., Groomes, T. E., Cook, E. W., DeLuca, S. C., et al. (1994). An operant approach to rehabilitation medicine: Overcoming learned nonuse by shaping. *Journal of the Experimental Analysis of Behavior, 61*(2), 281–293.

# CHAPTER 14

# Self-Management

Edward P. Sarafino, PhD

*Department of Psychology, College of New Jersey*

## Definitions

*Self-management* refers to the application of behavioral and cognitive principles to change one's own behavior by gaining control over conditions that encourage undesirable behaviors or discourage desirable ones. As such, self-management brings together many of the processes covered in this volume into a specifically targeted program of behavior change. This chapter provides a brief overview of these principles and processes, as well as ways that they can be used to create self-directed change. More detailed and extensive descriptions of self-management are available in books by Sarafino (2011) and Watson and Tharp (2014).

A self-management program focuses on changing a *target behavior*, which is the behavior that the person wants to change, and achieving a *behavioral goal*, which is the level of the target behavior the individual wants to reach. For example, for the target behavior of studying, a student might have the weekly behavioral goal of spending two hours in focused study for every hour of scheduled class time. By reaching the behavioral goal, the student is likely to achieve an important *outcome goal*, an intended abstracted or general result, such as improving the student's grades. Often, people think of an outcome goal to achieve and then determine what the target behavior and behavioral goal should be to accomplish the desired outcome.

Some target behaviors involve a *behavioral deficit*. For example, the person may not perform the activity often enough, long enough, well enough, or strongly enough. Other target behaviors involve a *behavioral excess*, in which the activity is performed too frequently, too strongly, or for too long. For many people, physical exercise is a behavioral deficit and smoking cigarettes is a behavioral excess. A person is likely to achieve her behavioral goal if she has a high degree of *self-efficacy*, the belief that she can succeed at a specific activity she wants to do, such as changing a behavior in a self-management program.

## Learning and Behavior

Experience leads to learning and plays a critical role in the development of almost all traits and behaviors. *Learning* is a relatively permanent change in behavioral tendency that results from experience. There are two main types of learning (see chapter 6):

- In *respondent (classical) conditioning*, a stimulus (the conditioned stimulus) gains the ability to elicit a response (the conditioned response) through association with a stimulus (the unconditioned stimulus) that already elicits that response. In respondent conditioning, *extinction* is a procedure or condition in which a conditioned stimulus is repeatedly presented without the unconditioned stimulus; this process reduces the strength of the conditioned response or the likelihood that it will occur.

- In *operant conditioning*, consequences change behavior. Positive and negative reinforcement (reward) increase the likelihood that the behavior will occur in the future, whereas punishment decreases the likelihood. In operant conditioning, extinction is the procedure or condition through which reinforcement is ended for a previously reinforced behavior, causing the behavior to decrease in likelihood and vigor. *Shaping* is a method of the differential reinforcement of successive target behavior. (This is discussed in detail in chapter 13.)

These types of learning can occur through direct experience or vicariously, such as by observing the learning experiences of other people—a process called *modeling*. When we see someone act afraid of snakes in a scary movie or see a plumber disassemble a faucet in our home, we may learn these behaviors through modeling. The learning process also establishes a behavior's *antecedents*: cues that precede and set the occasion for the behavior. For instance, if we notice that we are hungry and see appealing food (the antecedents), we reach for it and eat it, which is an operant behavior. For respondent behaviors, the antecedent is the conditioned stimulus. As I will discuss in more detail below, the conditioned response often functions to produce a consequence in everyday life.

Behaviors that are firmly established tend to become *habitual*—that is, they are performed automatically and without awareness, as when we reach absentmindedly for a candy and put it in our mouth. Habitual behaviors become less dependent on the consequences—for example, the reinforcement they receive—and more dependent on the antecedent cues, such as noticing the candy out of the corner of our eyes. The behavior has been linked to this cue in the past. Antecedents can be *overt*—that is, open to or directly observable through our

234

senses—or *covert*: internal and not open to observation. Negative emotions, such as anger or depression, can serve as covert antecedents, leading some people to buy things compulsively (Miltenberger et al., 2003). People often have more difficulty changing habitual behaviors, such as overeating or smoking cigarettes, than nonhabitual ones.

# Techniques for Managing Behavior

To modify a target behavior effectively, the behavior needs to be clearly defined in order to be measured accurately. Only by measuring the target behavior is it possible to determine whether it has changed. Casual observation of the behavior usually does not provide an accurate picture of the behavior's occurrence.

## *Assessing Behavior Change*

To evaluate a self-management program, data must be collected on the behavior's occurrence before and after the program. The data collected before trying to modify the target behavior is called *baseline* data; the term "baseline" also refers to the period of time during which those data are collected. The data collected when trying to modify the behavior is called *intervention* data; the term "intervention" also refers to the period of time during which those data are collected. Self-management programs generally include a baseline phase and an intervention phase, with data on the target behavior collected in each phase.

Because behavior can change in many ways, it is necessary to select the types of data that best reflect both the way you want the behavior to change and progress made toward the behavioral goal. Is the goal to modify how often the behavior occurs, how long it occurs, or how strongly it occurs? These measures form three types of data:

- *Frequency*—the number of times the behavior was observed. This type of data is best when each instance of the target behavior has a clear start and end and takes about the same amount of time to perform.

- *Duration*—how long an instance of the target behavior lasts from start to finish. Examples include measuring the duration of each session of physical exercise, watching TV, or studying.

- *Magnitude*—the intensity, degree, or size of an action or its product. Examples include measuring the loudness of your speech, the strength of an emotion you felt, and the weight of the dumbbells you lifted.

A less frequently used type of data in self-management is *quality*, or how well the target behavior is performed, such as playing a musical instrument or performing athletic skills. Sometimes it is useful and important to collect more than one type of data for a particular target behavior—for instance, you might design a self-management program to increase the frequency, duration, and magnitude of the physical exercise a client performs.

To assess changes in the target behavior, it is helpful to construct a *graph*—a drawing that depicts variations in the data—showing how one variable changes with another variable. A *variable* is a characteristic of people, objects, or events that can vary. The frequency, duration, and magnitude of a behavior are variables, and so is time. For self-management programs, the therapist creates a line graph with two axes: the horizontal (abscissa) line scales time, such as days, and the vertical (ordinate) line scales the target behavior's occurrence. Baseline data are plotted on the left side across time, and intervention data are plotted across time to the right of baseline. If the intervention data show a substantial improvement in the target behavior over its level in baseline, this is a clear sign that the self-management program was successful. For example, in a self-management program to reduce cigarette smoking, the level of the graph in baseline for smoking frequency would be sharply higher than in intervention.

## Assessing the Functions of Behavior

A *functional assessment* is a procedure that helps define the target behavior exactly and identifies connections between the behavior and its antecedents and consequences. The target behavior can be an operant behavior or a respondent behavior. In general, to carry out a functional assessment of a behavior, the client must observe and record each instance of the behavior and the antecedents and consequences she identifies. Several days of observation and record keeping will be needed before or overlapping with the baseline period. Using the information that is collected, the therapist can then determine how to alter the antecedents and consequences that have produced and maintained the behavior in the past. This plan will form the basis for the self-management program.

# Changing Operant Behavior

Behavior learned through operant conditioning follows a standard sequence: one or more antecedents lead to the behavior that produces one or more consequences. To change an operant behavior, the therapist must manage its antecedents and consequences.

## Managing Operant Antecedents

One strategy for managing operant antecedents is to develop or apply new ones. When applying a new antecedent, the appropriate behavior needs to be reinforced when it occurs. Three methods for developing new antecedents are prompting, fading, and modeling. A *prompt* is a stimulus that is added to the desired or normal antecedent for an appropriate behavior, and *prompting* is a procedure that adds the prompt. The function of prompting is to remind a client to perform a behavior he already knows how to do or to help him perform one that he doesn't do often or well enough. Some prompts involve physically guiding a behavior, such as grasping a client's hand to help her apply the frosting design on a fancy cake. Other prompts are verbal, telling a client what to do or not do, such as a sign in the kitchen that says "no snacking." And other prompts are pictorial or auditory, such as a photo of a client when he was slimmer or an alarm that reminds him to stop talking on the phone. Once the normal antecedents lead reliably to the desired behavior, the therapist can use *fading*, a procedure by which prompts are gradually removed. In *modeling*, people learn behaviors by watching someone else perform them.

Other methods to develop or apply new antecedents involve making environmental changes and using cognitive strategies. Because antecedents generally occur in the environment, desirable behavior can be encouraged by making environmental changes in three ways: first, by replacing the old environment with a new one (e.g., moving to a quieter location to study); second, by altering the availability of items that encourage undesirable behavior or discourage desirable behavior (e.g., removing cigarettes for someone trying to quit smoking); third, by *narrowing*, which is limiting the range of situations for an undesirable behavior, such as by limiting the places where or time of day when the behavior is allowed (e.g., reducing the amount of time spent watching TV by limiting the behavior to a specific place and time).

A cognitive strategy to apply as a new antecedent is *self-instruction*, which involves using a statement that helps a client perform a behavior or tells her how to perform it. A self-instruction is similar to a verbal prompt, only it is usually applied covertly. The instructions must be reasonable; a client telling herself that she can perform an impossible feat or that changing her behavior will have far-reaching effects on her life is not believable and will lead to failure.

## Managing the Consequences of Operant Behavior

To change operant behavior in self-management programs, two types of consequences—reinforcement and punishment—can be considered. Reinforcement can be classified as *positive*, which involves introducing or adding a stimulus after the behavior is performed, or *negative*, which involves reducing or removing an existing unpleasant circumstance if an appropriate behavior occurs. Reinforcement is most effective when it occurs immediately after the behavior rather than after a delay. To reduce a behavioral excess, extinction should be used when possible to decrease the likelihood and vigor of the target behavior. The technique of punishment can be used for reducing a behavioral excess, but it can have problematic side effects. Generally, positive reinforcement is the most commonly used and effective consequence in self-management programs and is the type on which I will focus.

When choosing positive reinforcers to apply for changing an operant behavior, it is important to use the ones that have a high level of *reward value*, the degree to which the reward is desirable. The greater the reward value, the more likely it will be to reinforce behavior (Trosclair-Lasserre, Lerman, Call, Addison, & Kodak, 2008). Two dimensions of a reinforcer that affect their reward value are quantity and quality. For example, when using candy as a reinforcer, a large amount and favorite flavor will be more effective than a small amount and merely acceptable flavor. A few types of positive reinforcers that therapists frequently apply in self-management programs include

tangible items, or material objects, such as money, articles of clothing, or musical recordings;

consumable items, or things the client can eat or drink, such as snacks, fruit, or soft drinks;

activities, or things the client likes to do, such as watching TV or checking for e-mail messages; and

tokens, or items that are symbolic of reward, such as tickets, small chips, or check marks on a chart that can be traded for tangible, consumable, or activity rewards.

Tokens have no reward value of their own; they become reinforcers by being associated with the backup reinforcers they can buy. They are useful in making reinforcement immediate, bridging the gap between behaving appropriately and getting the backup reinforcer. One way to select the reinforcers used in a self-management program is to have the client fill out a survey called the "preferred items and experiences questionnaire" (Sarafino & Graham, 2006). It is not advisable to use reinforcers that could work against the behavioral goal, such as using candy as a reward in a program to reduce caloric intake.

Once the reinforcers have been selected, the therapist has to plan how and when to apply them. In self-management programs, reinforcers are usually self-administered. This is convenient, but the reinforcer should not be too easily earned. If the person cannot objectively determine whether the behavior deserves a reward, other people may need to judge whether the reward has been earned. Whenever possible, the reinforcement should be administered immediately after the desired behavior occurs—the longer the delay, the less effective it is likely to be.

# Changing Emotional Behaviors

People learn emotional behaviors, such as avoidance behavior in response to fear, through direct or indirect respondent conditioning. The conditioning is direct when the conditioned stimulus (such as a dog) is paired with an unconditioned stimulus (such as growling and an attack by the dog); the conditioning is indirect when the learning is acquired through modeling, imagining it, or learning from others.

To start a self-management program, the therapist needs to construct a rating scale to assess the intensity of the emotional response. In addition, a functional assessment is needed to identify and describe the antecedents, behavior, and consequences (Emmelkamp, Bouman, & Scholing, 1992). The reason to identify the consequences of the emotional behavior is that respondent and operant conditioning usually occur together in real life—for instance, behaving in a fearful manner may lead to reinforcement, such as getting out of doing chores. The respondent behaviors can be managed by applying behavioral, affective, and cognitive methods.

## *Behavioral Methods for Managing Respondent Behaviors*

Behavioral methods can be useful in a self-management program to reduce an emotional behavior. One method is *extinction*: presenting the conditioned stimulus (for example, a flying insect) without the unconditioned stimulus (stinging) and associated response (pain), thereby weakening the emotion (fear). Fearful people anticipate the possibility of a conditioned stimulus, such as insects that can sting, and avoid situations where these insects might be. As a result, extinction does not occur, and fear persists (Lovibond, Mitchell, Minard, Brady, & Menzies, 2009). A self-management program to reduce fear can discourage avoidance and encourage extinction of the behavior.

Another behavioral method that can reduce emotional behavior is *systematic desensitization*, in which conditioned stimuli are presented while the therapist encourages the person to relax (Wolpe, 1973). To carry out this procedure, the therapist needs to create a list of conditioned stimuli that can elicit various levels of fear (e.g., of stinging insects), and then arrange the list as a *stimulus hierarchy*—that is, the conditioned stimuli are rank ordered, from very mild to very strong, for the intensity of the fear they would elicit. An example of a mild stimulus might be seeing a bee perched on a railing five feet away outside a closed window. A strong stimulus might be standing in a small room with a bee flying around (in this example, the client has enough room to stay away from it). Systematic desensitization combines these exposures with relaxation exercises. For example, the therapist might first present the client with the mildest stimulus in the hierarchy and ask her to rate the intensity of her fear on a rating scale. This series of steps constitutes a "trial" in the procedure. The trial would then be conducted repeatedly until the rating is zero for two successive trials. Then, repeated trials would be performed with the next-strongest stimulus in the hierarchy until the rating is zero for two successive trials. This procedure would continue until all of the stimuli in the hierarchy have been addressed. Reducing a moderately strong fear is likely to take at least several sessions lasting between fifteen and thirty minutes each.

## Affective and Cognitive Methods for Managing Respondent Behaviors

Relaxation techniques, including progressive muscle relaxation and meditation, can be useful for reducing emotional distress. In progressive muscle relaxation, the client may pay attention to bodily sensations while alternately tensing and relaxing specific muscle groups. For instance, the client might repeatedly tense and relax muscles in the arms, followed by muscles in the face, then shoulders, then stomach, and then legs; holding and releasing the breath can be included as well. In meditation sessions (see chapter 26), the client would contemplate or focus attention on an object, event, or idea. For example, he might focus attention on a meditation stimulus, such as a static visual object, spoken sound (a mantra), or his own breathing. After practicing the relaxation technique for many sessions and mastering it, the client can probably shorten the sessions; in meditation, he could simply quit earlier, and in progressive muscle relaxation, he might eliminate or combine certain muscle groups.

Cognitive methods, which modify one's thoughts that serve as antecedents to emotional behavior (see chapter 21), can also be used to reduce emotions and beliefs in self-management programs. For instance, the client might think *I can't protect myself against a bee*, which makes the fear stronger and more likely to occur. To combat this type of thinking, the therapist could instruct the client to make self-statements of two types. First, *coping statements* are declarations the client says to herself that emphasize her ability to tolerate unpleasant situations, such as "Relax, I'm in control because I can move away from the bee." Second, *reinterpretative statements* are things the client says to herself that redefine the circumstance, such as by giving herself a reason to view it differently. For example, she might say, "The bee's not interested in me and won't be as long as I leave it alone." Another cognitive method for reducing fear is distraction, such as shifting attention from a conditioned stimulus that elicits an emotional behavior to other overt or covert stimuli. For instance, if the client sees a bee while outside, she could shift her attention to a beautiful flower or tree.

# Implementation

To maximize the effectiveness of a self-management program, it should include methods to address the target behavior itself, its antecedents, and its consequences. The choice of methods to include in the plan will depend on the answers to two questions:

> Does the target behavior involve operant behavior, respondent behavior, or both?

> Is the program intended to modify a behavioral excess or a behavioral deficit?

For example, positive reinforcement is an essential method to correct an operant behavioral deficit, and extinction and punishment would be useful in decreasing a behavioral excess. The results of the functional assessment should inform the final plan.

## *Finalizing the Plan*

After selecting the techniques to apply, they should be designed to be most effective—for instance, choose reinforcers with high reward value, and make sure the client will not receive reinforcers he hasn't earned. Also, make sure the criteria for reinforcement are neither too stringent, making it unlikely the client will earn enough of them, nor too easy, making it unlikely that his behavior will improve enough to reach the behavioral goal. Suggest that the client involve friends and family, if they want to help.

Prepare the materials needed to carry out the self-management program. You don't want the client to run out of them in the middle of the process; this is especially important if the materials are reinforcers. In addition, it's a good idea to formalize the plan in a behavioral contract, which spells out clearly the target behavior, the conditions in which it should or should not be performed, and the consequences for performing the behavior (Philips, 2005). Have the client write out the contract and sign it; if the client has chosen to enlist the aid of other people to carry out the plan, have the client describe their role in the contract, and then have them sign it, too.

## Implementing the Plan

Collecting data is an essential part of implementing a self-management program. Before trying to change the target behavior, baseline data must be collected so the client can see the starting level of the behavior and compare it with these levels after the intervention begins. Be sure to have clients record each instance of the behavior as soon as it happens; stress that if they wait until later, their memory of it won't be as accurate. This means that clients must have recording materials on hand whenever the behavior could occur. If a client is trying to change a target behavior that occurs absentmindedly, such as cursing or nail-biting, have him devise a procedure that helps him remember to watch for the behavior and record the data. The client should plot the data in a graph during the baseline phase and continue doing so throughout the intervention. Check the graph during the intervention to see whether or not the client's behavior has improved from baseline and continues to improve across the weeks of intervention. If the improvements are not as strong as you or client would like, examine the methods being used and try to make them stronger.

## Maintaining Behavior Changes

People who change their behavior sometimes revert back to their old way of behaving over time. This process starts with a *lapse*, an instance of backsliding, such as when a client who has succeeded at exercising regularly skips a day. The client can probably bounce back from a lapse if she knows that backsliding is common and should be expected. If the client doesn't bounce back, a *relapse* may occur—the undesired behavior returns at its old level, such as not exercising at all. Many methods are available to maintain behavior changes. For example, the therapist can reintroduce parts of the intervention methods, such as prompts or reinforcers, or develop a buddy system in which the client and a friend or relative who has changed a similar behavior keep in touch and provide each other with encouragement and ideas for how to maintain the behavior.

# Summary

Self-management describes methods that individuals can use themselves to increase desirable and decrease undesirable behaviors. These methods are rooted in behavioral and cognitive principles. The most common behavioral principles include classical conditioning, operant conditioning, shaping, and modeling; the most common cognitive principles include self-statements (such as coping and reinterpretative statements) and distraction. Carrying out a self-management plan requires the accurate and frequent assessment of the target behavior, a clear behavioral goal, and a functional assessment of the antecedent and consequences of the target behavior. Self-management programs should be an integral part of many, if not all, treatments of psychological problems.

# References

Emmelkamp, P. M. G., Bouman, T. K., & Scholing, A. (1992). *Anxiety disorders: A practitioner's guide*. Chichester, UK: Wiley.

Lovibond, P. F., Mitchell, C. J., Minard, E., Brady, A., & Menzies, R. G. (2009). Safety behaviors preserve threat beliefs: Protection from extinction of human fear conditioning by an avoidance response. *Behaviour Research and Therapy, 47*(8), 716–720.

Miltenberger, R. G., Redlin, J., Crosby, R., Stickney, M., Mitchell, J., Wonderlich, S., et al. (2003). Direct and retrospective assessment of factors contributing to compulsive buying. *Journal of Behavior Therapy and Experimental Psychiatry, 34*(1), 1–9.

Philips, A. F. (2005). Behavioral contracting. In M. Hersen & J. Rosqvist (Eds.), *Encyclopedia of behavior modification and cognitive behavior therapy: Adult clinical applications* (vol. 1, pp. 106–110). Thousand Oaks, CA: Sage Publications.

Sarafino, E. P. (2011). *Self-management: Using behavioral and cognitive principles to manage your life.* New York: Wiley.

Sarafino, E. P., & Graham, J. A. (2006). Development and psychometric evaluation of an instrument to assess reinforcer preferences: The preferred items and experiences questionnaire. *Behavior Modification, 30*(6), 835–847.

Trosclair-Lasserre, N. M., Lerman, D. C., Call, N. A., Addison, L. R., & Kodak, T. (2008). Reinforcement magnitude: An evaluation of preference and reinforcer efficacy. *Journal of Applied Behavior Analysis, 41*(2), 203–220.

Watson, D. L., & Tharp, R. G. (2014) *Self-directed behavior: Self-modification for personal adjustment* (10th ed.). Belmont, CA: Wadsworth.

Wolpe, J. (1973). *The practice of behavior therapy* (2nd ed.). New York: Pergamon Press.

# CHAPTER 15

# Arousal Reduction

Matthew McKay, PhD

*The Wright Institute, Berkeley, CA*

## Background

The arousal reduction processes covered in this chapter target sympathetic nervous system arousal (Selye, 1955) and can be distinguished from arousal reduction targeting cognitive processes (Beck, 1976), attentional control (Wells, 2011), and decentering/distancing/defusion (Hayes, Strosahl, & Wilson, 2012), which are covered elsewhere in this volume. The history of modern arousal reduction strategies starts in the 1920s, when Jacobson (1929) introduced progressive muscle relaxation (PMR). Since that time, various breathing, muscle release, and visualization exercises have been added for a now complex armamentarium generally termed relaxation training.

In the 1930s, autogenics (Schultz & Luthe, 1959) provided a new form of arousal reduction that relied on *autosuggestion*: those seeking stress relief via autogenics repeat phrases using themes of warmth, heaviness, and other suggestions. Autogenics was practiced for years in Germany, and Kenneth Pelletier (1977) popularized it in the United States.

Mindfulness as a stress reduction technique was introduced in the West in the 1960s by Maharishi Mahesh Yogi (2001) as transcendental meditation, a secular form of which Benson (1997) later popularized and labeled the relaxation response. More recently, mindfulness-based stress reduction was introduced (Kabat-Zinn, 1990); it incorporates meditation and yoga into a stress reduction program taught in six-to-twelve-week classes around the world.

## Applications

Targets for arousal reduction processes include health problems and chronic pain; anger disorders; emotion dysregulation; and the majority of anxiety disorders, such as generalized anxiety disorder (GAD), specific phobia, social anxiety disorder, and post-traumatic stress disorder (PTSD).

## Health

A number of specific health problems associated with high levels of stress, such as hypertension, gastrointestinal disorders, cardiovascular problems, tension headaches, certain immune disorders, and the susceptibility to infection, appear to improve with either mindfulness or relaxation training (e.g., Huguet, McGrath, Stinson, Tougas, & Doucette, 2014; Krantz & McGeney, 2002). Autogenics has been found to reduce symptoms of asthma, gastrointestinal disorders, arrhythmias, hypertension, and tension headaches (e.g., Linden, 1990). In addition, chronic pain associated with lower back injury, fibromyalgia, cancer, irritable bowel syndrome, nerve damage, and other disorders has been treated with mindfulness (Kabat-Zinn, 1990, 2006), relaxation training (Kwekkeboom & Gretarsdottir, 2006), and autogenics (Sadigh, 2001).

## Emotion Disorders

Relaxation strategies are used in dialectical behavior therapy (Linehan, 1993) to target emotion dysregulation and enhance coping efficacy. Relaxation is also a core component of anger management protocols (e.g., Deffenbacher & McKay, 2000).

Perhaps the most extensive applications for relaxation and arousal reduction are for anxiety disorders. Craske and Barlow (2006) include relaxation training in their protocol for GAD, but Barlow (Allen, McHugh, & Barlow, 2008) has since dropped relaxation in his unified protocol for emotional disorders, arguing that it promotes unhealthy affect avoidance. Similarly, relaxation was commonly used in the exposure protocols for phobia (e.g., Bourne, 1998) but has since been found to reduce the extinction effects of exposure treatments (Craske et al., 2008).

Relaxation training for PTSD has had mixed results. Again, although relaxation appears to reduce the effectiveness of both brief and prolonged exposure treatments, it continues to have utility in managing PTSD symptoms, such as emotional volatility and flashbacks (Smyth, 1999).

All in all, while arousal reduction is no longer recommended for exposure—with the possible exception of anger exposure (Deffenbacher & McKay, 2000)—it continues to show utility for emotion regulation (Linehan, 1993) and stress-related health problems.

# Techniques

I recommend the six arousal reduction processes listed below for their research-supported effectiveness as well as the ease with which they can be taught or learned (Davis, Eshelman, & McKay, 2008). Step-by-step methods for teaching them follow:

- Breathing techniques

- PMR and passive relaxation

- Applied relaxation training

- Mindfulness techniques

- Visualization

- Autogenics

## *Breathing Techniques*

**Diaphragmatic breathing.** During periods of stress the diaphragm tightens to prepare for fight or flight (Cannon, 1915), sending a "danger" message to the brain. The object of diaphragmatic breathing is to stretch and relax the diaphragm, thus sending a signal to the brain that all is safe. Diaphragmatic breathing also tends to slow the breath rate, enhancing vagal tone (Hirsch & Bishop, 1981).

To practice this technique, have clients perform these steps:

1. Place one hand on the abdomen just above the belt line, and the other hand on the chest. Press down with the hand on the abdomen.

2. Inhale slowly in such a way that (1) the hand on the abdomen is pushed out, while (2) the hand on the chest remains still. (You should model diaphragmatic breathing while also monitoring the individual's ability to expand the diaphragm.)

If clients have difficulty (e.g., both hands move or the chest hand rises in a herky-jerky movement), you can suggest the following:

- Press harder with the hand on the abdomen.

- Imagine the abdomen to be a balloon that is filling with air.

- Recline (1) facedown, pressing the abdomen into the floor as you breathe, or recline (2) face up with a phone book or similar object draped over the abdomen that you can watch rise and fall.

Diaphragmatic breathing should be practiced five or ten minutes at a time a minimum of three times daily to acquire the skill. Thereafter, in addition to daily practice, encourage clients to use diaphragmatic breathing whenever they notice anxiety or physical tension.

A word of caution: Diaphragmatic breathing has been known to induce hypocapnia, paradoxically increasing anxiety for individuals with anxiety disorders, especially panic. Should this occur, capnometer-assisted breathing retraining (to measure carbon dioxide levels and help slow breath rate) is a viable alternative (Meuret, Rosenfield, Seidel, Bhaskara, & Hofmann, 2010).

**Breath control training.** This technique (Masi, 1993) has been used to slow breathing for relaxation purposes, as well as to manage hyperventilation in panic disorder. Encourage individuals to master the following steps:

1. Exhale deeply.

2. Inhale through the nose for three beats.

3. Exhale through the nose for four beats.

4. Once the pace is comfortably established, breathing can be slowed further: inhale for four beats; exhale for five beats.

5. Practice three times daily for five minutes; once mastered, use the method during stressful situations.

## Progressive Muscle Relaxation and Passive Relaxation

**Progressive muscle relaxation.** After Edmond Jacobson developed PMR in the 1920s, Joseph Wolpe (1958) subsequently borrowed the technique as a component of systematic desensitization, and other behavior therapists used it as an effective arousal reduction strategy. The process targets sympathetic nervous system arousal by reducing tension in motor muscles typically activated in the fight-or-flight stress response. Below is an instructional sequence for basic PMR, adapted from Davis, Eshelman, and McKay (2008).

*Tighten each muscle group for five to seven seconds.*

*Begin to relax as you take a few slow, deep breaths... Now as you let the rest of your body relax, clench your fists and bend them back at the wrist...feel the tension in your fists and forearms... Now relax... Feel the looseness in your hands and forearms... Notice the contrast with the tension... Repeat this, and all succeeding procedures, at least one more time. Now bend your elbows and tense your biceps... Observe the feeling of tautness... Let your hands drop down and relax... Feel that difference... Turn your attention to your head and wrinkle your forehead as tight as you can... Feel the tension in your forehead and scalp. Now relax and smooth it out. Now frown and notice the strain spreading throughout your forehead... Let go. Allow your brow to become smooth again... Squeeze your eyes closed...tighter... Relax your eyes. Now, open your mouth wide and feel the tension in your jaw... Relax your jaw. Notice the contrast between tension and relaxation... Now press your tongue against the roof of your mouth. Experience the strain in the back of your mouth... Relax... Press your lips now, purse them into an O... Relax your lips... Feel the relaxation in your forehead, scalp, eyes, jaw, tongue, and lips... Let go more and more...*

*Now roll your head slowly around on your neck, feeling the point of tension shifting as your head moves...and then slowly roll your head the other way. Relax, allowing your head to return to a comfortable upright position... Now shrug your shoulders; bring your shoulders up toward your ears...hold it... Drop your shoulders back down and feel the relaxation spreading through your neck, throat, and shoulders.*

*Now, tighten your stomach and hold. Feel the tension... Relax... Now place your hand on your stomach. Breathe deeply into your stomach, pushing your hand up. Hold... and relax... Feel the sensations of relaxation as the air rushes out... Now arch your back, without straining. Keep the rest of your body as relaxed as possible. Focus on the tension in your lower back... Now relax... Let the tension dissolve away.*

*Tighten your buttocks and thighs... Relax and feel the difference... Now straighten and tense your legs and curl your toes downward. Experience the tension... Relax... Straighten and tense your legs and bend your toes toward your face. Relax.*

*Feel the warmth and heaviness of deep relaxation throughout your entire body as you continue to breathe slowly and deeply.*

During PMR training, it's important to inquire what relaxation feels like for each muscle group. Do the muscles feel heavy, tingly, warm, and so forth?

Requiring clients to observe the relaxation experience will help them differentiate between tense and relaxed states. It will also facilitate the passive relaxation procedure explained later in this section.

Some individuals resist the above instructional sequence, finding it overly long and burdensome. If that's the case, introduce them to this shorthand version that takes less than five minutes.

- *Strongman pose:* Curl fists; tighten biceps and forearms. Hold for seven seconds, then relax. Repeat. Notice the feeling of relaxation.

- *Face like a walnut:* Frown; tighten eyes, cheeks, jaw, neck, and shoulders. Hold for seven seconds, then relax. Repeat. Notice the feeling of relaxation.

- *Head roll:* Roll head clockwise in a complete circle, then reverse.

- *Back like a bow:* Stretch shoulders backward while gently arching the back. Hold for seven seconds, then relax. Repeat. Notice the feeling of relaxation.

- *Take two:* Diaphragmatic breaths.

- *Head to toe:* Pull toes back toward the head while tightening the calves, thighs, and buttocks. Hold for seven seconds, then relax.

- *Ballerina pose:* Point toes while tensing the calves, thighs, and buttocks. Hold for seven seconds, then relax. Notice the feeling of relaxation.

**Passive relaxation.** This procedure, also known as passive tensing or relaxation without tension, follows the same sequence and relaxes the same muscle groups as the shorthand PMR. Instruct individuals to observe each target muscle group, noticing any areas of tension. Then have them take a deep, diaphragmatic breath. Just as they begin to exhale, they should say to themselves, "Relax," and proceed to relax away any tension in the target area. Each step should be repeated once, and individuals should be encouraged to seek the feeling of relaxation they achieved in PMR.

While most people are understandably reluctant to do the longer version of PMR in any public place, passive relaxation has the advantage that it can be done without anyone noticing, so it can be used anywhere. Furthermore, a client can streamline the procedure to focus on a single muscle group that habitually holds tension.

# Applied Relaxation Training

Öst (1987) developed applied relaxation training to rapidly relax severely phobic individuals, as well as people suffering from nonspecific stress disorders and sleep onset insomnia. The greatest advantage of Öst's method is that it provides fast stress relief. While applied relaxation takes several weeks of practice to learn, the technique itself can significantly reduce arousal in a minute or two.

*Step 1, PMR:* The training process begins with PMR—use of the shorthand version is recommended. This should be practiced three times daily for at least a week.

*Step 2, passive relaxation:* This technique should be practiced exclusively for another week. Encourage individuals to make sure each muscle group feels deeply relaxed before moving to the next target group. Furthermore, instruct them to notice if tension begins to creep back into previously relaxed muscles. If so, these should be relaxed again.

*Step 3, cue controlled relaxation:* This procedure should be initiated only after passive relaxation has been mastered. In fact, each cue controlled practice session begins with passive relaxation. Afterward, while in a state of deep muscle release, the focus shifts to the breath. While breathing deeply and regularly, individuals should now say to themselves "breathe in" as they inhale, and "relax" as they let go of the breath. Encourage them to let the word "relax" crowd every other thought from the mind, while each breath brings a deeper sense of calm and peace. Cue controlled breathing should continue for at least five minutes during each (twice-daily) practice session.

*Step 4, rapid relaxation:* For this technique, individuals choose a special relaxation cue—ideally something they see fairly often throughout the day. Examples might be a wristwatch, the hallway to the bathroom, a particular mirror or art object, and so on. Each time the cue object is noticed, instruct them to follow this sequence:

- Take deep breaths using the "breathe in/relax" mantra.

- Scan the body for tension, focusing on muscles that need to relax.

- Empty the target muscles of tension with each out-breath; progressively relax away tightness in every affected area of the body.

The goal is to use rapid relaxation fifteen times a day so individuals can train themselves to relax while in natural, nonstressful situations. If they don't see their relaxation cue often enough, they should add one or more cues until they reach fifteen practice opportunities a day.

*Step 5, applied relaxation:* The last stage of the training introduces using rapid relaxation in the face of threatening situations. Individuals will use the same techniques outlined above. They'll watch for their own physiological signs of stress—rapid heartbeat, neck tension, feeling hot, stomach knots, and so on—and use these as cues to initiate applied relaxation. Immediately upon noticing a cue, they will

- take deep breaths, saying to themselves "breathe in," and then "relax";

- scan the body for tension; and

- concentrate on relaxing *the muscles that aren't currently needed.*

Since a stress cue can occur at any time—while standing, sitting, walking—the focus must be on releasing tension in muscle groups not currently active. If one is standing, tension might be released in the chest, arms, shoulders, and face; if one is sitting, tension could be relaxed in the legs, abdomen, arms, and face.

Öst's relaxation procedure offers a versatile intervention to clinicians because it can be used anytime, anywhere—no matter what the current activity might be.

## Mindfulness Techniques

Mindfulness is a component of many newer behavior therapies (mindfulness-based stress reduction, acceptance and commitment therapy, dialectical behavior therapy, mindfulness-based cognitive therapy, and others). The common goal is to increasingly free individuals from a focus on the past and future—the source of rumination and worry—and anchor their awareness in the present moment (Kabat-Zinn, 1990, 2006). In essence, mindfulness processes initiate attention reallocation, from future threats or past losses and failures to present-moment sensory experience, and from cognitive processes to specific sensations.

**Body scan meditation.** This simple, present-moment exercise encourages individuals to nonjudgmentally observe inner sensations in the body—from toe to head. The following script, adapted from Davis, Eshelman, and McKay (2008), typifies the body scan process:

1.  Begin by becoming aware of the rising and falling of your breath in your chest and belly. You can ride the waves of your breath and let it begin to anchor you to the present moment.

2.  Bring your attention to the soles of your feet. Notice any sensation that is present there. Without judging or trying to make it different, simply observe the sensation. After a few moments imagine that your breath is flowing into the soles of your feet. As you breathe in and out you might experience an opening or softening and a release of tension. Just simply observe.

3.  Now bring your attention to the rest of your feet, up to your ankles. Become aware of any sensation in this part of your body. After a few moments imagine that your breath flows all the way down to your feet. Breathe into and out of your feet, simply noticing the sensations.

4.  Proceed up your body in this manner—lower legs, knees, thighs, pelvis, hips, buttocks, lower back, upper back, chest and belly, upper shoulders, neck, head, and face. Take your time to really feel each body part and notice whatever sensations are present, without forcing them or trying to make them be different. Breathe into each body area and let go of it as you move on to the next area.

5.  Notice any part of your body that has pain, tension, or discomfort. Simply be with the sensations in a nonjudgmental way. As you breathe, imagine your breath opening up any tight muscles or painful areas and creating more spaciousness. As you breathe out, imagine the tension or pain flowing out of that part of your body.

6.  When you reach the top of your head, scan your body one last time for any areas of tension or discomfort. Then imagine that you have a breath hole at the top of your head, much like the blowholes that whales or dolphins use to breathe. Breathe in from the top of your head, bringing your breath all the way down to the soles of your feet and then back up again through your whole body. Allow your breath to wash away any tension or uncomfortable sensations.

**Breath counting meditation.** This classic vipassana meditation has three components:

1. Observe the breath. This can be done either by sensing or watching the breathing process (cool air down the back of the throat, ribs and diaphragm expanding, etc.) or focusing attention on the moving diaphragm itself.

2. Count the breath. Each out-breath is counted, up to either four or ten, and the process is repeated for a set period of time. Thich Nhat Hahn (1989) suggests a simple alternative: just noting "in" on the in-breath and "out" on the out-breath.

3. As a thought arises, simply note the thought—perhaps saying to oneself, "thought"—and return to observing the breath.

When teaching this process, emphasize that thoughts will inevitably arise; this isn't a failure or mistake because the mind doesn't like to be empty. The object of this meditation is to notice thoughts as soon as possible, and then return attention to the breath.

**Mindfulness in daily life.** Attending to the present moment is a practice that individuals can develop by focusing on sensations associated with a particular daily experience:

- *Mindful walking* can include observing or counting one's strides and noticing sensations in the legs and swaying arms, the feeling of air moving against the face, the pressure of the feet against the ground, and so forth. When thoughts arise, attention is gently brought back to these physical sensations.

- *Mindful drinking* can include noticing the feeling of heat on one's hands, steam on the face, hot liquid touching the lips and tongue and passing down the back of the throat, and so on. Again, as thoughts arise, attention is redirected to the drinking experience.

- Additional mindful exercises can include brushing teeth, eating cereal, eating fruit, washing dishes, showering, driving, exercising, and many others. A new mindful activity should be added each week until a client has developed a substantial daily repertoire of such experiences.

## Visualization

Visualization processes induce attention reallocation, from fight or flight sensations and related cognitive processes to nonthreatening images that signal the parasympathetic nervous system to release tension. The most common imagery-based relaxation exercise is the special (or safe) place visualization (Achterberg, Dossey, & Kolkmeier, 1994; Siegel, 1990). It has been used extensively for arousal reduction, as well as for the management of extreme stress reactions following PTSD exposure trials.

Encourage individuals to select a place where they have felt safe and peaceful. It could be a beautiful beach, a mountain meadow, or a childhood bedroom where they were happy. If no such real place exists, encourage them to create a fictional but safe and relaxed environment. Some people, particularly those with an abuse history, may create images with extraordinary built-in protections. One sexually abused woman, for example, developed a safe place at the beach—but with thirty-foot walls, topped with glass shards, extending far out into the ocean.

Once the visualization has been selected, encourage individuals to fill in the details, including visual (shapes, colors, objects), auditory (voices, ambient sounds), and kinesthetic (sense of temperature, texture, weight, pressure) imagery. It's crucial to use the three sensory modalities noted above so the image will be rich enough to impact arousal level. Now lead several rehearsals of the special place visualization, taking stress readings (zero to ten) before and after to verify effectiveness. Encourage twice-daily practice sessions for the next week to achieve mastery.

The special place visualization can be combined with other relaxation exercises for an additive effect. Augmenting techniques can include diaphragmatic breathing, passive relaxation (focused on a particular tense muscle group), cue controlled relaxation, and others. For example, while conjuring a peaceful meadow, individuals may also be taking deep breaths or relaxing tension in the shoulder region.

## Autogenics

The autogenic technique targets the sympathetic adrenal system and vagal tone using autosuggestion to create deep relaxation. The following autogenic verbal formulas were developed and combined into five sets to reduce stress and normalize key body functions.

## SET 1

*My right arm is heavy.*

*My left arm is heavy.*

*Both of my arms are heavy.*

*My right leg is heavy.*

*My left leg is heavy.*

*Both of my legs are heavy.*

*My arms and legs are heavy.*

## SET 2

*My right arm is warm.*

*My left arm is warm.*

*Both of my arms are warm.*

*My right leg is warm.*

*My arms and legs are warm.*

## SET 3

*My right arm is heavy and warm.*

*Both of my arms are heavy and warm.*

*Both of my legs are heavy and warm.*

*My arms and legs are heavy and warm.*

*It breathes me.*

*My heartbeat is calm and regular.*

## SET 4

*My right arm is heavy and warm.*

*My arms and legs are heavy and warm.*

*It breathes me.*

*My heartbeat is calm and regular.*

*My solar plexus is warm.*

## SET 5

*My right arm is heavy and warm.*

*My arms and legs are heavy and warm.*

*It breathes me.*

*My heartbeat is calm and regular.*

*My solar plexus is warm.*

*My arms and legs are warm.*

*My forehead is cool.*

Individuals should learn one set at a time. The sets can be either recorded or memorized. It's generally recommended that clients practice twice daily and to give them a week to master each set. Because each set includes themes from previous sets, there's no need to repeat previous sets—the set an individual is working on can be his or her entire focus. (Other autogenic formulas for calming the mind and specific physical conditions are available; see Davis et al., 2008).

The guidelines for practicing autogenics are as follows:

- Close the eyes.

- Repeat each formula (suggestion) four times, saying it slowly (silently), and pausing a few seconds between formulas.

- While repeating a formula, individuals should "passively concentrate" on the part of the body it targets. This means staying alert to the experience without analyzing it.

- When the mind wanders—as is natural—attention should be returned to the formula as soon as possible.

- Symptoms of "autogenic discharge" (tingling, electric currents, involuntary movements, changes in perceived weight or temperature, etc.) are normal and transitory. Individuals are encouraged to note them and return to the formula.

# Choosing a Relaxation Protocol

People inevitably prefer some arousal reduction techniques over others, so it's advisable to teach four to five so they can decide what works best. For nonspecific stress, start with breathing techniques, including the breath counting meditation, and proceed to muscle relaxation and (to increase choices) visualization.

If an individual suffers significant health problems that are influenced by stress, begin with relaxation processes that directly target muscle tension—PMR, autogenics, or the body scan. For chronic pain and problems with specific muscle groups, try PMR (if tolerated) and, ultimately, passive relaxation, as well as the body scan meditation. If rumination or worry are part of the clinical picture, you could include mindfulness exercises to quiet mental activity.

Individuals who are beset with stress at work or in other public places are best served with applied relaxation training because it can be used in virtually any circumstance and quickly impacts arousal levels. Problems with emotion dysregulation, including GAD, can be treated with breathing techniques (diaphragmatic breathing, applied relaxation, and the breath counting meditation). Start by having the client use the breath counting meditation at regular intervals throughout the day to reduce baseline arousal. Then introduce either diaphragmatic breathing or applied relaxation for use during acute upsurges in emotion. The special place visualization can be used adjunctively for virtually any target problem, but it can be especially helpful with anxiety-based stress.

## Dose Considerations

Most relaxation techniques require two or three daily practice sessions—for at least a week—for mastery. Techniques designed to reduce general arousal (PMR, mindfulness, autogenics, special place visualization) should be scheduled at regular intervals throughout the day (tied to events like use of the restroom, or signaled by a smartphone alarm). Once mastered, techniques designed to address unpredictable surges in stress (diaphragmatic breathing, applied relaxation, and passive relaxation) can be used whenever the stress symptoms arise.

## Paradoxical Reactions

Some individuals, particularly people with trauma histories, will paradoxically respond to relaxation training with anxiety and hypervigilance. This is particularly true with PMR and some breathing exercises. When this happens, the best approach is to switch to a different arousal reduction strategy (autogenics and mindfulness are sometimes better tolerated), or titrate the relaxation dose, starting with ten to twenty seconds and increasing in small increments.

## References

Achterberg, J., Dossey, B. M., & Kolkmeier, L. (1994). *Rituals of healing: Using imagery for health and wellness.* New York: Bantam Books.

Allen, L. B., McHugh, R. K., & Barlow, D. (2008). Emotional disorders: A unified protocol. In D. Barlow (Ed.), *Clinical handbook of psychological disorders: A step-by-step treatment manual* (4th ed., pp. 216–249). New York: Guilford Press.

Beck, A. T. (1976). *Cognitive therapy and the emotional disorders.* New York: International Universities Press.

Benson, H. (1997). *Timeless healing: The power and biology of belief.* New York: Scribner.

Bourne, E. (1998). *Overcoming specific phobia: A hierarchy and exposure-based protocol for the treatment of all specific phobias.* Oakland, CA: New Harbinger Publications.

Cannon, W. (1915). *Bodily changes in pain, hunger, fear and rage: An account of recent researches into the function of emotional excitement*. New York: D. Appleton.

Craske, M. G., & Barlow, D. H. (2006). *Mastery of your anxiety and worry* (2nd ed.). New York: Oxford University Press.

Craske, M. G., Kircanski, K., Zelikowsky, M., Mystkowski, J., Chowdhury, N., & Baker, A. (2008). Optimizing inhibitory learning during exposure therapy. *Behaviour Research and Therapy, 46*(1), 5–27.

Davis, M., Eshelman, E. R., & McKay, M. (2008). *The relaxation and stress reduction workbook*. Oakland, CA: New Harbinger Publications.

Deffenbacher, J. L., & McKay, M. (2000). *Overcoming situational and general anger: A protocol for the treatment of anger based on relaxation, cognitive restructuring, and coping skills training*. Oakland, CA: New Harbinger Publications.

Hayes, S. C., Strosahl, K. D., & Wilson, K. G. (2012). *Acceptance and commitment therapy: The process and practice of mindful change* (2nd ed.). New York: Guilford Press.

Hirsch, J. A., & Bishop, B. (1981). Respiratory sinus arrhythmia in humans: How breathing pattern modulates heart rate. *American Journal of Physiology, 241*(4), H620–H629.

Huguet, A., McGrath, P. J., Stinson, J., Tougas, M. E., & Doucette, S. (2014). Efficacy of psychological treatment for headaches: An overview of systematic reviews and analysis of potential modifiers of treatment efficacy. *Clinical Journal of Pain, 30*(4), 353–369.

Jacobson, E. (1929). *Progressive relaxation*. Chicago: University of Chicago Press.

Kabat-Zinn, J. (1990). *Full catastrophe living: Using the wisdom of your body and mind to face stress, pain, and illness*. New York: Delacorte Press.

Kabat-Zinn, J. (2006). *Coming to our senses: Healing ourselves and the world through mindfulness*. New York: Hyperion.

Krantz, D. S., & McGeney, M. K. (2002). Effects of psychological and social factors on organic disease: A critical assessment of research on coronary heart disease. *Annual Review of Psychology, 53*(1), 341–369.

Kwekkeboom, K. O., & Gretarsdottir, E. (2006). Systematic review of relaxation interventions for pain. *Journal of Nursing Scholarship, 38*(3), 269–277.

Linden, W. (1990). *Autogenics training: A clinical guide*. New York: Guilford Press.

Linehan, M. M. (1993). *Cognitive behavioral treatment of borderline personality disorder*. New York: Guilford Press.

Mahesh Yogi, M. (2001). *Science of being and art of living: Transcendental meditation*. New York: Plume.

Masi, N. (1993). *Breath of life*. Plantation, FL: Resource Warehouse. Audio recording.

Meuret, A. E., Rosenfield, D., Seidel, A., Bhaskara, L., & Hofmann, S. G. (2010). Respiratory and cognitive mediators of treatment change in panic disorder: Evidence for intervention specificity. *Journal of Consulting and Clinical Psychology, 78*(5), 691–704.

Nhat Hahn, T. (1989). *The miracle of mindfulness: A manual on meditation*. Boston: Beacon Press.

Öst, L.-G. (1987). Applied relaxation: Description of a coping technique and review of controlled studies. *Behaviour Research and Therapy, 25*(5), 397–409.

Pelletier, K. R. (1977). *Mind as healer, mind as slayer: A holistic approach to preventing stress disorders*. New York: Delta.

Sadigh, M. R. (2001). *Autogenic training: A mind-body approach to the treatment of fibromyalgia and chronic pain syndrome*. Binghamton, NY: Haworth Medical Press.

Schultz, J. H., & Luthe, W. (1959). *Autogenic training*. New York: Grune and Stratton.

Selye, H. (1955). Stress and disease. *Science, 122*(3171), 625–631.

Siegel, B. S. (1990). *Love, medicine, and miracles: Lessons learned about self-healing from a surgeon's experience with exceptional patients*. New York: Harper and Row.

Smyth, L. D. (1999). *Overcoming post-traumatic stress disorder: a cognitive-behavioral exposure-based protocol for the treatment of PTSD and other anxiety disorders*. Oakland, CA: New Harbinger Publications.

Wells, A. (2011). *Metacognitive therapy for anxiety and depression*. New York: Guilford Press.

Wolpe, J. (1958). *Psychotherapy by reciprocal inhibition*. Stanford, CA: Stanford University Press.

# CHAPTER 16

# Coping and Emotion Regulation

Amelia Aldao, PhD
Andre J. Plate, BS
*Department of Psychology, The Ohio State University*

## Definitions and Background

*Emotion regulation* is the process by which individuals modify the intensity and/or duration of their emotions in order to respond to the various challenges posed by the environment (e.g., Gross, 1998). This construct stems from the coping literature, specifically that of emotion-focused coping (Lazarus & Folkman, 1984). Since the publication of Gross's process model of emotion regulation in 1998, there has been an exponential growth in the study of emotion regulation strategies in basic (Webb, Miles, & Sheeran, 2012) and clinical research (Aldao, Nolen-Hoeksema, & Schweizer, 2010). Two commonly discussed regulation strategies are *cognitive reappraisal* (i.e., reinterpreting thoughts or situations in order to change the intensity and/or duration of emotional experiences; see chapter 21) and *acceptance* (i.e., experiencing thoughts, emotions, and physiological sensations in the present moment and observing them in a nonjudgmental way; see chapter 24). Clients can sometimes encounter difficulties when seeking to implement these emotion regulation strategies in their everyday lives, however, in part because their effectiveness varies as a function of context (e.g., Aldao, 2013).

## Reappraisal and Acceptance

The idea that specifically changing the way we think can alter our emotional experiences was conceptualized by Aaron Beck in the early 1960s as he began to formalize his highly influential cognitive therapy for depression (A. T. Beck, 1964). Through cognitive restructuring and reappraisal, the client is encouraged to modify maladaptive thinking by critically evaluating the evidence for and against an automatic thought or overarching belief, and by generating cognitive alternatives. Studies have found that reappraisal increases from pre- to post-treatment (Mennin, Fresco, Ritter, & Heimberg, 2015), and that these changes mediate improvement following treatment (Goldin et al., 2012).

A growing number of practitioners and researchers have focused on the importance of *accepting*, rather than changing, difficult emotions, physical sensations, or other experiences. For example, acceptance and commitment therapy (ACT; Hayes, Strosahl, & Wilson, 1999) is based on the idea that avoiding emotional experience tends to be toxic, especially when it becomes fixed across contexts (i.e., disconnected from long-term values), fostering a pattern of psychological inflexibility that may lead to the onset, maintenance, and/or exacerbation of psychopathology. For instance, a person who drinks alcohol after work every day may do so to reduce tension, to increase pleasurable feelings, or both. Regardless of context, this person may more readily engage in behavioral patterns (i.e., drinking) that conflict with his personal values (e.g., being emotionally available to his spouse and children). ACT and related therapies, such as dialectical behavior therapy (Linehan, 1993), teach acceptance skills that in this instance may help the client experience alcohol cravings with openness and curiosity, without having to act on them. Acceptance skills are readily increased from pre- to post-treatment, and these changes commonly mediate long-term clinical improvement (e.g., Gifford et al., 2011).

By teaching reappraisal and acceptance, a clinician might help a woman suffering from generalized anxiety disorder and depression increase her awareness of the presence and function of her distressing emotions and worries. Doing so might help her notice that her experience of anxiety is characterized by specific patterns of thinking (e.g., worrying), physiological sensations (e.g., muscle tension), and maladaptive behaviors (e.g., irritability, rigid avoidance of situations that elicit anxiety). By developing awareness and acceptance of emotional experiences, she might be better equipped to adopt flexible patterns of thinking later on in treatment. For example, she might come to view her worries as merely thoughts that she can detach from or feelings that are temporary and will pass with time. She might also nonjudgmentally acknowledge her muscle tension as a bodily sensation that is uncomfortable, yet not harmful. This, in turn, might reduce her avoidance, enhance her abilities to reappraise her maladaptive cognitions, and increase her engagement in long-term adaptive behaviors.

It is worth noting, however, that teaching these emotion regulation strategies to clients can be challenging. It is particularly common for clients to easily learn to implement reappraisal and/or acceptance within therapy sessions but then struggle when utilizing them in response to real-life stressors. In order to effectively teach clients to use emotion regulation strategies flexibly in their everyday lives—and, consequently, enhance the effectiveness of cognitive behavioral approaches—it becomes essential that we help clients generalize learning from the therapy room to the outside world. To that end, we turn to the latest work in the field of affective science, which has increasingly focused on the contextual factors that regulate the use and impact of emotion regulation strategies (e.g., Aldao, 2013; Aldao, Sheppes, & Gross, 2015; Kashdan & Rottenberg, 2010).

# The Role of Context

There are two main sources of contextual variability that might shed light on the general use of regulation strategies. First, each strategy (e.g., reappraisal, acceptance) can be implemented in different ways by employing a wide range of regulatory tactics, such as focusing on positive aspects of the situation, reconceptualizing future consequences, distancing from the situation, and even accepting aspects of the experience (McRae, Ciesielski, & Gross, 2012). We refer to this as *regulatory drift*. Second, a given strategy might have different functions in each context. We refer to this as *multifinality*.

## *Regulatory Drift*

Meta-analytic findings suggest that even small variations in how a strategy is implemented can have diverging consequences on affect (Webb et al., 2012). In this respect, Webb and colleagues identified three types of reappraisal commonly given as instructions in laboratory studies: (1) reappraising the emotional stimulus (e.g., reinterpreting a negative situation to view it more positively), (2) reappraising the emotional response (e.g., reframing an emotional reaction to minimize its negative consequences), and (3) adopting a different perspective (e.g., observing emotions and events from a third-person perspective or detaching from one's thoughts through cognitive defusion). Each of these reappraisals produced differential effects on emotional arousal. For example, reappraising the emotional stimulus was more effective at reducing emotional outcomes than reappraising the emotional response.

Individuals who suffer from psychopathology tend to experience difficulty recognizing that different situations might call for different regulatory goals (e.g., Ehring & Quack, 2010). Clients tend to have difficulty identifying and labeling their emotions (e.g., Vine & Aldao, 2014), which may reduce their awareness of what emotions might need to be regulated in the first place. This may help explain why problems in emotional identification are associated with a variety of maladaptive behaviors, such as binge drinking, aggression, and self-injury (Kashdan, Barrett, & McKnight, 2015). Lastly, even when clients are aware of the goals of a situation and the emotions experienced there, they may still drift toward utilizing regulation strategies that provide quick and easy short-term relief, even if it comes at the expense of longer-term outcomes (e.g., Aldao et al., 2015; Barlow, 2002; Hayes, Luoma, Bond, Masuda, & Lillis, 2006). For example, a client with obsessive-compulsive disorder might learn to reappraise her contamination concerns about touching the subway handrails from "I touched something dirty. I'm going to contract a disease" to "I touched something dirty but the chances of me actually contracting a disease are very low." Doing so would allow her to embrace uncertainty. However, when the subway train suddenly speeds up, throws her off balance, and she needs to grasp onto the railing so that she does not fall, she might drift toward using a more maladaptive form of reappraisal. She may respond to her obsessional thoughts by saying, "I touched something dirty and contaminated, but my friend is here, so as long as I ask for reassurance that I won't contract a disease, then I will be safe." This type of reappraisal might result in a similar reduction of anxiety in the short term as the first one, but over time it will result in the mistaken belief that the client needs to depend on a friend and engage in reassurance seeking (e.g., maladaptive safety behaviors) that may preclude opportunities for corrective learning (i.e., that touching the handrail does not mean she will contract an illness). It is worth noting, however, that the use of safety behaviors might not always be detrimental (e.g., Rachman, Radomsky, & Shafran, 2008), which suggests that conducting a careful functional analysis of their long-term consequences—and potential for interfering with values—is essential.

## Multifinality

A given strategy has different functional relationships with emotional, cognitive, and behavioral outcomes in different contexts—what is called *multifinality* (Nolen-Hoeksema & Watkins, 2011). For example, social stressors may alter the link between stress and adaptive emotion regulation. This is not surprising given that a substantial amount of emotion regulation happens in relation to other people (e.g., Hofmann, 2014; Zaki & Williams, 2013). For example, in a recent study we found that the use of reappraisal by adolescents was associated with flexible physiological reactivity (i.e., vagal withdrawal) in response to stress *only* with high levels of interpersonal stressors (i.e., peer victimization). When interpersonal stressors were low, reappraisal was associated with maladaptive physiological responding (Christensen, Aldao, Sheridan, & McLaughlin, 2015). In another study, reappraisal was associated with reduced depression symptoms *only* when participants were experiencing uncontrollable stressors. If stressors were controllable, the use of reappraisal led to higher levels of depression (Troy, Shallcross, & Mauss, 2013).

In addition, there is evidence suggesting that the link between acceptance and mental health might be a function of context. Shallcross, Troy, Boland, and Mauss (2010) found that when community participants reported experiencing high levels of stress, their habitual use of acceptance was associated with marginally lower levels of depression symptoms four months later. For participants reporting low levels of stress, there was no association between acceptance and depression symptoms.

If the usefulness of a given strategy hinges on the particular context in which it is implemented (e.g., Aldao, 2013), it may be important to match strategies to a given type of situation (e.g., Cheng, Lau, & Chan, 2014). Clients might experience difficulties with this matching for a number of reasons. As we discussed above, it is possible that they might have a difficult time identifying the goals of a situation and/or the emotions they experience and, consequently, which regulation strategy to use. In addition, they might perseverate and use the same strategy across vastly different contexts. It is possible that clients might perseverate when *selecting* which strategies to use. In this respect, one recent study with a sample of firefighters found that lower levels of switching between strategies (reappraisal, distraction) as a function of various emotional intensities (low, high) was associated with a positive relationship between trauma exposure and PTSD symptoms. That is, in participants with low regulatory flexibility, the link between trauma and symptoms was strong. Conversely, in participants with greater regulatory flexibility, such a link was nonexistent (Levy-Gigi et al., 2016). Thus, these findings suggest that regulatory flexibility might be a critical factor underlying the relationship between exposure to trauma and experience of psychological symptoms.

Perhaps this low regulatory flexibility involving reappraisal might be the result of individuals having low confidence in their ability to effectively modify emotions. In this respect, a recent study found that in the context of a social stressor, healthy participants who were told that emotions were malleable were more likely to spontaneously use reappraisal than those who were told that emotions were not malleable (Kneeland, Nolen-Hoeksema, Dovidio, & Gruber, 2016).

It is also likely that clients might have inflexibility even when explicitly instructed to use different regulation strategies. In this respect, Bonanno and colleagues have shown that individuals with psychological disorders (e.g., trauma, complicated grief) have a difficult time following instructions to enhance or suppress their facial expressions in response to emotion-eliciting pictures (e.g., Bonanno, 2004; Gupta & Bonanno, 2010).

Clients might further have difficulty incorporating feedback about their utilization of regulation strategies. A recent study examined switching from reappraisal to distraction in response to viewing pictures that were emotionally evocative. It found that when participants were highly responsive to internal feedback (defined as high corrugator activity, which reflects frowning) while viewing the pictures in trials in which they ultimately switched strategies, more switching was associated with higher life satisfaction. Conversely, when participants were less responsive to internal feedback, more switching was linked to lower life satisfaction (Birk & Bonanno, 2016). In other words, switching that was based on internal feedback was linked with high life satisfaction, whereas switching that was loosely coupled with feedback (i.e., was haphazard) was associated with low life satisfaction. These findings underscore the importance of incorporating meaningful information about the environment and our reactions to it before making regulatory choices. Thus, psychopathology is linked to difficulties identifying and labeling emotional reactions (e.g., Vine & Aldao, 2014) and physical sensations (e.g., Olatunji & Wolitzky-Taylor, 2009).

# Teaching Emotion Regulation Flexibility

Based on the affective science research reviewed above, in this section we provide a series of recommendations for helping clients enhance their regulatory flexibility and generalize what they learn in psychotherapy to their own lives outside the therapy room.

The first step is to track how varying emotions, thoughts, goals, and affective and behavioral outcomes characterize different situations. It is essential to help clients balance short- and long-term outcomes of emotion regulation. Otherwise, they might drift toward utilizing strategies that provide immediate relief but might interfere with their long-term functioning. To do this, it can be helpful to modify the "daily dysfunctional thought record" (A. T. Beck, 1979; J. S. Beck, 2011) and turn it into an "emotion regulation map"; this worksheet (provided at the end of the chapter) can help clients become more aware of their emotional reactions and subsequent consequences. We recommend starting with the following columns for this map: (1) situation description, (2) emotions experienced (both helpful and unhelpful) and their intensity, (3) regulation strategies used, (4) short-term outcomes of regulation, and (5) long-term outcomes of regulation. You can also use this emotion regulation map to set up exercises to help your clients flexibly regulate their emotions (see also Aldao et al., 2015). Here are a few flexibility techniques to develop this map.

**Practice different types of reappraisals.** The classic daily dysfunctional thought record (A. T. Beck, 1979) contains a series of questions that clients can ask themselves in order to reappraise distorted thoughts (e.g., "What is the evidence that this thought is true?" and "Are there any alternative explanations that may be more helpful and realistic ways of thinking?"). These questions can help clients to create their personalized emotion regulation map by responding to *each* maladaptive thought.

**Practice different types of acceptance.** Encourage clients to practice accepting and learning from different experiential aspects of difficult situations, such as bodily sensations, behavioral urges, memories, or emotions. For example, clients may sit with unpleasant physiological sensations with dispassionate curiosity, not seeking to change or manipulate them, but then shift to memories those sensations bring to mind (see chapter 24).

**Regulate a wide range of emotions.** Repeat the previous steps with emotional situations that are less problematic for clients. For example, you can ask clients who are primarily anxious, and who experience low levels of anger, to reappraise and accept anger-eliciting situations. This too will facilitate the growth of their repertoire of strategies across many different areas of their lives that elicit emotional responses.

**Counterregulate.** Most of the time, clients want to be able to down-regulate negative emotions and up-regulate the positive ones. However, this reflects a narrow approach to emotion regulation. At times, it can be quite helpful to increase negative emotions (e.g., increase anger to be assertive during communication) and/or to reduce positive ones (e.g., resist the temptation to laugh during a serious work meeting; e.g., Tamir, Mitchell, & Gross, 2008). Thus, it is important to practice up- and down-regulating all kinds of emotions.

**Regulate across social contexts.** Given the evidence suggesting that social stressors are particularly important moderators of emotion regulation and adaptive functioning (e.g., Christensen et al., 2015; Troy et al., 2013), and the recent work linking rigid interpersonal emotion regulation to psychopathology (e.g., Hofmann, 2014; Hofmann, Carpenter, & Curtiss, 2016), you can ask clients to practice different emotion regulation strategies in contexts that vary in the amount of social stress they produce. You can also ask them to recruit friends and/or family to help them implement certain forms of strategies in certain contexts. Although eventually clients need to regulate on their own, this type of social scaffolding might be particularly helpful in the early stages of treatment. It might also be useful for clients to identify whether certain individuals and/or relationships make them more or less likely to implement different forms of regulation. In addition, it might be helpful for them to identify whether they rely too much on a given individual or type of interaction. This might be indicative of an inflexible safety behavior.

**Switching among strategies.** Encourage clients to set up experiments in which they try out an emotion regulation strategy that, based on their regulation map, might not work as well in a given situation. Ask them to select another strategy from their repertoire and to repeat the experiment using the new strategy. Does this new strategy produce similar or different effects? For this exercise, you might want to start with situations that are less emotionally evocative or use strategies the client feels more self-efficacy using in less distressing situations. That way clients can explore different regulation options in a safer context until they have developed more refined regulation skills that can be gradually expanded to more challenging environments. Down the line, you can also expand to monitoring the long-term effects and adaptiveness of using each strategy.

## Conclusions

Cognitive behavioral approaches teach clients to use strategies such as reappraisal and acceptance to manage their emotional experiences in more adaptive and functional ways. However, using these strategies flexibly in the real world can be quite difficult, and these difficulties might help account for the fact that cognitive behavioral therapy is not effective for everyone (Vittengl, Clark, Dunn, & Jarrett, 2007). In this chapter, we turned to the latest research on affective science for answers. This growing literature suggests that the difficulties our clients encounter generalizing emotion regulation knowledge from the clinic to their everyday lives might stem from the context-dependent nature of emotion regulation. By helping our clients to regulate their emotions more flexibly, therapists are targeting processes that should lead to greater success and to the enhanced efficacy of evidence-based therapy approaches.

# Emotion Regulation Map

Use this worksheet to keep track of your emotions in distressing situations, as well as the strategies that you used to manage your emotions. Refer back to this sheet to evaluate the short- and long-term consequences of using these emotion regulation strategies. Afterward, evaluate how effective each strategy was and adjust which strategies you will use in the future accordingly. Remember, it is important to try out and practice different strategies for different emotions that you experience. Doing so will improve your ability to manage a variety of emotions across many situations.

| 1. SITUATION DESCRIPTION | 2. EMOTIONS EXPERIENCED AND THEIR INTENSITY | 3. REGULATION STRATEGIES USED | 4. SHORT-TERM OUTCOMES OF REGULATION | 5. LONG-TERM OUTCOMES OF REGULATION |
|---|---|---|---|---|
| Be as specific as possible. | Describe the emotions that you experienced. | List which emotion regulation strategies you used. | What happened immediately after you used these strategies? | Did using these strategies help you achieve your long-term goals? How so? |
| What were you doing? | Rate the intensity of each emotion (0–100). | Be very detailed in how you used each specific strategy. | How did your emotions change? Did they increase or decrease in intensity? | How might you manage your emotions differently in the future? |
| What triggered your emotional reaction? | | | How did your thoughts, physical sensations, and behaviors change? | |
| When was it? | | | | |
| Who were you with? | | | | |
| Where were you? | | | | |

# References

Aldao, A. (2013). The future of emotion regulation research: Capturing context. *Perspectives on Psychological Science, 8*(2), 155–172.

Aldao, A., Nolen-Hoeksema, S., & Schweizer, S. (2010). Emotion-regulation strategies across psychopathology: A meta-analytic review. *Clinical Psychology Review, 30*(2), 217–237.

Aldao, A., Sheppes, G., & Gross, J. J. (2015). Emotion regulation flexibility. *Cognitive Therapy and Research, 39*(3), 263–278.

Barlow, D. H. (2002). *Anxiety and its disorders: The nature and treatment of anxiety and panic* (2nd ed.). New York: Guilford Press.

Beck, A. T. (1964). Thinking and depression: II. Theory and therapy. *Archives of General Psychiatry, 10*(6), 561–571.

Beck, A. T. (1979). *Cognitive therapy of depression.* New York: Guilford Press.

Beck, J. S. (2011). *Cognitive behavior therapy: Basics and beyond* (2nd ed.). New York: Guilford Press.

Birk, J. L., & Bonanno, G. A. (2016). When to throw the switch: The adaptiveness of modifying emotion regulation strategies based on affective and physiological feedback. *Emotion, 16*(6), 657–670.

Bonanno, G. A. (2004). Loss, trauma, and human resilience: Have we underestimated the human capacity to thrive after extremely aversive events? *American Psychologist, 59*(1), 20–28.

Cheng, C., Lau, B. H.-P., & Chan, M.-P. S. (2014). Coping flexibility and psychological adjustment to stressful life changes: A meta-analytic review. *Psychological Bulletin, 140*(6), 1582–1607.

Christensen, K. A., Aldao, A., Sheridan, M. A., & McLaughlin, K. A. (2015). Habitual reappraisal in context: Peer victimization moderates its association with physiological reactivity to social stress. *Cognition and Emotion, 31*(2), 384–394.

Ehring, T., & Quack, D. (2010). Emotion regulation difficulties in trauma survivors: The role of trauma type and PTSD symptom severity. *Behavior Therapy, 41*(4), 587–598.

Gifford, E. V., Kohlenberg, B. S., Hayes, S. C., Pierson, H. M., Piasecki, M. P., Antonuccio, D. O., et al. (2011). Does acceptance and relationship focused behavior therapy contribute to bupropion outcomes? A randomized controlled trial of functional analytic psychotherapy and acceptance and commitment therapy for smoking cessation. *Behavior Therapy, 42*(4), 700–715.

Goldin, P. R., Ziv, M., Jazaieri, H., Werner, K., Kraemer, H., Heimberg, R. G., et al. (2012). Cognitive reappraisal self-efficacy mediates the effects of individual cognitive-behavioral therapy for social anxiety disorder. *Journal of Consulting and Clinical Psychology, 80*(6), 1034–1040.

Gross, J. J. (1998). The emerging field of emotion regulation: An integrative review. *Review of General Psychology, 2*(3), 271–299.

Gupta, S., & Bonanno, G. A. (2010). Trait self-enhancement as a buffer against potentially traumatic events: A prospective study. *Psychological Trauma: Theory, Research, Practice, and Policy, 2*(2), 83–92.

Hayes, S. C., Luoma, J. B., Bond, F. W., Masuda, A., & Lillis, J. (2006). Acceptance and commitment therapy: Model, processes, and outcomes. *Behaviour Research and Therapy, 44*(1), 1–25.

Hayes, S. C., Strosahl, K. D., & Wilson, K. G. (1999). *Acceptance and commitment therapy: An experiential approach to behavior change.* New York: Guilford Press.

Hofmann, S. G. (2014). Interpersonal emotion regulation model of mood and anxiety disorders. *Cognitive Therapy and Research, 38*(5), 483–492.

Hofmann, S. G., Carpenter, J. K., & Curtiss, J. (2016). Interpersonal Emotion Regulation Questionnaire (IERQ): Scale development and psychometric characteristics. *Cognitive Therapy and Research, 40*(3), 341–356.

Kashdan, T. B., Barrett, L. F., & McKnight, P. E. (2015). Unpacking emotion differentiation: Transforming unpleasant experience by perceiving distinctions in negativity. *Current Directions in Psychological Science, 24*(1), 10–16.

Kashdan, T. B., & Rottenberg, J. (2010). Psychological flexibility as a fundamental aspect of health. *Clinical Psychology Review, 30*(7), 865–878.

Kneeland, E. T., Nolen-Hoeksema, S., Dovidio, J. F., & Gruber, J. (2016). Emotion malleability beliefs influence the spontaneous regulation of social anxiety. *Cognitive Therapy and Research, 40*(4), 496–509.

Lazarus, R. S., & Folkman, S. (1984). *Stress, appraisal, and coping.* New York: Springer.

Levy-Gigi, E., Bonanno, G. A., Shapiro, A. R., Richter-Levin, G., Kéri, S., & Sheppes, G. (2016). Emotion regulatory flexibility sheds light on the elusive relationship between repeated traumatic exposure and posttraumatic stress disorder symptoms. *Clinical Psychological Science, 4*(1), 28–39.

Linehan, M. M. (1993). *Cognitive behavioral treatment of borderline personality disorder.* New York: Guilford Press.

McRae, K., Ciesielski, B., & Gross, J. J. (2012). Unpacking cognitive reappraisal: Goals, tactics, and outcomes. *Emotion, 12*(2), 250–255.

Mennin, D. S., Fresco, D. M., Ritter, M., & Heimberg, R. G. (2015). An open trial of emotion regulation therapy for generalized anxiety disorder and co-occurring depression. *Depression and Anxiety, 32*(8), 614–623.

Nolen-Hoeksema, S., & Watkins, E. R. (2011). A heuristic for developing transdiagnostic models of psychopathology: Explaining multifinality and divergent trajectories. *Perspectives on Psychological Science, 6*(6), 589–609.

Olatunji, B. O., & Wolitzky-Taylor, K. B. (2009). Anxiety sensitivity and the anxiety disorders: A meta-analytic review and synthesis. *Psychological Bulletin, 135*(6), 974–999.

Rachman, S., Radomsky, A. S., & Shafran, R. (2008). Safety behaviour: A reconsideration. *Behaviour Research and Therapy, 46*(2), 163–173.

Shallcross, A. J., Troy, A. S., Boland, M., & Mauss, I. B. (2010). Let it be: Accepting negative emotional experiences predicts decreased negative affect and depressive symptoms. *Behaviour Research and Therapy, 48*(9), 921–929.

Tamir, M., Mitchell, C., & Gross, J. J. (2008). Hedonic and instrumental motives in anger regulation. *Psychological Science, 19*(4), 324–328.

Troy, A. S., Shallcross, A. J., & Mauss, I. B. (2013). A person-by-situation approach to emotion regulation: Cognitive reappraisal can either help or hurt, depending on the context. *Psychological Science, 24*(12), 2505–2514.

Vine, V., & Aldao, A. (2014). Impaired emotional clarity and psychopathology: A transdiagnostic deficit with symptom-specific pathways through emotion regulation. *Journal of Social and Clinical Psychology, 33*(4), 319–342.

Vittengl, J. R., Clark, L. A., Dunn, T. W., & Jarrett, R. B. (2007). Reducing relapse and recurrence in unipolar depression: A comparative meta-analysis of cognitive-behavioral therapy's effects. *Journal of Consulting and Clinical Psychology, 75*(3), 475–488.

Webb, T. L., Miles, E., & Sheeran, P. (2012). Dealing with feeling: A meta-analysis of the effectiveness of strategies derived from the process model of emotion regulation. *Psychological Bulletin, 138*(4), 775–808.

Zaki, J., & Williams, W. C. (2013). Interpersonal emotion regulation. *Emotion, 13*(5), 803–810.

# CHAPTER 17

# Problem Solving

Arthur M. Nezu, PhD
Christine Maguth Nezu, PhD
Alexandra P. Greenfield, MS
*Department of Psychology, Drexel University*

## Definitions and Background

*Problem-solving therapy* (PST) is a psychosocial intervention that trains individuals to adopt and effectively apply adaptive problem-solving attitudes (e.g., enhanced self-efficacy) and behaviors (e.g., planful problem solving) in order to help them effectively cope with the exigencies of stressful events (Nezu, 2004). The goal is not only to reduce psychopathology, but also to enhance psychological functioning in a positive direction in order to prevent relapse and the development of new distressing problems. Originally outlined by D'Zurilla and Goldfried (1971), the theory and practice of PST has been refined and significantly revised to assimilate recent research in psychopathology, cognitive science, and affective neuroscience. Because the therapy protocol has changed significantly from its earlier roots, we use the term *contemporary* problem-solving therapy to highlight these changes (Nezu, Greenfield, & Nezu, 2016).

Based on a biopsychosocial diathesis-stress model of psychopathology, PST involves training people to cope effectively with life stressors hypothesized to engender negative health and mental health outcomes (Nezu et al., 2016). These include major negative life events (e.g., death of a loved one, chronic illness, job loss) and ongoing daily problems (e.g., continuous tension with coworkers, reduced finances, marital difficulties). PST theory suggests that much of what is conceptualized as psychopathology is a function of ineffective coping with such stressors. As such, teaching individuals to become better problem solvers is hypothesized to lead to decreased extant physical and mental health problems, as well as improved resilience to future stressors. Scores of randomized controlled trials and meta-analyses (e.g., Barth et al., 2013; Bell & D'Zurilla, 2009; Cape, Whittington, Buszewicz, Wallace, & Underwood, 2010; Kirkham, Seitz, & Choi, 2015; Malouff, Thorsteinsson, & Schutte, 2007) indicate that PST is an effective treatment for a diverse population of individuals experiencing a wide range of psychological, behavioral, and health disorders.

## Tool Kits

According to the PST approach, certain major obstacles can impede effective problem resolution, including (a) cognitive overload, (b) emotional dysregulation, (c) biased cognitive processing of emotion-related information, (d) poor motivation, and (e) ineffective problem-solving strategies. To overcome such barriers, PST provides training in the following four major problem-solving "tool kits": (a) problem-solving multitasking, (b) the stop, slow down, think, and act (S.S.T.A.) method of approaching problems, (c) healthy thinking and positive imagery, and (d) planful problem solving (see Nezu, Nezu, & D'Zurilla, 2013, for a detailed PST treatment manual).

Note that an individualized case formulation of a client's specific problem-solving strengths and weaknesses should determine whether *all* strategies in *all* tool kits are taught and emphasized. In other words, it is not mandatory to employ all materials across all four tool kits during treatment. Rather, therapists should use assessment and outcome data to inform which tools to emphasize and include.

To help illustrate this overall approach, we first introduce Jessica, a client for whom PST was assessed as appropriate and potentially helpful. The remainder of the chapter provides brief descriptions of the PST tools with some illustrations of how they were applied to her case.

## Case Study

Jessica was a thirty-year-old medical student with a family history of anxiety and depression. She came to treatment with the view that she was incapable of meeting her goals in life. She believed that other people were always "happier" and less worried about their achievements, relationships, or value. When focused on academic goals, she would become obsessive and convinced that she could never achieve them. Further, if she became somewhat successful in her career, she felt that her personal life was certain to suffer, and that she would never have quality relationships or be able to experience enjoyable leisure activities simultaneously.

Jessica's personal and romantic relationships generally focused on sexual excitement or nurturing others. This frequently engendered obstacles to pursuing her own important life goals. The resulting sense of failure and comparison with others who were moving forward in their lives created a vicious cycle of stressful problems.

As a function of a formal assessment, the therapist determined that Jessica possessed a strong sense of purpose, a creative and skilled mind, and a desire for a loving connection with others. Her means of trying to solve problems or meet goals, however, was continually thwarted by her negative problem orientation (shame, worry, and pessimism) and her avoidance of meaningful connections. For example, when the one-sided relationships she had selected and created were not reciprocated, she experienced a sense of neediness, anger, failure, and dread. Due to her strong reactions to stress (i.e., feeling overwhelmed, depressed, and anxious), as well as her unsuccessful attempts to move toward her values and life dreams, the therapist determined that PST would be an appropriate therapeutic approach.

As we describe the major PST tools next, we also include relevant examples from Jessica's treatment sessions.

## Tool Kit 1: Overcoming Cognitive Overload

One of the barriers to effective problem solving is the limited capacity of the brain to successfully perform multiple tasks simultaneously, especially when under stress. To overcome this barrier, the first PST tool kit involves training individuals to use three multitasking enhancement skills: externalization, simplification, and visualization.

*Externalization* involves displaying information externally. This procedure relieves the mind from having to actively hold information to be remembered. Externalization can include writing ideas down, drawing a diagram, making a list, creating an audio recording, or talking aloud.

*Simplification* involves breaking a problem down into more manageable pieces. To use this strategy, clients are taught to focus only on the most relevant information: to identify smaller, concrete steps to reach one's goal and to translate complex, vague, and abstract concepts into more simple, specific, and concrete language. One way for individuals to practice using this skill is to write down a brief description of the problem (i.e., applying the externalization strategy), and then ask or imagine asking a friend to read the description and give feedback regarding its clarity.

*Visualization* may be used for a variety of purposes to aid the problem-solving process. When using visual imagery, clients are taught to engage all their senses (where relevant) to imagine seeing, smelling, tasting, touching, and hearing the experience they are creating in their mind. One form of visualization is *problem clarification*, in which clients create a visual representation of a problem they face or a goal they wish to achieve in order to gain clarity about it. A second form of visualization is *imaginal rehearsal*, in which clients practice planned solutions in their mind. This form of visualization can be especially useful when people are overwhelmed with considering how they will carry out a solution or personal action plan at a later time. A third form is *guided imagery*, a type of stress management that reduces one's negative arousal. In this activity, the therapist provides detailed instructions that foster the client's ability to take a mental trip to a relaxing "safe place," such as a favorite vacation spot.

**Related session excerpt.** This excerpt demonstrates how Jessica applied some of the multitasking tools to handle anxiety.

*Jessica*  I felt overwhelmed. My chest started to tighten when I thought about meeting this guy—who I had just started to date—for drinks.

*Therapist:*  Were you able to use any of the multitasking tools to manage this feeling of being overwhelmed, as we discussed?

*Jessica:*  Yeah, I decided to use externalization combined with visualization—I listed some of my concerns, especially wanting to spend more time with him. I then wrote down my goals for changing the way I used to relate to men—I really want to be more honest in disclosing the things that are important to me. I visualized myself expressing to him that I wanted to be able to spend more time with him. I used the visualization to practice trying to be honest, but also fair and empathic, not demanding like before, saying that I understood his schedule was busy and taking responsibility for my schedule also being an obstacle, but that I did want to get more time to hang out—some day activities, and the like. He expressed some things about how it was difficult because our schedules didn't always match up, that he really is trying to save more money this year, and so that means working more, etc. He didn't necessarily say that he would meet me halfway, but I guess just me expressing this to him was important for me—as I was being honest. Overall, the actual date turned out pretty nice. I did feel less overloaded, more relaxed.

## *PST Tool Kit 2: Overcoming Emotional Dysregulation and Maladaptive Problem Solving Under Stress*

Stressful stimuli can engender significant neurobiological arousal that leads to an immediate negative emotional reaction. Given the speed with which these responses can be generated, such negative arousal can impact one's problem-solving attempts in ways that can be detrimental, such as by being avoidant or impulsive rather than planful or rational. Applying the second PST tool kit—stop, slow down, think, and act (S.S.T.A)—can help individuals overcome the difficulties with managing such negative emotional reactions.

**Related session excerpt.** This excerpt demonstrates how to describe the S.S.T.A. tool kit, and why it is important.

*Jessica:* Why can't I ever just go into a situation without constant self-doubt? Other people are able to take a test or give a presentation without withdrawing to their room and continually worrying about everyone knowing how inadequate they are. I'm dreading taking the medical boards—what if I just lose it and freeze?

*Therapist:* Let's see if we can use the simplification tool to first break down this situation, and then consider ways to help "retrain your brain" in order for you to focus on problem solving rather than the worry. The answer to your first question is simply that you are human. Everyone has self-doubt. The difference between you and someone else is that your self-doubt leads to more worry, which leads to more self-doubt, and so forth. In a matter of seconds, your arousal goes from zero to sixty—more like thirty to one hundred because you start off being aroused. It's important for you to turn down the volume on this arousal long enough to allow your brain to start problem solving. The goal of this new tool kit is to buy some time, become more aware of your feelings, and minimize their negative impact on problem solving. It's important to have emotions work in your favor by learning to become more aware, to better manage or regulate your negative emotions, and to embrace the lesson that your emotions are telling you. This set of tools is represented by the acronym S.S.T.A., which stands for stop, slow down, think, and act. It is best learned by continued practice.

*Jessica:* How can this help me get through my medical boards?

*Therapist:* Let's first use visualization—put yourself in this situation right now. Imagine that you are in your den, studying for the board exam. You begin to experience self-doubt. What's next?

*Jessica:* I think that I may not pass this… I start to feel sick to my stomach, and I keep saying over and over again: "Why can't I be different, like everyone else? Why do I have to worry so much? Why am I so messed up?"

*Therapist:* Now *stop!* Start to breathe slowly, which, by the way, is one of several different slow-down techniques that I will teach you. Use this slow-down strategy to become aware of what is happening and what you are feeling.

*Jessica:* I'm scared and I feel inferior to everyone else.

*Therapist:* See what you discovered here by observing your inner experience? You *feel* the normal discomfort of fear that you could fail; but based on your past, you have learned to automatically tell yourself that this feeling means that there is something wrong with you. Because this is untrue and not helpful, we're going to have you train your own brain to turn down the volume on that arousal, so that your brain can get back to focusing on studying without such interference from your worries. It's like applying the brakes to the train early on, rather than letting the train leave the station and then trying to stop it.

(Note: Jessica found the slow-down techniques of S.S.T.A. and breathing slowly helpful and reported that she used them approximately ten times during her actual board examination, which, parenthetically, she successfully passed.)

When practicing the S.S.T.A. procedure, the therapist instructs clients to select a current problem, to use visualization to reexperience the situation in which the problem arose, and then to follow these steps.

**Step 1: Stop and be aware.** Clients first learn to *stop* when they become aware of a significant change in emotion, so they can be more mindful of the experience. A variety of behaviors (e.g., shouting out loud, visualizing a STOP sign or a flashing red traffic light, raising one's hands) can help them to "put on the brakes" so they can identify and interpret their emotions.

This initial step helps individuals become more aware of their reactions to stressful stimuli and more attuned to the meaning and nature of their emotional experiences. The therapist teaches clients to identify unique triggers and increase their emotional awareness by stopping to notice their feelings throughout the day; the events that led to any change in emotions, physical sensations, and behavior; as well as the intensity of their feelings. They are further taught to use externalization to write these observations down, which can help them remember as well as clarify what they are feeling.

**Step 2: Slow down.** Because regulating one's negative emotions can be very difficult, this tool kit provides clients with a variety of ways to slow down so they can continue putting on the brakes. Additionally, these strategies can help individuals to better accept or tolerate such arousal, as well as better understand that such emotions basically denote that a problem is occurring and needs to be solved. The strategies include counting from ten to one, diaphragmatic breathing, guided imagery or visualization, smiling, yawning, meditation, deep muscle relaxation, exercise, talking to others, and prayer. Clients are also encouraged to use approaches that have been helpful in the past.

**Steps 3 and 4: Think and act.** Once individuals are better able to approach the problem with less arousal and emotional interference, they learn to apply a series of critical-thinking steps in order to more systematically and rationally handle the problem situation. These steps are contained in tool kit 4. However, when relevant and necessary, the therapist may provide some clients with a third tool kit, one that addresses negative thinking and low motivation.

## Tool Kit 3: Overcoming Negative Thinking and Low Motivation

The third problem-solving tool kit—healthy thinking and positive imagery—is aimed at individuals for whom dealing with negative thinking and feelings of hopelessness interferes with effective problem solving. The ABC model of healthy thinking is one approach that draws heavily on other cognitive and behavioral strategies that help individuals to cognitively restructure their negative thinking by detecting irrational beliefs, by testing the validity of negative cognitions behaviorally, and by modifying maladaptive dysfunctional beliefs. According to this approach, clients are asked to identify the (A) activating event or stressful problem, (B) beliefs or thoughts about the problem, and their (C) consequential emotional reaction, and then they examine the accuracy and inaccuracy of the thoughts. These thoughts can be replaced with more positive self-statements. In addition, cognitive defusion, acceptance, and mindfulness methods (see chapters 23, 24, and 26) may be deployed at this point of PST.

The in-session activity called reverse advocacy role-play is another tool that can help individuals overcome negative thinking. In this activity, the therapist temporarily adopts a negative attitude toward a stressful problem and asks the client to assume the role of the therapist, whose objective is to provide reasons for why the negative statement is incorrect, irrational, or maladaptive. The process of verbalizing a more appropriate set of beliefs helps the individual to begin to personally adopt a more positive problem orientation and to become more aware of the possibility of greater cognitive flexibility during well-practiced patterns of negative thinking. This activity can also be used in a group setting, as participants can take turns representing both maladaptive and adaptive responses to a given problem.

To increase hopefulness and the adoption of a more positive problem orientation, a fourth form of visualization can be an effective tool. Individuals are asked to visualize the experience of having solved the problem (as compared to focusing on *how* to solve the problem). These images can also be linked to client values (see chapter 25) to further increase the client's motivation. Additionally, by visualizing the simplification of large goals into smaller, more manageable objectives, individuals may become more engaged in planful problem solving.

## Tool Kit 4: Fostering Effective Problem Solving

The final tool kit focuses on teaching four planful problem-solving skills. The first is *problem definition*, whereby clients learn to take the opportunity to fully understand the nature of the problem before attempting to solve it. In describing this process to clients, it may be helpful to use the analogy of laying out a route for travel as being similar to the process of defining problems. In addition, successful problem definition involves seeking all available information about the problem and discriminating between facts and assumptions. A useful exercise to demonstrate this latter principle is to show clients a picture of an ambiguous situation taken from a magazine or newspaper. The therapist directs individuals to view the picture for a few moments, put it aside, and then write down everything they saw or thought was happening in the picture. They then look through the list, and along with feedback from the therapist, differentiate statements that describe facts from those that describe assumptions.

Problem definition also involves describing the facts about a problem in clear and unambiguous language, which clients can do using the externalization and simplification strategies from the multitasking tool kit. It's very important that clients identify goals that are realistic and attainable. If a goal seems initially too large to accomplish, the client can use simplification to break the problem down into smaller ones while still keeping the final destination in mind. Once the clients have articulated a goal or set of goals, they are taught to identify the barriers to reaching such goals. This last activity is particularly important, as a client is unlikely to successfully resolve a given problem unless most of these barriers are overcome.

**Related session excerpt.** This excerpt demonstrates how to help a client better define a problem.

*Jessica:*   With my medical school rotations I have no time for myself. I don't do well with having to work nights at the hospital—afterward, I feel so tired that I just want to sleep. I start thinking that I'll never have any quality relationships or a personal life.

After spending some time reviewing Jessica's sense of feeling overwhelmed, and her assumption that the very existence of obstacles represents valid evidence that she will never have a personal life, she and her therapist began to collaborate on identifying goals for increasing satisfying personal time.

*Jessica:*   It would give me more hope if I could get out once a week to do something for myself and feel more balanced.

*Therapist:*   Great. So, let's break this down to be more specific about what "balance" means to you.

*Jessica:*   Not having to do with school or medicine, but something that makes me feel stronger, healthier, and more connected to people.

*Therapist:*   Okay…so the goal is to once a week do something for yourself and feel more *balanced*, defined as "feeling stronger, healthier, and more connected to people"?

*Jessica:*   Right, but with my schedule, I just don't see…

*Therapist:*   See what you're doing? You are way ahead of me; we haven't even finished defining this problem yet before you want to become negative. We do need to identify obstacles to your goal in order to identify solutions to overcome such obstacles. I know that your barriers are stressful and real… If they didn't exist, you could go and simply achieve your goal. Sometimes, I think one of the biggest hurdles for you is to respect and validate that such obstacles are significant. Let's start to list these barriers.

| | |
|---|---|
| *Jessica:* | Okay, so I have very little time. Maybe just two or three times a week that I could carve out a couple hours away from the hospital. |
| *Therapist:* | Okay, very limited time…that certainly presents a challenge. |
| *Jessica:* | And my few friends are often on different schedules. |
| *Therapist:* | Another significant obstacle, especially for people at your age who are in the midst of building careers. |
| *Jessica:* | I have no men in my life and don't have time to set up a whole lot of dates. |
| *Therapist:* | Right—no significant other, at this time, who you can rely on for support to set things up. |
| *Jessica:* | Money. |
| *Therapist:* | Limited finances provide one more obstacle. Any others? |
| *Jessica:* | I'm tired when I get off call, and that puts me in such a crappy mood that I'm not even motivated to make plans. |
| *Therapist:* | That list provides us with a comprehensive problem definition. Let's recap the obstacles, which really underscore how stressful this problem is for you to work through. I'm really proud of you for trying. Obstacles include limited time, friends with different schedules, no significant other to rely on, limited finances, and negative mood when you are first off call. |
| *Jessica:* | So you do seem to get why this is a tough problem. (*Sighs.*) |

At the end of this problem-definition step, Jessica had a sense of being heard, of her goals being supported, and of her obstacles being both identified and validated. It was important for both her and the therapist to recognize that when going on to the next aspect of the problem-solving tool kit, Jessica would be generating creative ways to approach her goals and address her obstacles. For example, one way to manage the obstacle of low mood following being on call is to plan to sleep for several hours and to avoid planning activities for that particular time (as her mood may sabotage her best intentions and add to her feeling of being overwhelmed).

The second planful problem-solving skill is *generating alternatives*, which involves brainstorming a range of possible solutions to get closer to goals and to overcome identified obstacles, thus increasing cognitive flexibility (see chapter 21). Creating a pool of solution options can increase clients' chances of arriving at the best solution, help them feel more hopeful, minimize black-and-white thinking, and reduce the tendency to act impulsively. There are three major brainstorming principles used to foster one's creativity: quantity leads to quality (i.e., the more the better), defer judgment (i.e., withhold judgment until after a pool of ideas is generated), and variety enhances creativity (i.e., think of a wide variety of ideas). When clients feel stuck, the therapist might suggest combining two or more ideas to make a new one, taking one idea and slightly modifying it to generate a new approach, thinking of how others might solve the problem, or visualizing oneself or others overcoming the various obstacles to the goal. Clients can practice this basic creativity skill with a variety of hypothetical problems, such as generating ideas about what one might do with a single brick. It may also be helpful to create a more realistic problem with specific barriers, such as how one might meet new people after moving to another neighborhood while addressing barriers such as shyness or limited finances. By applying the brainstorming principles to scenarios that aren't laden with emotion, clients can practice them to improve the generating-alternatives skill before applying it to the more emotionally charged real-world problems they came to therapy to overcome.

*Decision making* is the third planful problem-solving task. It involves initially screening out obvious ineffective solutions, predicting a range of possible consequences for the remaining solutions, conducting a cost-benefit analysis of the predicted outcomes, and developing a solution plan geared to achieving the articulated problem-solving goal. In weighing the pros and cons of the various solution ideas, individuals are taught to use the following criteria: the likelihood that the solution can overcome the major obstacles, the likelihood that the individual can carry out the solution, various personal consequences (e.g., time, effort, physical health), and various social consequences (e.g., effects on family and friends). They are also instructed to consider both short-term and long-term consequences. A solution plan, then, would include alternatives that are rated highly.

In the last planful problem-solving activity, *solution implementation and verification*, clients observe and monitor the effects of the chosen solution, determine if the problem is successfully resolved, and troubleshoot areas of difficulty when problem-solving efforts are not successful. In addition, it is important for clients to reinforce themselves for engaging in the planful problem-solving process, particularly individuals who believe they are poor problem solvers and doubt their ability to successfully resolve stressful problems. Examples include going to one's favorite restaurant, buying a new dress, or simply "patting oneself on the back."

# Implementing the Tool Kits

Although each tool kit is introduced and learned in a linear fashion, the majority of PST sessions are aimed at integrating these strategies so a client can apply them to current, stressful life challenges. In actual practice, PST is applied less as a standard protocol and more as a flexibly implemented strategy—based on sound clinical judgment—that concentrates on an individual client's targeted areas of practice and improvement. For example, extensive time was spent helping Jessica to better regulate her negative arousal when confronted with problems, to manage cognitive overload, and to decrease feelings of hopelessness.

# References

Barth, J., Munder, T., Gerger, H., Nüesch, E., Trelle, S., Znoj, H., et al. (2013). Comparative efficacy of seven psychotherapeutic interventions for patients with depression: A network meta-analysis. *PLoS Medicine, 10*(5), e1001454.

Bell, A. C., & D'Zurilla, T. J. (2009). Problem-solving therapy for depression: A meta-analysis. *Clinical Psychology Review, 29*(4), 348–353.

Cape, J., Whittington, C., Buszewicz, M., Wallace, P., & Underwood, L. (2010). Brief psychological therapies for anxiety and depression in primary care: Meta-analysis and meta-regression. *BMC Medicine, 8*(Article 38).

D'Zurilla, T. J., & Goldfried, M. R. (1971). Problem solving and behavior modification. *Journal of Abnormal Psychology, 78*(1), 107–126.

Kirkham, J., Seitz, D. P., & Choi, N. G. (2015). Meta-analysis of problem solving therapy for the treatment of depression in older adults. *American Journal of Geriatric Psychiatry, 23*(3), S129–S130.

Malouff, J. M., Thorsteinsson, E. B., & Schutte, N. S. (2007). The efficacy of problem solving therapy in reducing mental and physical health problems: A meta-analysis. *Clinical Psychology Review, 27*(1), 46–57.

Nezu, A. M. (2004). Problem solving and behavior therapy revisited. *Behavior Therapy, 35*(1), 1–33.

Nezu, A. M., Greenfield, A. P., & Nezu, C. M. (2016). Contemporary problem-solving therapy: A transdiagnostic approach. In C. M. Nezu & A. M. Nezu (Eds.), *The Oxford handbook of cognitive and behavioral therapies* (pp. 160–171). New York: Oxford University Press.

Nezu, A. M., Nezu, C. M., & D'Zurilla, T. J. (2013). *Problem-solving therapy: A treatment manual.* New York: Springer.

# CHAPTER 18

# Exposure Strategies

Carolyn D. Davies, MA
Michelle G. Craske, PhD

*Department of Psychology, University of California, Los Angeles*

## Definitions and Background

*Exposure* refers to the process of helping a client repeatedly face a feared stimulus in order to learn new, more adaptive ways of responding and to reduce the anxiety and fear associated with the stimulus. A stimulus targeted by exposure can include animate or inanimate objects (e.g., spiders, elevators), situations or activities (e.g., public speaking), cognitions (e.g., intrusive thoughts about contamination), physical sensations (e.g., heart racing), or memories (e.g., distressing memories of an assault).

Exposure is recognized as a highly effective behavioral strategy for treating a range of anxiety and fear-related problems, including panic disorder, agoraphobia, social anxiety disorder, post-traumatic stress disorder (PTSD), and obsessive-compulsive disorder (OCD; Stewart & Chambless, 2009). From its earliest days, exposure has been central to the behavioral and cognitive therapies through the use of systematic desensitization to treat phobias and anxiety disorders (Wolpe, 1958).

## Theoretical Basis

*Fear* (an emotional response to imminent threat) and *anxiety* (an emotional response to anticipated or potential threat) can develop after a person has a direct, negative experience with an object or situation (through a process called *classical conditioning*), observes the aversive experiences or fearful behavior of others (called *vicarious conditioning*), or receives threat-laden information from others. Following these experiences, a previously neutral object or situation can become associated with danger, leading to fear responses and anxiety, negative expectations about the feared stimulus, and associated behaviors (e.g., avoidance) upon subsequent encounters with the stimulus. Furthermore, the fear can generalize to include other associated objects or situations. For example, a woman who got stuck in an elevator for several hours as a child became extremely fearful of enclosed places, to the point that she would have a panic attack in an array of situations if she felt trapped. She avoided taking elevators at all costs, and her fear and avoidance of elevators generalized to other similar situations, such as being in a small room, sitting in the middle of the row in an auditorium, and even being stuck in traffic.

Avoidance behaviors are central to the maintenance of fear and anxiety. While avoidance or escape behaviors can temporarily reduce distress, they maintain anxiety and fear in the long run by preventing new learning from occurring. In effect, exposure is designed to remove avoidance behaviors so that maladaptive beliefs are not reinforced and new learning can occur.

## How Does Exposure Work?

Exposure relies on processes that facilitate new learning. One of these processes is called inhibitory learning, which has been extensively examined through studies using extinction. Akin to exposure, *extinction* involves presenting a feared stimulus repeatedly without its associated aversive outcome. Through extinction, an individual forms a new association with the stimulus so that two competing associations exist: one *excitatory* association that connotes danger and one *inhibitory* association that connotes safety. Thus, following an extinction procedure, an individual will have memories of the stimulus associated with both danger and safety (Bouton, 2004). Using the elevator example, after completing several exposures of riding an elevator without getting stuck, the client would now have two different associations tied to elevators: one that signals danger or getting trapped (excitatory association) and another that signals safety (inhibitory association). Much of the research on improving exposure focuses on examining ways to enhance inhibitory learning in order to strengthen and promote the retrieval of inhibitory associations (Craske, Treanor, Conway, Zbozinek, & Vervliet, 2014). A number of strategies for enhancing inhibitory learning have been tested and are described in the section "Enhancement Strategies."

The reduction of fear responses during exposure sessions does not appear to be necessary for improvement (Craske et al., 2008), however, and thus may not be the primary driver of change. Psychological acceptance (see chapter 24) and cognitive defusion (see chapter 23) may facilitate exposure outcomes (Arch et al.,

2012), particularly among people with multiple problems (Wolitzky-Taylor, Arch, Rosenfield, & Craske, 2012) or high levels of behavioral avoidance (Davies, Niles, Pittig, Arch, & Craske, 2015). Finally, increases in self-efficacy as a result of completing exposures may also play a role in facilitating an individual's engagement in and improvement from exposure therapy (Jones & Menzies, 2000).

# Types of Exposure

Exposure can be implemented as a component within a treatment plan or as a treatment by itself. A number of treatment protocols and manualized treatments include exposure, including prolonged exposure therapy for PTSD (Foa, Hembree, & Rothbaum, 2007) and exposure and response prevention for OCD (e.g., Foa, Yadin, & Lichner, 2012), but the basic principles of exposure are the same, regardless of diagnosis or treatment manual.

Exposures are highly individualized to the client's own fears and avoidance behaviors and therefore must be collaboratively designed by the therapist and client. Typically, the therapist and client agree upon a hierarchy of feared situations and work through this list of exposures over the course of approximately twelve to fifteen sessions, with both in-session and between-session exposures assigned for homework. In-session exposures allow the therapist to help design and model exposures, guide and reinforce behaviors, and gauge progress. Between-session exposures are critical for increasing learning and improving clinical outcomes, as they allow for an increased frequency and a variety of exposures in settings without the therapist. There are three main types of exposure.

*In vivo exposure* involves direct exposure to live situations or objects. For example, a therapist with a client who fears public speaking might ask him to give a speech in front of an audience; for a client with a phobia of blood and/or injections, the therapist might ask her to look at pictures or videos of a blood draw and eventually have the client have her blood drawn at a clinic. Virtual reality exposure therapy can be used for situations that are difficult to access.

*Interoceptive exposure* refers to the deliberate induction of physical sensations, such as increased heart rate, light-headedness, or shortness of breath. Interoceptive exposure is relevant for clients who experience any type of panicky sensations or heightened concern with bodily sensations. Common interoceptive exposures include running in place, hyperventilation, staring in a mirror, breathing through a straw, and spinning in a circle.

*Imaginal exposure* is most helpful when it is not possible or feasible to access a feared situation in vivo or when an image itself is the feared stimulus (such as in OCD or PTSD). During imaginal exposure, clients vividly imagine and describe a feared scenario in detail, using first-person, present-tense language. Clients then record and repeatedly listen to the scenario. A variation on imaginal exposure is *written exposure*, which involves writing out, in detail, a feared scenario and repeatedly reading it. Examples of imaginal exposure include imagining getting fired from a job (for a client who worries excessively about making a mistake at work and getting fired) or imagining a traumatic event that occurred during combat (for a soldier with PTSD).

# Implementation

Before beginning exposure therapy, the therapist must have a clear understanding of how exposure will be helpful for the client. Thoroughly assessing fear and anxiety, including the role that avoidance behaviors play in the client's distress, will help the therapist and client develop and stick to an exposure treatment plan. Furthermore, because exposure is inherently anxiety provoking, providing a strong rationale and obtaining a client's agreement to the treatment plan is a critical element of exposure.

When providing the rationale for exposure, the primary point to relay is that avoidance behaviors, though temporarily anxiety relieving, can increase distress and maintain fear and anxiety in the long run. In the example dialogue below, the therapist first assesses avoidance behaviors with a client who experiences panic attacks.

*Therapist:* When we feel anxious or afraid, our natural response is to try to avoid or get away from whatever is making us feel that way. What are some situations that you avoid?

*Client:* I think it's mainly around driving for me. I used to be able to at least drive in the right lane on the highway, but now I can only drive on side streets. I also avoid driving over bridges.

*Therapist:* Okay, so driving on highways and bridges. What about other situations? Are there any activities or places you avoid?

*Client:* Well, I don't like big crowds either. My son wanted me to take him to see a movie that just came out last week, but the thought of standing in line and then sitting in that crowded theater… I couldn't bring myself to do it. My sister took him instead.

*Therapist:* These behaviors—avoiding crowds and driving only in certain areas—are very common responses to anxiety and panicky feelings.

Avoidance is a natural response to situations that we think are threatening or scary. Unfortunately, too much avoidance can interfere with our lives and prevent us from doing things we want to do. In what ways do you think avoidance behaviors have impacted you?

*Client:* It's impacted me a lot. The hardest part has been with my son. I feel terrible that I can't take him places he wants to go or enjoy things with him. That's definitely the worst part about all of this.

A few important points should be noted from this dialogue. First, the therapist provided some psychoeducation about avoidance behaviors. Second, the therapist began to identify avoidance behaviors as the problem (rather than anxiety or fear per se), as these behaviors will be the target of exposure. Third, the therapist elicited examples of how avoidance behaviors interfere in the client's life. After responding with appropriate validation, the therapist can then provide an introduction to exposure.

*Therapist* In addition to interfering with our lives, avoidance also prevents us from learning that bad outcomes don't always occur or aren't as bad as we first thought. So even though avoidance can sometimes provide temporary relief from anxiety, in the long run it can actually make anxiety worse, which can then lead to even more avoidance. For this reason, the focus of this treatment is to decrease avoidance by approaching or confronting situations and sensations that you avoid. I know this can be difficult, so we are going to start gradually and work our way toward situations that are more difficult. How does this sound to you?

After checking with the client to make sure she understands the rationale for exposure, the therapist and client can begin to create a plan for exposures using the following steps.

**1. Create a hierarchy.** The first step to designing exposures is to create a list of feared situations (also called a fear hierarchy) and their associated fear ratings (on a scale of 0 to 10, with 10 being the most extreme). This list should include a variety of situations that elicit mild (3 to 4), moderate (5 to 7), and high (8 to 10) levels of fear or anxiety. Additionally, the hierarchy should include situations that can be targeted with in vivo, interoceptive, and imaginal exposure. The therapist and client work together to create this list and can continue adding to it as needed.

As part of the list-generation step, the therapist can complete an assessment of interoceptive exposures in order to identify the physical sensations that need to be targeted. The therapist models each interoceptive exercise (running in place, spinning in a circle, etc.), then the client completes the exercise, aiming to continue for approximately one minute. After each exercise, the therapist gathers two ratings from the client: level of fear or anxiety and level of similarity to sensations experienced when anxious. Interoceptive exposures that elicit high levels of similarity and moderate to high levels of fear or anxiety should be added to the exposure hierarchy.

**2. Choose a first exposure.** Strictly adhering to the order of the hierarchy is not necessary, but initial exposures should start at the lower end, at a fear level of approximately 3 or 4. This allows the client to understand the procedure of exposure and to build some self-efficacy, which may help the client engage in more difficult exposures later on.

**3. Identify the anticipated negative outcomes.** Before beginning an exposure, the therapist elicits the client's expected or anticipated outcomes. This allows the therapist and client to "test out" a hypothesis about the outcome of an exposure and encourages the client to become a "scientist" who tests predictions and gathers evidence. Importantly, an expected outcome must be testable and observable. For example, for the client with the panic attacks described above, a hypothesis she might test out during interoceptive exposure is, "If I spin in a circle for more than half a minute, I will faint." Once a testable outcome is obtained, the therapist can then ask, "On a scale of 0 to 100, how likely is this to occur?"

A second piece of information that is helpful to gather prior to an exposure is a rating of how bad it would be if the anticipated negative outcome did occur. For example, the therapist can ask, "On a scale of 0 to 100, how bad would it be if you did pass out as a result of the exposure?" This question can be especially helpful for situations in which the anticipated outcome may actually occur (e.g., rejection in the case of a social anxiety exposure), after which clients may learn that the outcome was not as bad as they had initially anticipated.

**4. Test out the anticipated negative outcome.** The therapist and client then decide on the best exposure to test out the client's anticipated negative outcome. Importantly, the amount of time the client engages in the exposure is predetermined, based not on the level of fear reduction during the exposure but on what the client needs to learn. For example, for the client who experiences panic attacks, the exposure might consist of spinning in a circle for one minute (see table 1). This approach not only helps maximize expectancy violation (see the "Test it out" strategy for enhancing exposure in the following section), but it also encourages the client to focus on behavioral outcomes as the goal rather than fear reduction.

**5. Ask follow-up questions following exposure.** Following each exposure, the therapist asks the client targeted questions about what happened. For example, "Did what you were most worried about happening actually occur?" or "What did you expect to happen versus what actually happened?" or "Were you able to handle the distress or discomfort?" Throughout exposure work, the therapist identifies and reinforces *approach behaviors* (behaviors that move toward previously avoided situations) with the goal of helping the client engage in behaviors *despite* feelings of anxiety.

## Table 1. First-exposure exercise for a client with panic disorder

An example of a first-exposure exercise for a client with panic disorder. Additional exposures are designed in this same way, usually increasing in difficulty as sessions proceed.

| Before Exposure | |
|---|---|
| Goal: | *Spin in a circle for one minute.* |
| What are you most worried will happen? | *I will faint.* |
| On a scale of 0 to 100, how likely is it that this will happen? | *85* |
| On a scale of 0 to 100, how bad would it be if this did happen? | *95* |
| **After Exposure** | |
| Yes or no, did what you were most worried about occur? | *No.* |
| How do you know? | *I remained conscious.* |
| What did you learn? | *Feeling dizzy doesn't necessarily mean I am going to faint.* |

# Enhancement Strategies

Research on inhibitory learning during exposure has led to the identification of strategies that therapists can use to refine and enhance exposure. These strategies, along with their theoretical bases, detailed in a previous paper from our lab (Craske et al., 2014), are summarized below.

**Expectancy violation—"Test it out."** The basic idea of this strategy is to maximize the difference between the anticipated negative outcome and the actual outcome during an exposure; it's based on the premise that the mismatch between expectancy and outcome is critical for new learning (Hofmann, 2008). The therapist should attempt to emphasize this mismatch as much as possible by (1) having the client identify specific expectations about an aversive outcome prior to an exposure; (2) designing the exposure to test out this expectancy; (3) determining the duration of the exposure based on what is needed to violate expectancies, not based on the reduction of fear levels; and (4) asking clients, after each exposure trial, to judge what they learned (for example, "What surprised you about doing the exposure? What did you learn from doing this exposure?") Furthermore, therapists should refrain from using cognitive restructuring strategies prior to exposures, as these interventions are designed to reduce the expectancy of a negative outcome and may thereby reduce the mismatch between the client's initial expectancy and the actual outcome.

**Deepened extinction—"Combine it."** This strategy combines multiple feared stimuli, or cues, in one exposure. After conducting exposure to each cue individually, both cues can then be combined to deepen the learning process. For example, imaginal exposure to an obsession, such as the obsession to stab a loved one, and in vivo exposure to a cue that triggers the obsession, such as holding a knife, would then be followed by exposure to the obsession of stabbing a loved one while holding a knife. Interoceptive exposure can also be incorporated into in vivo or imaginal exposure. For example, a client with social anxiety may run in place to elevate her heart rate prior to delivering a speech.

**Reinforced extinction—"Face your fear."** This strategy involves occasionally including aversive or deliberately negative outcomes during an exposure. Examples include adding social rejection in exposures to social situations or deliberately inducing a panic attack. In these examples, the exposure may not only enhance learning by heightening the salience of the exposure, but it may offer the client the opportunity to learn new coping strategies for negative outcomes. This strategy should not be used in situations in which a negative outcome would be dangerous (e.g., you would not conduct an exposure to a car accident).

**Variability—"Vary it up."** Including variability in exposures enhances inhibitory learning during exposure and better represents the situations the client will face outside of therapy. Therapists can vary exposures in a number of ways, such as by including exposures to a wide range of diverse stimuli, varying the time and intensity of exposures, completing exposures in both familiar and unfamiliar places and at varying times of the day, and completing exposures from varying levels of the client's hierarchy rather than steadily progressing from easier to more difficult exposures.

**Remove safety behaviors—"Throw it out."** This strategy removes or prevents *safety signals* or *safety behaviors*, which are objects or behaviors that reduce or minimize fear or anxiety. Common safety signals include the presence of another person (including the therapist), medication, a cell phone, and food or drink; common safety behaviors include asking another person for reassurance, averting eye contact, overpreparing, escaping, and engaging in compulsive behaviors (e.g., hand washing or checking). Safety signals and behaviors can be detrimental to exposure therapy and can also lead to interference or distress with the signals and behaviors themselves (e.g., excessively calling one's friend for reassurance may interfere with the friendship). Therefore, therapists should encourage clients to eliminate or gradually reduce the use of safety signals and behaviors.

**Attentional focus—"Stay with it."** This strategy helps clients maintain attentional focus during exposure. Attending to exposure stimuli helps clients observe the outcome of the exposure and prevents them from being distracted and engaging in safety behaviors. The therapist might encourage clients to "stay with it" by directing their gaze during in vivo exposure or redirecting their descriptions during imaginal exposure.

**Affect labeling—"Talk it out."** *Affect labeling* refers to using words to describe the content of an exposure (e.g., "ugly spider") or one's emotional response during exposure (e.g., "anxious" or "scared"). This strategy is based on social neuroscience research showing that linguistic processing can attenuate affective responses (Lieberman et al., 2007). To use this strategy, the therapist should encourage clients to label their emotion in the moment or describe the current object or situation without engaging in any strategies to alter or change their cognitions.

**Mental reinstatement/retrieval cues—"Bring it back."** The final strategy uses reminders (also called retrieval cues) to help clients remember what they learned during previous exposures. This strategy is best used as a relapse-prevention skill rather than at the beginning of treatment because retrieval cues may become safety signals. As part of relapse prevention, the therapist may encourage clients to remind themselves of what they learned during exposure therapy each time they encounter a previously feared stimulus, or have them carry an item (e.g., a wristband) that serves as a tactile reminder.

# Applications and Contraindications

Exposure is effective for treating most anxiety and fear-related problems. Therapists can evaluate whether exposure is needed by conducting a diagnostic assessment or a functional analysis to determine why the client is engaging in a certain problematic behavior. For example, the therapist might ask, "What types of situations trigger your fear or anxiety? What do you do when you experience anxiety or fear? What are you most concerned will happen if you do not engage in this behavior?" Overestimation of threat and engagement in safety or avoidance behaviors indicate that exposure is likely needed. Exposure is generally very safe and effective for addressing fear, anxiety, and associated maladaptive avoidance. However, there are certain cases in which exposure is contraindicated or must be used with caution:

- *Recent suicidal or nonsuicidal self-injury.* Little data exist on the use of exposure with highly suicidal or self-injuring clients, but delaying exposure until suicidality or self-injury has abated is recommended.

- *Environmental danger.* Exposures should not be conducted in situations where there is actual danger. For example, don't conduct in vivo exposure with a client's abusive partner.

- *Interoceptive exposures with certain medical conditions.* Some interoceptive exposures could aggravate certain medical conditions (e.g., seizure disorder). In such cases, the therapist should consult with the client's medical doctor to adapt interoceptive exposures.

# Tips for Success

As with any therapeutic strategy, problems can arise. Below are tips to help address the most common issues.

**Redirect predictions about emotional responses.** Commonly, clients will identify a predicted outcome about their emotional response during an exposure, such as "I will panic" or "I will get anxious." In these cases, further probing may be required to elicit observable or behavioral predictions. For example, the therapist might ask, "What are you most concerned will happen if you panic?" If a client's biggest concern is that the anxiety will be overwhelming, she may predict, for example, "I will be so anxious that I won't be able to do anything." An exposure designed to test this prediction would involve having the client complete some activity immediately following the exposure.

**Avoid mind-reading predictions.** *Mind-reading predictions* are predictions about what others will think. For example, a client completing a public-speaking exposure may predict, "The audience will notice that I am nervous," or "They will think I'm stupid and incompetent." To elicit a behavioral outcome, try one of the following:

- *Probe for observable behaviors from others.* Using the example above, the therapist might ask, "What specifically will the audience *do* if they think you are stupid and incompetent?"

- *Ask for feedback from other individuals involved in the exposure.* For example, following a public-speaking exposure, the client can ask the audience, "How did I sound? Did I seem nervous to you?" When feasible and appropriate, this approach can be helpful. However, it should not be overused, as asking for feedback can become a safety behavior.

- *Use video feedback.* Video feedback can be used to test out specific predictions about a client's appearance (e.g., "My face will be bright red") or performance (e.g., "I will stumble over my words") during an exposure. This approach is most helpful for public-speaking exposures, but, as with asking for feedback, it should not be overused.

**Do not let anxiety—yours or your client's—interfere with exposure work.** Therapists new to exposure may be uncomfortable with the notion of purposely provoking fear and anxiety during therapy, perhaps due to the belief that the client's symptoms will worsen or that the client will drop out. Therapists who avoid their own emotions tend to avoid doing exposure (Scherr, Herbert, & Forman, 2015), at the expense of their clients' improvement. Though exposure can be difficult, we know from decades of research that despite its temporarily anxiety- or fear-producing effects, exposure is very effective for providing long-term relief from anxiety and fear-based problems. The following suggestions may help prevent your client's or your own anxiety from interfering with effective exposure treatment:

- *Practice, practice, practice.* As with any new behavior, conducting exposures requires practice. Practicing exposures that you are going to ask a client to complete prior to a session is one way to increase your comfort and skill with new exposures.

- *Use therapist modeling.* Modeling exposures for your client can be very helpful, especially in initial sessions.

- *Reiterate rationale for exposure.* If you get stuck, try to get back on track by discussing with the client the reasons for doing exposures.

- *Work your way up.* If an exposure is too difficult for a client, do not give up. Start with an easier exposure to help your client build self-efficacy, and then build up to the more challenging exposures.

- *Watch out for safety signals and behaviors.* These behaviors and signals can sometimes be hard to spot. If your client is reporting low fear levels during a difficult exposure, that may be a clue that the client is utilizing safety behaviors or signals.

- *Keep in mind that anxiety means the exposure is working.*

**Do not overemphasize fear reduction.** While fear reduction may occur during the course of exposure therapy, it is not the primary goal. Instead:

- *Reinforce approach behaviors.* Use encouragement and praise to reinforce approach behaviors and the completion of exposures, regardless of whether there was a change in fear or anxiety.

- *Focus on actual outcomes.* After completing an exposure, ask the client specific follow-up questions in order to highlight the actual outcomes of the exposure instead of the fear level.

- *Keep in mind that fear reduction during exposure is not necessary for a client to improve.* In fact, learning to tolerate fear and to act despite difficult emotions is likely a more important component of exposure than fear reduction.

**Consider cultural adaptations of exposure.** Using culturally informed approaches to adapt exposures for diverse populations can improve outcomes (e.g., see Pan, Huey, & Hernandez, 2011).

# References

Arch, J. J., Eifert, G. H., Davies, C., Plumb Vilardaga, J. C., Rose, R. D., & Craske, M. G. (2012). Randomized clinical trial of cognitive behavioral therapy (CBT) versus acceptance and commitment therapy (ACT) for mixed anxiety disorders. *Journal of Consulting and Clinical Psychology, 80*(5), 750–765.

Bouton, M. E. (2004). Context and behavioral processes in extinction. *Learning and Memory, 11*(5), 485–494.

Craske, M. G., Kircanski, K., Zelikowsky, M., Mystkowski, J., Chowdhury, N., & Baker, A. (2008). Optimizing inhibitory learning during exposure therapy. *Behaviour Research and Therapy, 46*(1), 5–27.

Craske, M. G., Treanor, M., Conway, C. C., Zbozinek, T., & Vervliet, B. (2014). Maximizing exposure therapy: An inhibitory learning approach. *Behaviour Research and Therapy, 58*(1), 10–23.

Davies, C. D., Niles, A. N., Pittig, A., Arch, J. J., & Craske, M. G. (2015). Physiological and behavioral indices of emotion dysregulation as predictors of outcome from cognitive behavioral therapy and acceptance and commitment therapy for anxiety. *Journal of Behavior Therapy and Experimental Psychiatry, 46,* 35–43.

Foa, E. B., Hembree, E. A., & Rothbaum, B. O. (2007). *Prolonged exposure therapy for PTSD: Emotional processing of traumatic experiences therapist guide.* Oxford: Oxford University Press.

Foa, E. B., Yadin, E., & Lichner, T. K. (2012). *Exposure and response (ritual) prevention for obsessive compulsive disorder: Therapist guide* (2nd ed.). Oxford: Oxford University Press.

Hofmann, S. G. (2008). Cognitive processes during fear acquisition and extinction in animals and humans: Implications for exposure therapy of anxiety disorders. *Clinical Psychology Review, 28*(2), 199–210.

Jones, M. K., & Menzies, R. G. (2000). Danger expectancies, self-efficacy and insight in spider phobia. *Behaviour Research and Therapy, 38*(6), 585–600.

Lieberman, M. D., Eisenberger, N. I., Crockett, M. J., Tom, S. M., Pfeifer, J. H., & Way, B. M. (2007). Putting feelings into words: Affect labeling disrupts amygdala activity in response to affective stimuli. *Psychological Science, 18*(5), 421–428.

Pan, D., Huey Jr., S. J., & Hernandez, D. (2011). Culturally-adapted versus standard exposure treatment for phobic Asian Americans: Treatment efficacy, moderators, and predictors. *Cultural Diversity and Ethnic Minority Psychology, 17*(1), 11–22.

Scherr, S. R., Herbert, J. D., & Forman, E. M. (2015). The role of therapist experiential avoidance in predicting therapist preference for exposure treatment for OCD. *Journal of Contextual Behavioral Science, 4*(1), 21–29.

Stewart, R. E., & Chambless, D. L. (2009). Cognitive-behavioral therapy for adult anxiety disorders in clinical practice: A meta-analysis of effectiveness studies. *Journal of Consulting and Clinical Psychology, 77*(4), 595–606.

Wolitzky-Taylor, K. B., Arch, J. J., Rosenfield, D., & Craske, M. G. (2012). Moderators and non-specific predictors of treatment outcome for anxiety disorders: A comparison of cognitive behavioral therapy to acceptance and commitment therapy. *Journal of Consulting and Clinical Psychology, 80*(5), 786–799.

Wolpe, J. (1958). *Psychotherapy by reciprocal inhibition.* Stanford, CA: Stanford University Press.

# CHAPTER 19

# Behavioral Activation

## Christopher R. Martell, PhD, ABPP

*Department of Psychological and Brain Sciences,
University of Massachusetts, Amherst*

## Background

Behavioral activation (BA) is both a single behavioral strategy used as part of a broader cognitive behavioral therapy (CBT) treatment for depression and a full treatment on its own. When used as part of broader CBT, it is most appropriately referred to as activity scheduling or pleasant events scheduling (MacPhillamy & Lewinsohn, 1982). As a stand-alone treatment, it has come to be known from two well-known protocols. One protocol is based on a large study conducted at the University of Washington (Dimidjian et al., 2006), which began with the original protocol (Martell, Addis, & Jacobson, 2001) and resulted in an updated clinician's guide (Martell, Dimidjian, & Herman-Dunn, 2010). This protocol allows for an average twenty-four sessions of BA and is presented as a flexible treatment, with strategic priorities and client goals based on each client's particular needs. Behavioral activation for depression (BATD; Lejuez, Hopko, Acierno, Daughters, & Pagoto, 2011), a briefer BA approach, was developed independently and contemporaneously. My primary focus in this chapter will be on broad-based BA (Martell et al., 2001, 2010), as it provides a comprehensive methodology for conducting the treatment, but there are many shared elements between it and the two stand-alone versions, and I will mention some features of BATD.

## Basic Clinical Skills

It may seem straightforward from the very name "behavioral activation" that getting people active is easily accomplished. There is an ironic quality to conducting BA, however, in that the very thing that depressed individuals often find extremely difficult is what we are asking our clients to do: engage in activity. It is therefore important that therapists demonstrate adequate clinical skill and maintain a certain stance with clients in order to encourage activation.

**Empathy and warmth.** While it may go without saying that therapists should have empathy for their clients, it bears repeating that the work of BA can often drain therapists. Because we're asking clients to do what is difficult for them, therapists may need to imagine themselves in their clients' situations in order to help them break down tasks into manageable steps. Furthermore, the therapist who empathizes with clients can keep them from becoming frustrated when they have difficulty completing assignments. BA is a directive therapy, with therapists collaborating with clients but also making suggestions for possible activities a client may attempt, and it's always easier to have a good working relationship when the therapist expresses genuine warmth and concern.

**Attending to the present moment.** Therapists working with depressed clients will recognize how the clients' mood pervades all aspects of their life, including therapy sessions. BA therapists therefore need to be awake to opportunities during sessions to activate and engage clients. By attending to the present moment of the session, therapists can strategically respond to examples of improvement in behavior. While therapists do not need formal mindfulness training (Kabat-Zinn, 1994), this work of attending to the present moment certainly has much in common with mindfulness-based approaches to treatment in relation to helping clients manage unhelpful rumination (Segal, Williams, & Teasdale, 2001). For example, if a client tells a story that demonstrates hopefulness, the therapist can meet it with an enthusiastic but natural response. Similarly, the therapist may shift his body posture to match the client who is making better eye contact, providing natural social reinforcement for engagement.

In BA, clients are taught to attend to the present moment. Rather than focus on past failures or future worries, activation requires that they engage with whatever they are currently doing. Even people who are not depressed sometimes go about an activity without paying much attention. How often do we complete a mundane task like washing dishes or folding laundry and basically forget what we'd done because our mind was elsewhere during the process? When depressed individuals are trapped in patterns of negative thinking, practicing attending to the details of each activity and the environmental context in which the activity occurs can help to increase the likelihood that getting active will improve their mood and pull them out of the morass of depression.

**Validating.** Depressed individuals are not just whining or complaining about nothing; they are experiencing a life that can feel absent of pleasure and can have difficulty doing even basic activities. Thus, therapists need to validate client experiences while encouraging clients to engage in activities differently so they can move beyond the blues. Martell and colleagues (2010) define "validation" in BA as "demonstrating an understanding of the client's experience…and communicating that you understand the client's experience, based on their history or current context" (pp. 51–52).

**Implicit acceptance.** BA is considered a contemporary behavioral therapy that is contextually based (Martell et al., 2001), and as with other contextual behavioral methods (e.g., Hayes, Strosahl, & Wilson, 2012), modern forms of BA emphasize accepting emotion and life's difficulties (see chapter 24 in this volume). In BA, acceptance is implicit rather than explicit; it is not a direct goal. However, when clients are asked to engage in activity without first modifying how they feel, the implicit idea is that they can accept negative feelings and act in constructive ways even when they are feeling bad. There is a strong focus in BA on acting in accordance with a goal rather than a mood.

# Techniques and Processes

BA intentionally does not include many techniques. It is a parsimonious treatment with the sole purpose of getting people to reengage in activity so they are more likely to have their behavior positively reinforced in their daily environment. The idea is that the more active clients become, the more likely they are to have their behavior reinforced positively, which means they will be more likely to continue to engage in the activity under similar conditions. Thus, the entire program of BA, whether it's the highly structured protocol used by Lejuez and colleagues (2011) or the more idiographic approach advocated by Martell and colleagues (2001, 2010), revolves around structuring and scheduling reinforcing activities that the client engages in throughout the treatment.

**Values, reinforcement, and activity monitoring.** It's most possible to get clients in contact with natural reinforcers when they engage in activity that is consistent with the things they highly value in life (e.g., being a good parent, maintaining strong friendships, having career success, and so on) or when they engage in activities previously associated with an improvement in mood. Thus, the therapist-client collaboration to increase activity and engagement focuses on identifying activities that are likely to be positively reinforced in the natural environment. In order to try to optimize this, therapists structure tasks so that clients can achieve them in their current state of depression, and they troubleshoot the barriers that keep clients from engaging in and accomplishing those activities. Lejuez and colleagues have rightly highlighted the reality that activities that are consistent with client values will be reinforced naturally in the environment. In their BATD revised manual (Lejuez et al., 2011), the authors state that

> Establishing values prior to identifying activities helps ensure that selected activities (healthy behaviors) will be positively reinforced over time, by virtue of being connected to values as opposed to being arbitrarily selected. Patients are asked to consider multiple life areas when identifying values and activities to ensure that they increase their access to positive reinforcement in several areas of life rather than in one or two, the latter of which can narrow the opportunities for success. (p. 114)

Thus, some conversation about what clients value, or what is important to them in their life, is an important first step when beginning to identify activities that are likely to be antidepressant (Martell et al., 2010) for clients (see chapter 25 on values work in this volume; see also Hayes et al., 2012). An initial assignment for structuring and scheduling activities is to have clients monitor activities for at least one week between sessions.

Activity monitoring consists of having clients note what they have done, what emotion was associated with a particular activity, and how intensely they experienced the emotion. By having clients note activities and emotions, the therapist and client can discuss the connection between activity and mood, and more detailed monitoring helps highlight how various activities and contexts—even those that occur for just a few hours—can result in shifts in mood; this information may be useful in assessing the function of an activity. Clients can record every hour of every day, although that is not usually practical. Therefore, I ask clients to record activities either roughly three times a day—for example, at lunch, dinner, and bedtime—noting what they did and how they felt for the previous few hours, or at specified periods of time during the week.

It is easier for clients to accomplish activity monitoring if they are told that they need to write only a word or two that will jog their memories for review with the therapist during session. When therapists review the activity monitoring with clients, they can learn what activities and situations may be associated with worsened mood, and therefore may initially be avoided, and what activities are associated with improvements in mood, and thus may be good candidates for increasing. The review is also useful for assessing the components that have led to improvements. It is important to keep in mind, however, that just because an activity makes someone feel worse or better, this information alone is not enough to decide whether an activity should be avoided or increased. For example, some clients may engage in activities to avoid feelings of sadness or grief that could, ultimately, be important for them to face in order for treatment to have lasting benefit.

**Activity structuring and scheduling.** Some form of activity scheduling has been used in behavioral and cognitive behavioral therapies for depression for decades. Pleasant events scheduling (MacPhillamy & Lewinsohn, 1982) and mastery/pleasure ratings and scheduling (Beck, Rush, Shaw, & Emery, 1979) have been standard types of activity scheduling. As stated previously, identifying activities that are consistent with a client's values, or that have been associated with improvement in a client's mood, is a good place to begin activity scheduling. Lejuez and colleagues (2011) also have clients develop a hierarchy of activities, based on their predicted difficulty, and then set goals for the week. Martell and colleagues (2010) have worked with clients under the premise that change is easier when it is accomplished incrementally, and thus BA therapists using this model pay significant attention to structuring an activity so it is likely to happen; they also make sure that there is sufficient detail about what, when, where, and with whom the activity will happen to increase the likelihood that the client will actually be able to do it. Activity scheduling is not just telling clients to do things they don't do, which is frequently what depressed clients have heard from friends and family.

Novice BA therapists can make the mistake of assigning activities that seem to be pleasant activities but are not consistent with a client's values or may not be the right activities to target initially. They frequently jump on opportunities to suggest that clients take walks or have coffee with friends. Without a functional analysis or assessment to understand how various activities will serve a client, suggesting an activity that might be good for a client is risky; it may just result in her acquiescing to a rule rather than engaging in behaviors that will be reinforced naturally in her environment and have a high likelihood of increasing and ultimately improving depressed mood.

The following example demonstrates how a therapist and client reviewed an activity monitoring chart and constructed an initial activation exercise together. During the week following this therapy session, the client was to undertake the activity.

*Daphne had completed three days' worth of activities and had recorded the emotions she felt during each activity on her monitoring chart before arriving at her therapy appointment. The therapist talked through each notation with Daphne. Two patterns emerged that the therapist highlighted for Daphne. First, when Daphne spent time alone, she typically had a beer or two and brooded over her losses and failures, and her depression ratings were at their highest.*

*While brooding could be a focus of attention, during this initial assignment the therapist noted another pattern. When Daphne called her friend Anna, her mood lifted. She had called Anna several times during the week, each time rating her depression much lower. In one notation, Daphne listed her emotion while talking with Anna as "happy."*

*The therapist and Daphne had discussed before what she valued most in social relationships, and Daphne had reported that she valued "sharing in mutual help and understanding with friends." When the therapist asked what Daphne and Anna had discussed during the telephone conversations the previous week, Daphne reported that Anna was planning to move to a new apartment closer to where Daphne lived, and she was excited to have such a close friend living nearby. Anna currently lived across town. Daphne and her therapist then discussed activities in which she could engage over the next week. Daphne thought that she would feel better about herself if she offered Anna help with moving, but she also feared that she would fail at this task, as she had been failing at a number of planned activities recently.*

*The therapist asked Daphne to describe some activities that she thought would be manageable over the next week. She said that she lived near a rental shop that sold moving boxes, and she thought that it would be a nice gesture to get some boxes and bring them to Anna. Given the reality that Daphne had not accomplished many tasks away from home recently, her therapist asked how they could break the task down so that she would be more successful. Daphne noted that buying the boxes and then driving them to Anna might be ambitious. She stated also that she needed to find out what kind of boxes Anna needed. Daphne and her therapist broke the activity into three smaller tasks. First, Daphne would call Anna on Tuesday, after work, to ask what type of boxes she could use. Second, Daphne would drive to the rental shop on Thursday morning and purchase as many boxes as she could afford and fit in her small car. Third, on Friday evening Daphne would call Anna again and tell her what she got, and then make arrangements for the following week to meet Anna for coffee and to bring the boxes to her.*

Therapists and clients may use activity diaries or charts throughout treatment, or they may use them only during the initial sessions and then agree to other methods for tracking client activities. Some clients prefer to simply list activities and check them off when completed. While I believe it increases the likelihood of success if clients can dedicate a specific time to doing an activity, I have not found it helpful to force this upon clients if they prefer to simply commit to doing the activities as a weekly goal without specifying times in advance. BA is a pragmatic therapy, and practitioners use what works, following basic behavioral principles and the BA formulation. Therapists also individualize treatment by understanding the situations and consequences likely to increase client activity and engagement.

**Functional analysis.** Behavioral activation therapists are more concerned with the function of a client's behavior than with its topography. In other words, BA is not about increasing activities that look positive or pleasant from the perspective of an outside observer, or even from the perspective of the client. Rather BA is concerned with the functional consequences of behavior, and with the conditions under which a behavior is more likely to increase in frequency over time as it is reinforced by its consequences. Thus, BA therapists use a clinical functional analysis or, more technically, a functional assessment (A-B-C, or antecedent, behavior, consequence) to understand client behavior, and they teach clients to understand their behavior in this way as well. The following points illustrate several uses of the functional analysis in BA:

- *To understand a client's behavioral repertoire.* Functional analysis is used in BA to gain a better understanding of clients, in the service of helping them to activate and engage in potentially reinforcing activities or in antidepressant behaviors (Martell et al., 2010) that will ultimately be reinforced. The therapist can gain a general understanding of the contingencies that may control the client's behavior. Broadly speaking, it is useful to understand whether the client behaviors that are targeted in session are under aversive control, such as when a client engages in an activity mostly to avoid feelings or situations that she experiences as unpleasant, or if behaviors that maintain depression are being positively reinforced, such as when a client immediately lies down when returning home from work because family members then sit with him and give him attention he would not otherwise receive (Lejuez et al., 2011).

- *To identify barriers to activation.* Functional assessment is also used in the service of specific activation assignments. It is common for clients to have difficulty engaging in activities. If this were not the case, they would likely not be in treatment. Teaching clients to understand a simple three-term contingency, the A-B-C, can help both therapist and client better understand the difficulties in activation. Usually the therapist should change the jargon of "antecedent, behavior, consequence" to something more accessible. The same process can be described to clients as "situation, and action, and a consequence," or even "What happened?" or "What did you do?" and "Then what happened next?"

# Barriers

Activating is difficult. This is true for everyone. Some mornings we are tired and don't really want to get out of bed. Each time we press the snooze button, we have had a barrier to activating. Barriers can be external, or public: for example, planning to attend an event but having a car break down on the same day. Or they can be internal, or private: for example, not wanting to get out of bed because of feeling tired.

Barriers to activation are idiosyncratic, and identifying what is particularly problematic for an individual is important. However, there are two relatively common barriers that are identified and targeted in BA: avoidance behaviors and rumination. Wolpe (1982) suggests that many behaviors of people whom we would currently diagnose with depression or anxiety function as avoidance. Many of the behaviors of depressed clients are negatively reinforced and allow them to escape or avoid, such as aversive feelings or situations that they dread. The acronym TRAP can help clients identify avoidance. Clients are asked to identify "triggers," a "response" (which therapists often simplify by suggesting that clients notice their emotional response), and an "avoidance pattern." The word "pattern" indicates that avoidance is common, but clients don't need to identify a specific pattern of behavior in each situation. Once clients have identified avoidance, the therapist asks them to "get out of the TRAP and get back on TRAC," in the same trigger (T) situation and with the same feelings (R), to find an alternative coping (AC) behavior (Martell, et al, 2001).

In BA, thoughts are approached as private behaviors, and rather than attend to the content, as one would rightly do in cognitive therapy, BA therapists consider the function of ruminative processes of thinking. When clients tell a therapist that they are thinking about things repeatedly, or when the therapist notices this occurring, clients are invited to try one of two alternative behaviors. The therapist first asks clients to use a brief problem-solving skill to state a problem, to brainstorm solutions, to decide on one to attempt, and then to assess the outcome. If clients cannot identify a solution to a problem or are brooding over things that happened in the past, the therapist invites them to attend to the experience of an activity. This is suggested so that they refocus attention from brooding to paying attention to sights, sounds, smells, and other sensations, or to elements of a task. This is also a way to help clients actually engage in behaviors they are attempting, rather than just going through the motions while brooding on other disturbing things that pull them out of the moment.

# Summary

Behavioral activation is a straightforward procedure that has primarily been used with depressed clients, or with clients who are depressed and have comorbid medical problems (Hopko, Bell, Armento, Hunt, & Lejuez, 2005). The key process focus is reinforcement, but related processes of attention to the present moment, emotional acceptance, and values clarification are also involved. The goal of BA is to have clients actively engage in behaviors that they value, have meaning for them, and are likely to be naturally reinforced in the environment.

Research indicates that BA can successfully be conducted in a less formal fashion, following a clear behavioral formulation (Dimidjian et al., 2006), or in a very structured, brief format (Lejuez et al., 2011). BA can be used as a strategy in a broader cognitive behavioral intervention (Beck et al., 1979); in this case it usually consists of simply identifying activities that give clients a sense of pleasure or accomplishment, and it is conducted following a case conceptualization that serves to change unhelpful beliefs and behaviors.

Though BA was initially studied for the treatment of depression, several studies suggest that BA has shown promise with other problems, and research is under way to expand its use. It is hoped that future research will clarify cultural adaptations that may be necessary with diverse populations, the physiological processes that are impacted with BA, and BA's uses with different age-groups.

# References

Beck, A. T., Rush, A. J., Shaw, B. F., & Emery, G. (1979). *Cognitive therapy of depression*. New York: Guilford Press.

Dimidjian, S., Hollon, S. D., Dobson, K. S., Schmaling, K. B., Kohlenberg, R. J., Addis, M. E., et al. (2006). Randomized trial of behavioral activation, cognitive therapy, and antidepressant medication in the acute treatment of adults with major depression. *Journal of Consulting and Clinical Psychology, 74*(4), 658–670.

Hayes, S. C., Strosahl, K. D., & Wilson, K. G. (2012). *Acceptance and commitment therapy: The process and practice of mindful change* (2nd ed.). New York: Guilford Press.

Hopko, D. R., Bell, J. L., Armento, M. E. A., Hunt, M. K., & Lejuez, C. W. (2005). Behavior therapy for depressed cancer patients in primary care. *Psychotherapy: Theory, Research, Practice, Training, 42*(2), 236–243.

Kabat-Zinn, J. (1994). *Wherever you go, there you are: Mindfulness meditation in Everyday life*. New York: Hyperion.

Lejuez, C. W., Hopko, D. R., Acierno, R., Daughters, S. B., & Pagoto, S. L. (2011). Ten year revision of the brief behavioral activation treatment for depression: Revised treatment manual. *Behavior Modification, 35*(2), 111–161.

MacPhillamy, D. J., & Lewinsohn, P. M. (1982). The pleasant events schedule: Studies in reliability, validity, and scale intercorrelation. *Journal of Consulting and Clinical Psychology, 50*(3), 363–380.

Martell, C. R., Addis, M. E., & Jacobson, N. S. (2001). *Depression in context: Strategies for guided action*. New York: W. W. Norton.

Martell, C. R., Dimidjian, S., & Herman-Dunn, R. (2010). *Behavioral activation for depression: A clinician's guide*. New York: Guilford Press.

Segal, Z. V., Williams, J. M. G., & Teasdale, J. D. (2001). *Mindfulness-based cognitive therapy for depression: A new approach to preventing relapse*. New York: Guilford Press.

Wolpe, J. (1982). *The practice of behavior therapy* (3rd ed.). New York: Pergamon Press.

# CHAPTER 20

# Interpersonal Skills

Kim T. Mueser, PhD

*Center for Psychiatric Rehabilitation and
Departments of Occupational Therapy, Psychology,
and Psychiatry, Boston University*

## Background

People are by nature gregarious creatures. Most individuals live with others with whom they share household tasks, work with other people, engage in leisure and recreational activities with others, and share or strive for close, personally and physically intimate relationships with a select few. Humans' unique capacity for communication and cooperative behavior has led to the development of complex social systems, mastery over the environment, and the ability to prolong and improve the quality of their lives.

Given the importance of communication to cooperative behavior, it is no surprise that interpersonal skills for expressing thoughts, feelings, needs, preferences, and desires, and for responding to others, play a key role in functioning across the broad range of social and other life domains. Problems in functioning naturally lead to unhappiness, frustration, and dissatisfaction. The ability to recognize when poor social skills in specific areas are contributing to a client's problems or are limiting the individual's potential for growth, and to teach more effective skills, is a critical competency for cognitive and behavioral therapists serving any clinical population.

## Understanding Problems with Interpersonal Skills

The desire for more effective interactions with others can be used to motivate change and improve interpersonal skills. People often seek therapy because they are unhappy with their relationships. A person may lack friends and feel anxious in social situations, or he may yearn for closeness and intimacy with a romantic companion. People in close relationships may feel unhappy due to a variety of problems, such as conflict over money or child-rearing; lack of engagement or affection; difficulty expressing or responding to feelings or desires; or destructive interpersonal behaviors, such as verbal or physical abuse.

Problematic interpersonal skills can also contribute to issues at work, such as difficulties interacting with customers or responding to feedback from a supervisor. Limited interpersonal skills for situations such as shopping, requesting repairs from a landlord, or resolving a disagreement with a neighbor or roommate can also interfere with daily living and independence. When people lack adequate skills, the ability to obtain proper treatment and to manage physical and mental health conditions can also be jeopardized due to their avoidance of health care providers, the limited effectiveness of their interactions with providers, and their reduced ability to obtain social support for illness management.

A strong evidence base supports the effectiveness of interpersonal skills training for improving social and community functioning (Kurtz & Mueser, 2008; Lyman et al., 2014). Using these methods to improve interpersonal skills is especially important for clinical populations with poor psychosocial functioning, such as people with schizophrenia spectrum disorders, or for those with developmental disorders, such as autism spectrum disorders or an intellectual disability.

# Definitions

*Interpersonal skillfulness* can be defined as the smooth and seamless integration of specific behaviors that are necessary for effective communication and are critical to achieving social and instrumental goals (Liberman, DeRisi, & Mueser, 1989). Four different types of skills are commonly distinguished: nonverbal skills, paralinguistic features, verbal content, and interactive balance. Therapists usually teach complex interpersonal skills by focusing on specific components, which are built up gradually through extensive practice and feedback.

*Nonverbal skills* are behaviors other than speech, such as eye contact, facial expression, use of gestures, interpersonal proximity, and body orientation, that convey interest, feelings, and meaning during social interactions. *Paralinguistic features* are the vocal characteristics of speech, such as loudness, fluency, and affect expressed through tone and pitch (prosody). *Verbal content* is the appropriateness of what is said, including choice of words and phrasing, regardless of how it is said. *Interactive balance* pertains to the interplay of communication between two people, including the latency of time in responding to the partner's utterance, the proportion of time spent talking, and the relevance and responsiveness to what the partner said.

Nonverbal and paralinguistic behaviors are sometimes inconsistent with the verbal content of a communication, which can undermine the person's intent. For example, expressing a negative feeling in a quiet, faltering voice tone with an apologetic facial expression could be interpreted to mean that the person is not really upset, and that the concern can be ignored. Problems with interactive balance, such as long latencies of response due to reduced information-processing capacity in schizophrenia (Mueser, Bellack, Douglas, & Morrison, 1991), can interfere with the ebb and flow of a conversation and make it feel awkward and unrewarding to the partner. Conversely, frequently interrupting or responding too quickly can make the conversation feel rushed or hurried and can be interpreted to mean that the speaker isn't really interested in what the other person has to say.

Effective social interactions also require social cognition skills, including the ability to accurately perceive and respond to relevant information in different social situations and to understand common "unwritten rules" of communication within a culture and setting (Augoustinos, Walker, & Donaghue, 2006). Important social information must be gleaned from the situational context in which the interaction takes place (e.g., setting, such as public, private, work, home; relationship to the individual, such as stranger, coworker, boss, friend, family member) and from the other person's behavior. Accurately perceiving the conversational partner's emotions from nonverbal paralinguistic cues, and understanding the person's perspective (called theory of mind), are key social cognition skills that are frequently impaired in people with serious mental illness (Penn, Corrigan, Bentall, Racenstein, & Newman, 1997).

# Nonskill Factors That Can Affect Social Functioning

Aside from interpersonal skills, a variety of other factors can influence social functioning. Depression and associated beliefs of hopelessness, helplessness, and worthlessness often compromise social drive and reduce the effort people expend connecting with others. Just looking sad can make someone appear less attractive and less appealing to others (Mueser, Grau, Sussman, & Rosen, 1984), and living with a depressed person can induce depression (Coyne et al., 1987). Anxiety can lead to social avoidance or result in such preoccupation with worry that people are unable to use available skills. Anger or frustration can inhibit the ability of people to listen to the perspectives of others, leading to unrestrained expressions of negative feelings and increased interpersonal conflict.

Other psychiatric symptoms can also be problematic. Negative symptoms of schizophrenia, such as apathy and anhedonia, can reduce social drive when people expect that social interactions will require too much effort or will be unrewarding (Gard, Kring, Gard, Horan, & Green, 2007). *Blunted affect* (diminished facial and paralinguistic expressiveness) and *alogia* (poverty of speech) may make people appear less engaged during social interactions than they actually feel. Psychotic symptoms, such as hallucinations and delusions, can distract or preoccupy people, making them inattentive, unresponsive, or inappropriate during social interactions. Hypomania and mania can take a toll on an individual's social relationships due to symptoms such as pressured speech, irritability, grandiosity, and increased involvement in activities with potentially harmful consequences (e.g., sexual liaisons, spending money). Substance use and dependency can have a major impact on social functioning, ranging from the disinhibiting effects of alcohol on aggression to the manipulation of close relationships in order to maintain a drug dependency.

The environment can also influence the ability of people to use interpersonal skills and to benefit from skills training. When there are limited opportunities for meaningful social activity, as is often the case for people institutionalized for extended periods of time (Wing & Brown, 1970), continued impaired social functioning is a foregone conclusion, regardless of the person's interpersonal skills. Similarly, if efforts to use appropriate interpersonal skills, such as expressing feelings or preferences, are thwarted, as in the example of a depressed person living with a domineering partner, the depressed person may give up on trying to use those skills and consequently remain dissatisfied and unhappy in the relationship.

# History and Theoretical Foundations of Interpersonal Skills Training

Interpersonal skills training methods date back to the 1950s and 1960s, and their clinical foundations are found in the early work of Salter (1949), Wolpe (1958), and Lazarus (1966), which focused on helping individuals overcome shyness and anxiety in close relationships. The theoretical origins of some of this work drew from previous research on operant conditioning, shaping, and social learning modeling. Skinner's (1953) work on the use of positive reinforcement and shaping (see chapters 11 and 13) showed that it was possible to teach complex behaviors by breaking them down into simpler ones. Bandura's (Bandura, Ross, & Ross, 1961) work on social modeling demonstrated the power of observing others in learning new social behaviors. The development of behavioral rehearsal in role-plays as a technique for facilitating the initial practice and refinement of skills further enhanced the benefits of combining social modeling and shaping to teach interpersonal skills. The systematic use of role-plays to first model skills, and then to engage individuals in behavioral rehearsals of those skills, followed by shaping feedback, resulted in an efficient method for teaching interpersonal skills under relatively controlled conditions. Clients could then practice those skills in naturally occurring situations.

In a nutshell, clinicians provide interpersonal skills training by first breaking a skill down into its constituent elements, reviewing them with the client, and then modeling the skill through role-play. After discussing the demonstration, the clinician engages the client in role-play to practice the skill, followed by positive and then corrective feedback about the client's performance. The clinician then engages the client in another role-play to further improve his or her performance, followed by additional feedback to shape the skill. Several role-plays are conducted with the client, each followed by feedback to further hone the person's skill. Finally, the client and clinician agree on a homework assignment for a skill the client will try in real-life situations.

# Format and Logistics of Interpersonal Skills Training

Skills training can be provided in individual, group, family, or couples formats. In a group format the number of participants is usually limited to six to eight in order to permit enough time for everyone to practice the skills. Skills training in a group format is generally more efficient, and it provides access to multiple role models and the support and encouragement from other group members to try new skills.

Interpersonal skills training is sometimes the primary focus of the intervention and covers a preplanned curriculum of skills addressing a specific topic area. Such programs are typically provided in a group format, such as conversations skills for people with serious mental illness (Bellack, Mueser, Gingerich, & Agresta, 2004), substance-use refusal skills for people with an addiction (Monti, Kadden, Rohsenow, Cooney, & Abrams, 2002), or conflict management skills for people with anger or aggression problems (Taylor & Novaco, 2005). Sessions typically last 1 to 1.5 hours and are conducted 1 to 3 times per week, with programs lasting from 2 to 3 months to more than a year.

Interpersonal skills training may also be part of a multicomponent program, such as dialectical behavior therapy for people with borderline personality disorder (Linehan, 1993) or a program teaching self-management skills (see chapter 14). The illness management and recovery program (Mueser & Gingerich, 2011) provides skills training to help people with serious mental illness interact more effectively with treatment providers and to increase the social support for managing their illness. Family therapy programs designed to teach families how to help a loved one manage a mental illness such as schizophrenia or bipolar disorder often incorporate communication and problem solving to reduce family stress, in addition to psychoeducation about the nature of the psychiatric illness (Miklowitz, 2010; Mueser & Glynn, 1999).

Interpersonal skills may also be taught, as the need arises, during individual psychotherapy. In these circumstances, the skills training can range from as little as ten to fifteen minutes per session over several sessions to a more extended focus over a longer period of time.

# Training Methods

Regardless of the treatment modality used or the prominence in treatment, interpersonal skills training uses a systematic method, which table 1 summarizes. Interpersonal skills training is defined most basically by the integrated use of four techniques, described below.

## Table 1.    Steps of common interpersonal skills

ACTIVE LISTENING

- Look at the person.

- Show you are listening by nodding your head, smiling, or saying something like "uh-huh" or "okay."

- Ask questions to find out more information or to make sure you understand.

- Repeat back the person's main points or make a comment about something he said.

EXPRESSING A POSITIVE FEELING

- Look at the person with a positive facial expression.

- Describe what you are pleased about.

- Tell her how it made you feel.

MAKING A REQUEST

- Look at the person.

- Explain what you would like him to do.

- Tell him how it would make you feel.

EXPRESSING A NEGATIVE FEELING

- Look at the person with a serious facial expression.

- Explain what you are upset about.

- Tell her how it made you feel.

- Suggest a way that it could be prevented in the future.

COMPROMISE AND NEGOTIATION

- Explain your viewpoint.

- Listen to the other person's viewpoint.

- Repeat back or paraphrase the other person's viewpoint.

- Suggest a compromise.

- Talk it over until you reach a compromise that you both agree on.

GIVING A COMPLIMENT

- Look at the person.

- Use a positive, sincere voice tone.

- Be specific about what it is that you like.

**Focus on core components of specific interpersonal skills.** In order to use a shaping approach to teaching skills, the clinician must first pay attention to the specific components of the targeted skill. Nonverbal and paralinguistic skills should be consistent with the verbal content of the communication. People often get stuck on what they should say in particular situations, and to address this it is useful to break down the verbal content of specific skills into several steps. These steps, which can be combined with nonverbal or paralinguistic elements, can then be highlighted when modeling the skill and providing feedback after the role-plays. Table 2 provides examples of steps for training common interpersonal skills; extensive curricula for a broad range of skills are readily accessible elsewhere to clinicians (e.g., Bellack et al., 2004; Monti et al., 2002).

# Table 2.   General approach to interpersonal skills training

1. **Establish a rationale for the skill.**

   - Briefly introduce the skill.

   - Elicit reasons for learning the skill by asking questions.

   - Acknowledge all reasons given.

   - Provide additional rationale as needed.

2. **Discuss the steps of the skill.**

   - Break the skill down into three to five component steps.

   - Use handouts, posters, and so forth when feasible.

   - Briefly discuss the reasons for each step.

3. **Model the skill in a role-play.**

   - Explain that you will demonstrate the skill.

   - "Set up," or explain, the context of the role-play situation.

   - Model the skill in a role-play.

   - Keep the role-play brief and to the point.

4. **Review the role play with the client(s).**

   - Discuss which specific steps of the skill were used in the role-play.

   - Ask the client(s) to evaluate the effectiveness of the role-play.

5. **Engage the client in a role-play of the same or a similar situation.**

   - Ask the client to try to use the skill in a role-play.

- Modify the situation as needed to make it plausible for the person.

- For groups, ask other members to observe the client in order to provide feedback.

6. **Provide positive feedback.**

- Provide specific, positive feedback about what the person did well in the role-play.

- Praise all efforts.

- Include feedback about the steps of the skill and other aspects of the performance that were done well.

- If in a group format,
    - elicit positive feedback first from group members before providing additional positive feedback, and
    - cut off any negative feedback or criticism.

7. **Provide corrective feedback.**

- Give (or elicit first from group members) suggestions for how the client could do the skill better.

- Limit feedback to one or two suggestions.

- Communicate suggestions in an upbeat, positive manner.

8. **Engage the client in one to three more role-plays of the same situation.**

- Request that the person change one or two behaviors per role-play.

- Focus on behaviors that are most salient and changeable.

- Use additional modeling if needed to highlight specific behaviors the person is trying to change.

9. **After each role-play, provide additional feedback and suggestions for improved performance.**

- Focus first on the behaviors that were to be changed.

- Use additional teaching strategies as needed to facilitate behavior change (e.g., coaching, prompting, modeling).

- Be generous but specific when providing feedback.

- Skip corrective feedback for the last role-play the client performs.

- Elicit the client's self-appraisal of performance after the last role-play.

- If skills training is conducted in a group or family format, follow steps 5–8 for each member.

10. **Develop an assignment for the client (or group members) to practice the skill on her own.**

- Develop the assignment collaboratively with the client.

- Aim for the client to practice the skill at least twice before the next session.

- Tailor the assignment to maximize relevance to the client and the likelihood of follow-through.

- Troubleshoot possible obstacles to the client following through on the assignment.

- Review the home assignment at the beginning of the next session.

**Use modeling in role-plays to demonstrate interpersonal skills.** Although underutilized in routine practice, the routine modeling of interpersonal skills is a powerful skills training technique. Modeling a skill before engaging the client in role-play to practice it puts the person at ease, reducing anxiety and normalizing role-playing as a normal part of the psychotherapeutic process, as something used by the clinician and client alike.

Some clients have difficulty improving their skills over successive role-plays from verbal feedback and instructions alone. In such cases, additional modeling by the clinician can be useful. Prior to demonstrating the skill again, the clinician can draw the client's attention to specific component behaviors (e.g., voice loudness, a feeling statement), followed by the client trying the skill again in role-play. In some situations it can be helpful to highlight the importance of a particular component skill by modeling it in two successive role-plays, one showing poor performance and the other good performance of the component, followed by discussion and then a role-play in which the client tries the skill again.

**Use positive and corrective feedback to shape social skills over multiple role-plays.** The primary assumption underlying the skills training approach is that improving an individual's competence at performing a skill in simulated situations will facilitate the transfer of that skill to naturally occurring interactions. Repeatedly practicing and honing skills is different from "trying" a skill once in a role-play. Some learning may occur the first time the client practices a skill in a role-play. However, the greatest learning occurs in successive role-plays of the same situation, with the clinician targeting specific nuances of the skill, and the client experimenting with making those changes and developing comfort and familiarity with the skill in the safety of the session. Thus, when initially training an interpersonal skill, the clinician should engage the client in a minimum of two role-plays, with three being even better, and four or more role-plays often leading to the greatest benefit.

The sine qua non of skills training is engaging the client in multiple role-plays of the same skill and situation within a session, combined with clinician modeling, feedback, and instructions to shape the person's performance of the skill. The nature of the feedback provided for each role-play is critical to ensuring that the client's learning experience is a positive one, and to making the skills training as effective as possible. In order to reinforce the person's effort to learn new skills, and to maximize her willingness to try again, genuine, positive feedback should always be given immediately following the client's role-play, before any negative feedback is given. Feedback should be behaviorally specific, draw attention to specific aspects of the skill done well, and begin with any component skills that improved from one role-play to the next.

The primary purpose of corrective feedback is to identify specific areas of the client's performance that could be improved upon, and to then engage the person in another role-play focusing on changing those component skills. The choice of which areas to focus on changing is determined by the salience of the deficit and the ease with which the client may change it. For example, when the client's voice volume is very low or his tone is soft or meek, then vocal loudness, firmness, or expressivity may be an initial priority. When a simple verbal-content step of a skill is omitted from a role-play, such as describing a feeling or not being specific about something, it is often easy for clients to add that step in during the next role-play.

The clinician needs to be able to shift to providing corrective feedback without negating the warm feelings engendered by the positive feedback. The clinician can accomplish this by being brief; by providing specific, matter-of-fact corrective feedback; and by moving quickly to suggesting, in a positive, upbeat manner, how the person could improve her performance in the next role-play. It is also helpful to avoid using "but" statements after giving positive feedback (e.g.,

"Nice job! You had a pleasant facial expression, and you were clear about what you were pleased with in that role-play, *but* you left out how it made you feel").

**Develop home-practice assignments.** The artificial nature of role-playing provides a unique opportunity for people to learn, practice, and refine their interpersonal skills without concern for the social repercussions of their behavior. This differs from practicing skills in real-world social situations, where the consequences of skillfulness, or lack thereof, are naturally experienced. However, if clients are to realize the benefits of improved interpersonal skills, regular efforts need to be made to help them use these skills on their own.

Follow through on home assignments. First, after establishing the rationale for practicing skills outside of session, the clinician and client should collaboratively develop home assignments to ensure understanding, buy-in, and feasibility. Second, assignments should be specific and include plans, such as how many times the client will use the skill, with whom and in what situations the client will use the skill, and how the client will remember the assignment. Third, the clinician and client should anticipate possible obstacles to follow-through on home assignments and identify solutions to those obstacles.

Although home assignments are the standard method for facilitating the generalization of skills, additional strategies are necessary for clients with major cognitive or symptoms challenges. One strategy is to use in vivo practice trips designed to provide clients with a supportive experience when trying newly learned skills in natural settings (Glynn et al., 2002). Clinicians usually provide these trips when conducting skills training in a group format, and they involve regularly scheduled group excursions to community settings where clients can try their skills.

Another strategy for facilitating generalization is to involve indigenous supporters (Wallace & Tauber, 2004). *Indigenous supporters* are people close to clients who usually have a nonprofessional relationship with them (e.g., family member, close friend), although paraprofessional staff may serve for people who live in residential or long-term hospital settings. By virtue of their involvement with the client outside of sessions, these people are in an ideal position to prompt and reinforce the client's use of skills. In order to involve such people, the clinician needs to reach out (with client permission) and engage indigenous supporters so they can understand the nature of the skills training program and support its goals. Then, in regular meetings, the clinician shares information with the supportive person about recently targeted skills, identifies suitable situations for using the skills, and obtains feedback about the client's use of skills or the person's efforts to prompt their use.

# Processes of Change

There are likely multiple processes of change involved in how interpersonal skills training improves social functioning. The dominant conceptualization that led to the skills training model was that effective social relationships require the integration of component social skills, and that the failure to learn these skills or the loss of them through disuse contributes to poor social functioning. Based on this conceptualization, the skills training approach was developed with the aim of increasing an individual's repertoire of interpersonal skills, through shaping and extensive practice, and helping clients reach the point where they can perform skills automatically when desired. Although interpersonal skills are stable over time in the absence of intervention, poor social skills are associated with worse psychosocial functioning, and skills training increases both social skills and social functioning (Bellack, Morrison, Wixted, & Mueser, 1990; Kurtz & Mueser, 2008); it remains to be seen if improved social skills mediate gains in social functioning.

Some people who are capable of performing interpersonal skills but fail to use them when opportunities arise appear to benefit from interpersonal skills training. For example, some clients have low self-efficacy in their ability to have successful social interactions (Pratt, Mueser, Smith, & Lu, 2005) due to factors such as depression or anticipation of social defeat (Granholm, Holden, Link, McQuaid, & Jeste, 2013). The positive, validating nature of skills training, combined with the process of collaboratively agreeing to try skills in different situations, may encourage clients to use their skills, leading to positive social experiences that challenge their inaccurate beliefs. The cognitive behavioral social skills training program seeks to capitalize on both of these processes by combining skills training with cognitive behavioral therapy aimed at challenging inaccurate perceptions of the self and others, both of which interfere with pursuing social goals (Granholm, McQuaid, & Holden, 2016).

Other processes of change that may contribute to the effects of interpersonal skills training are exposure and greater emotional acceptance (see chapters 18 and 24). Role-plays elicit small amounts of discomfort in a safe environment, and repeated exposure to these situations as clients pursue their social goals may reduce their avoidance of social situations that likewise produce some discomfort.

# Case Study

Juan was a thirty-two-year-old Latino man with schizotypal personality disorder. His presenting concern was problems at work. Juan was a computer technology consultant who worked for a large firm, where he provided repairs and software updates for the laptops and personal computers of employees. He expressed concern that he often felt uncomfortable at work and was afraid of losing his job. The clinician spent two sessions with Juan obtaining background information and a more thorough work history before delving into specific situations at work that Juan found difficult to manage.

The clinician learned that Juan had difficulty interacting with employees whose computers he fixed, responding to feedback from his supervisor, and socializing with his other consultant coworkers. With Juan's help, the clinician set up and engaged him in a series of role-plays to evaluate his interpersonal skills in these situations. This assessment indicated that Juan had difficulty engaging in small talk with employees when he came to fix their computers, as well as with coworkers during informal interactions or breaks. He also found it hard to respond to employees who were anxious about getting their computer fixed. Juan didn't see why he had to interact so much with employees and coworkers, and he thought they should just leave him alone so he could do his work. Finally, Juan had difficulty listening to negative feedback from his supervisor and eliciting suggestions for improving his job performance.

To address these problems, the clinician identified several skills to teach Juan, initially using the same role-play situations developed for the assessment to teach the skills, and then developed additional role-play situations to facilitate further in-session practice. The clinician also spent time talking with Juan about the importance of informal (or "trivial") social interactions at work and helped him conceptualize "interpersonal skills" in those situations as being similar to his technological expertise—just another part of his job. The clinician targeted improving conversational skills to reduce Juan's discomfort interacting with coworkers and employees; these skills included identifying suitable topics for informal socializing (e.g., sports, the weather, local news), active listening to others, responding to the comments of others by providing his own perspective, and gracefully ending brief conversations.

To address situations in which employees were anxious about the repair of their computers, the clinician taught Juan to acknowledge their concerns by paraphrasing back to them their concerns, and to then provide reassurance that he would address their concerns with a timely repair. To improve Juan's ability to respond to his supervisor's feedback, the clinician taught him to reflect back what he heard his supervisor say to ensure he had proper understanding, to seek clarification regarding how he could improve his performance, and to request feedback following attempts to implement the desired changes.

Skills training was provided in twenty-four sessions over a six-month period. They spent most of each session role-playing newly learned skills, which were introduced every two or three sessions; developing plans for Juan to practice these skills at work; using role-plays to review practice assignments and conduct additional training as needed; and reviewing previously taught skills. Juan was readily engaged in the skills training, and over the course of treatment his interpersonal skills improved across the targeted situations, with notably less discomfort at work. Toward the end of treatment, Juan reported that he had been recommended for a raise because his supervisor had noted significant improvements in his work.

# Conclusions

Effective interpersonal skills play an important role in the quality of close relationships, and they have a strong bearing on other life domains, such as work, school, or parenting, as well as self-care and independent living. Poor interpersonal skills in specific areas are a common factor contributing to distress and maladjustment, and they underlie many of the problems for which people seek psychotherapy. Teaching interpersonal skills is a core competency required of all practicing cognitive and behavioral clinicians. Clinicians can teach interpersonal skills by using a systematic training method that involves breaking down complex skills into simpler components or steps, modeling the skill in role-plays, engaging the client in role-plays to practice the skill, providing positive and corrective feedback after each role-play to hone client performance, and developing home assignments for clients to practice skills outside of session. Interpersonal skills training improves social functioning and community adjustment and can help with problems of vocational functioning, substance abuse, family and/or couples conflict, and collaboration with treatment providers.

# References

Augoustinos, M., Walker, I., & Donaghue, N. (2006). *Social cognition: An integrated introduction.* London: Sage Publications.

Bandura, A., Ross, D., & Ross, S. A. (1961). Transmission of aggression through the imitation of aggressive models. *Journal of Abnormal and Social Psychology, 63*(3), 575–582.

Bellack, A. S., Morrison, R. L., Wixted, J. T., & Mueser, K. T. (1990). An analysis of social competence in schizophrenia. *British Journal of Psychiatry, 156*(6), 809–818.

Bellack, A. S., Mueser, K. T., Gingerich, S., & Agresta, J. (2004). *Social skills training for schizophrenia: A step-by-step guide* (2nd ed.). New York: Guilford Press.

Coyne, J. C., Kessler, R. C., Tal, M., Turnbull, J., Wortman, C. B., & Greden, J. F. (1987). Living with a depressed person. *Journal of Consulting and Clinical Psychology, 55*(3), 347–352.

Gard, D. E., Kring, A. M., Gard, M. G., Horan, W. P., & Green, M. F. (2007). Anhedonia in schizophrenia: Distinctions between anticipatory and consummatory pleasure. *Schizophrenia Research, 93*(1–3), 253–260.

Glynn, S. M., Marder, S. R., Liberman, R. P., Blair, K., Wirshing, W. C., Wirshing, D. A., et al. (2002). Supplementing clinic-based skills training with manual-based community support sessions: Effects on social adjustment of patients with schizophrenia. *American Journal of Psychiatry, 159*(5), 829–837.

Granholm, E., Holden, J., Link, P. C., McQuaid, J. R., & Jeste, D. V. (2013). Randomized controlled trial of cognitive behavioral social skills training for older consumers with schizophrenia: Defeatist performance attitudes and functional outcome. *American Journal of Geriatric Psychiatry, 21*(3), 251–262.

Granholm, E. L., McQuaid, J. R., & Holden, J. L. (2016). *Cognitive-behavioral social skills training for schizophrenia: A practical treatment guide.* New York: Guilford Press.

Kurtz, M. M., & Mueser, K. T. (2008). A meta-analysis of controlled research on social skills training for schizophrenia. *Journal of Consulting and Clinical Psychology, 76*(3), 491–504.

Lazarus, A. A. (1966). Behaviour rehearsal vs. non-directive therapy vs. advice in effecting behaviour change. *Behaviour Research and Therapy, 4*(3), 209–212.

Liberman, R. P., DeRisi, W. J., & Mueser, K. T. (1989). *Social skills training for psychiatric patients.* Needham Heights, MA: Allyn and Bacon.

Linehan, M. M. (1993). *Cognitive behavioral treatment of borderline personality disorder.* New York: Guilford Press.

Lyman, D. R., Kurtz, M. M., Farkas, M., George, P., Dougherty, R. H., Daniels, A. S., et al. (2014). Skill building: Assessing the evidence. *Psychiatric Services, 65*(6), 727–738.

Miklowitz, D. J. (2010). *Bipolar disorder: A family-focused treatment approach* (2nd ed.). New York: Guilford Press.

Monti, P. M., Kadden, R. M., Rohsenow, D. J., Cooney, N. L., & Abrams, D. B. (2002). *Treating Alcohol dependence: A coping skills training guide* (2nd ed.). New York: Guilford Press.

Mueser, K. T., Bellack, A. S., Douglas, M. S., & Morrison, R. L. (1991). Prevalence and stability of social skill deficits in schizophrenia. *Schizophrenia Research, 5*(2), 167–176.

Mueser, K. T., & Gingerich, S. (2011). *Illness management and recovery: Personalized skills and strategies for those with mental illness* (3rd ed.). Center City, MN: Hazelden Publishing.

Mueser, K. T., & Glynn, S. M. (1999). *Behavioral family therapy for psychiatric disorders* (2nd ed.). Oakland, CA: New Harbinger Publications.

Mueser, K. T., Grau, B. W., Sussman, S., & Rosen, A. J. (1984). You're only as pretty as you feel: Facial expression as a determinant of physical attractiveness. *Journal of Personality and Social Psychology, 46*(2), 469–478.

Penn, D. L., Corrigan, P. W., Bentall, R. P., Racenstein, J. M., & Newman, L. (1997). Social cognition in schizophrenia. *Psychological Bulletin, 121*(1), 114–132.

Pratt, S. I., Mueser, K. T., Smith, T. E., & Lu, W. (2005). Self-efficacy and psychosocial functioning in schizophrenia: A mediational analysis. *Schizophrenia Research, 78*(2–3), 187–197.

Salter, A. (1949). *Conditioned reflex therapy.* New York: Creative Age Press.

Skinner, B. F. (1953). *Science and human behavior.* New York: Simon and Schuster.

Taylor, J. L., & Novaco, R. W. (2005). *Anger treatment for people with developmental disabilities: A theory, evidence and manual based approach.* Chichester, UK: John Wiley and Sons.

Wallace, C. J., & Tauber, R. (2004). Supplementing supported employment with workplace skills training. *Psychiatric Services, 55*(5), 513–515.

Wing, J. K., & Brown, G. W. (1970). *Institutionalism and schizophrenia: A comparative study of three mental hospitals 1960–1968.* Cambridge, UK: Cambridge University Press.

Wolpe, J. (1958). *Psychotherapy by reciprocal inhibition.* Stanford, CA: Stanford University Press.

# CHAPTER 21

# Cognitive Reappraisal

## Amy Wenzel, PhD, ABPP
### *University of Pennsylvania School of Medicine*

## Definitions and Background

Over 2,000 years ago, the Greek philosopher Aristotle noted, "It is the mark of an educated mind to be able to entertain a thought without accepting it." In the present day, mental health professionals from all theoretical orientations work with clients whose lives are stymied by negative and judgmental thoughts and beliefs that they regard as absolute truth. To address the needs of such clients, treatment packages in the family of cognitive behavioral therapies (CBTs) have incorporated strategies for recognizing and addressing negative thoughts and beliefs.

*Cognitive reappraisal* is a strategy in which people reinterpret the meaning of a stimulus in order to alter their emotional response (Gross, 1998). One traditional approach to cognitive reappraisal used in many cognitive behavioral treatment packages is *cognitive restructuring*, or the guided and systematic process by which clinicians help clients to recognize and, if necessary, modify unhelpful thinking associated with emotional distress. It is a key strategic intervention in Aaron T. Beck's cognitive therapy approach (e.g., A. T. Beck, Rush, Shaw, & Emery, 1979). In contrast to reinterpreting and changing thinking, *cognitive defusion* is the ability to distance oneself from one's thoughts and continue on even in the presence of those thoughts (Hayes, Strosahl, & Wilson, 2012), which allows people to let go of the significance that they attach to their thoughts (see chapter 23 of this volume for further discussion). Regularly using cognitive reappraisal and defusion promotes *psychological flexibility*, or the ability to live fully in the present moment and engage in valued activity, regardless of the thoughts one may be experiencing. In this chapter, I illustrate cognitive reappraisal through a description of techniques for delivering cognitive restructuring. However, this chapter also demonstrates the way in which foci on defusion and present-moment awareness can be used in conjunction in order to achieve psychological flexibility.

A growing body of research devotes attention to the mechanisms by which cognitive reappraisal achieves desired outcomes in treatment. Perhaps the most central tenet of Beckian CBT is that cognition mediates the association between experiences in life and one's emotional and behavioral reactions (cf. Dobson & Dozois, 2010). There certainly exist some data to support this notion (Hofmann, 2004; Hofmann et al., 2007). At the same time, there also exists research that does not support this premise, either because (a) the studies did not include the necessary variables and statistical tests to demonstrate mediation unequivocally (cf. Smits, Julian, Rosenfield, & Powers, 2012); (b) the change in symptoms of emotional distress occurred before the change in mediators (e.g., Stice, Rohde, Seeley, & Gau, 2010); (c) the change in problematic cognition simply did not predict outcome (e.g., Burns & Spangler, 2001); or (d) the change in problematic cognition was just as great in a non-CBT condition (e.g., pharmacotherapy) as in CBT (e.g., DeRubeis et al., 1990). More recent research raises the possibility that cognitive reappraisal exerts its effects through the process of *decentering*, or the ability to recognize that thoughts are simply mental events rather than truths that necessitate a particular course of action (Hayes-Skelton & Graham, 2013).

Cognitive behavioral therapists who use cognitive reappraisal with their clients can target three levels of cognition: (a) thoughts that arise in specific situations (i.e., automatic thoughts); (b) conditional rules and assumptions (i.e., intermediate beliefs) that guide the characteristic way in which people interpret events and respond behaviorally; and (c) core beliefs, or fundamental beliefs that people hold about themselves, others, the world, or the future (cf. J. S. Beck, 2011). Consider the case of Lisa, a client who describes an upsetting situation in which she was not invited to a friend's baby shower. Her automatic thought might be something like "My friend doesn't like me." This automatic thought might be associated with a conditional assumption, like "If someone is truly a friend, then she would invite me to an important social event," and a core belief, like "I'm undesirable." Over time, through cognitive reappraisal, clients are able to see that the automatic thoughts they experience in specific situations are reflective of underlying beliefs they hold. Cognitive reappraisal helps clients to slow down their thinking to recognize maladaptive thinking (i.e., thinking that is either inaccurate, exaggerated, or simply unhelpful even if accurate) and either (a) take strategic action to ensure that their thinking is as accurate and as helpful as possible, or (b) recognize that their thinking is simply mental activity that has no bearing on reality and their ability to live their lives in the ways they want. In the next section, I describe the techniques for delivering cognitive restructuring: the cognitive reappraisal approach that is often used by cognitive behavioral therapists.

# Implementation

Cognitive restructuring typically occurs in three steps: the identification, evaluation, and modification of automatic thoughts or underlying beliefs. The following sections provide guidance for implementing each of these steps.

## Identifying Maladaptive Thinking

When clinicians notice a distinct negative shift in clients' affect, they ask, "What was running through your mind just then?" When clients identify a thought, clinicians ask what emotion they were experiencing. These steps serve to further reinforce the association between cognition and emotion, and they also give clients practice in slowing down their thinking enough so they can recognize key thoughts associated with their emotional distress. Once clients have identified one or more emotions, clinicians typically ask them to rate the intensity of the emotions on a 0-to-10 Likert-type scale (e.g., 0 = very low intensity; 10 = the most intense emotional distress imaginable) or using percentages (e.g., 30%, 95%). In some instances, clinicians ask clients to rate (using a similar type of scale) the degree to which they believe the automatic thought. It is important to socialize clients to rating the intensity of their emotions early in the process of cognitive restructuring, as they will use those ratings later to evaluate the degree to which cognitive restructuring has been effective.

Although this exercise appears to be straightforward, in reality it can be difficult for many clients. Most people have not practiced slowing down their thinking to identify key thoughts associated with emotional distress. Thus, the simple act of thoughtfully identifying cognition, in and of itself, has the potential to be therapeutic for three reasons: it (a) reinforces the cognitive model and illustrates the way in which it has continued relevance in clients' lives, (b) creates awareness of psychological processes that are exacerbating mental health problems, and (c) interrupts the "runaway train" of negative thinking that can happen for some clients. When clients experience difficulty identifying thoughts, cognitive behavioral therapists can ask them what they "guess" they were thinking in light of their emotional reaction, or they can provide a menu of options from which a client can choose. They can also assess for the presence of images rather than thoughts in the form of verbal language, as some clients report having images of terrible future outcomes or upsetting memories from the past.

Over time, clients gain skill in identifying and working with automatic thoughts. At this point, many cognitive behavioral therapists will move toward a focus of working at the level of underlying beliefs (i.e., intermediate-level conditional rules and assumptions, core beliefs). There are many ways to identify underlying beliefs. Clients can identify themes inherent in the automatic thoughts that they have shaped over the course of treatment. Therapists can use the *downward arrow technique*, in which they repeatedly probe a client about the meaning associated with an automatic thought until the client gets to a meaning that is so fundamental that there is no additional meaning underneath it (Burns, 1980). Recall the earlier example of Lisa, who identified the automatic thought "My friend doesn't like me" when she realized that she was not invited to her friend's baby shower. Using the downward arrow technique, her therapist asked her, "What does it mean that you weren't invited?" Lisa responded, "It means that we were never friends in the first place." The therapist continued, "What does it mean about you if you were never friends in the first place?" Lisa responded, "It means that I'm more invested in my friends than they are in me." The therapist continued, "What does that say if you are more invested in your friends than they are in you?" Lisa became tearful, began shaking, and responded with a core belief: "It means that I'm totally undesirable." When clients demonstrate significant affect in session, such as tearfulness, shaking, aversion of eye contact, and so on, it provides yet another clue that they have identified a powerful belief that underlies their automatic thoughts.

## Evaluating Maladaptive Thinking

Once clients have recognized the thoughts and beliefs that have the potential to exacerbate emotional distress, they can begin to consider the accuracy and helpfulness of their thinking, as well as the degree to which they are attaching excessive significance to their thinking. Although many clinicians describe this process as "challenging" maladaptive thinking, it is preferable to approach it from a more neutral stance, such that the clinician and client are detectives jointly examining the evidence, or scientists evaluating the data and then drawing a conclusion (i.e., a hypothesis-testing approach). Most clinicians find that with the vast majority of clients, there is a grain of truth in their thinking (if not several grains of truth), so it is important not to presuppose that their thinking is altogether abnormal. Many clinicians prefer to aim for "balanced" thinking, with balance being achieved by acknowledging and tolerating the accuracies of the clients' thinking and by modifying the inaccuracies (though it should be noted that other clinicians, particularly those who practice from the stance of acceptance-based approaches, use cognitive defusion to intervene in a way that promotes distance from maladaptive thinking, rather than changing the content of the thinking).

There is no one formula that clinicians use to evaluate maladaptive thinking. Rather, clinicians are mindful that they are practicing from a stance of *collaborative empiricism*, or the joint enterprise between the clinician and client in which they take a scientific approach to examining and drawing conclusions about the client's thinking and behavior. Rather than telling clients how to think, clinicians use *guided discovery*, in which they ask guided but open-ended questions (i.e., Socratic questioning) and set up new experiences in order to prompt clients to evaluate their thinking and develop an alternative approach to viewing life circumstances. In the following paragraphs, I describe typical lines of Socratic questioning.

Perhaps the most versatile way to evaluate maladaptive thinking is to ask, "What evidence supports this thought or belief? What evidence is inconsistent with this thought or belief?" Clients who engage in this line of Socratic questioning often find that they are focused exclusively on evidence that supports maladaptive thinking, ignoring a vast array of evidence that is inconsistent with the thought or belief. Once they consider the full spectrum of evidence that is relevant to their thinking, they often see that their original thought or belief is overly pessimistic, self-deprecating, or judgmental. Although many clinicians have great success with this tool, two notes of caution are in order. First, clients sometimes identify evidence that supports their thinking but is not truly factual, or to which they are attaching excessive significance. For example, when Lisa was asked to supply evidence that her friend does not like her, she listed the fact that she was not invited to the baby shower. Although this statement might be factual, she is attaching a negative interpretation to it by equating being invited to a baby shower with being liked by her friend, and then concluding that her friend does not like her. Thus, at times evidence that clients identify might need to be subjected to cognitive restructuring. Second, clinicians who work with clients with obsessive-compulsive disorder are encouraged to use the examination of evidence judiciously (Abramowitz & Arch, 2013), as this tool itself can become a compulsion they use to minimize the anxiety associated with their obsessive automatic thoughts.

When clients experience adversity in life, they often attribute it to a personal shortcoming, which in turn can exacerbate their emotional distress. *Reattribution* is a cognitive restructuring technique in which clients learn to consider many explanations for why an event occurred, rather than focusing exclusively (and incorrectly) on something being wrong with them or what they did. Clinicians who use this technique pose the Socratic question "Are there any other explanations for this unfortunate situation?" When Lisa's therapist used reattribution and encouraged her to consider viable explanations for the fact that she was not invited to the baby shower, she acknowledged that her friend has a big family, and often only family is invited to events like this; that it was likely another person, rather than her friend per se, who organized the shower and invited guests; and that she and her friend had recently gone on a lunch date that was filled with warmth and good conversation. Clinicians who use reattribution sometimes draw a pie chart with their clients, allowing them to allocate various explanations for adversity in a graphical format.

All clinicians encounter clients who *catastrophize*, or worry that horrible things will happen to them or their family members in the future. It has been a tradition in CBT to initiate a line of Socratic questioning in which clinicians ask these clients to identify the worst, the best, and the most realistic outcomes. In many cases, clients see that the most realistic outcome is much more closely aligned with the best outcome than with the worst outcome. However, some clients, particularly those with anxiety disorders, do not experience a corresponding decrease in emotional distress when they use this tool, claiming that the remote possibility of the worst outcome is too difficult for them to tolerate. However, many of these clients respond well to evaluating how they could cope with the worst outcome, perhaps even developing a *decatastrophizing plan* outlining how they would proceed if the worst outcome were to occur. Although this tool can be helpful in managing anxiety and promoting a problem-solving orientation, it should be noted that it also serves to decrease uncertainty, even when the tolerance of risk and uncertainty might be the very skill that would best serve these clients.

At times, clients are wrapped up in their own internal experience and have difficulty separating logic from emotional distress. To get some distance from the problematic situation, the clinician can pose the Socratic question "What would you tell a friend if he or she were in this situation?" Clients often find that they would tell a friend something different, and much more balanced, than what they are telling themselves, which can prompt them to evaluate why they are treating themselves differently than they would treat others.

It is important for clinicians to recognize that not all automatic thoughts are negative and inaccurate; in some instances, automatic thoughts represent a very real and difficult reality. In these cases, it is contraindicated to ask guided questions to evaluate the accuracy of these thoughts. Clinicians can, nevertheless, encourage clients to evaluate how helpful their thinking is for their mood, for others, for problem solving, and for acceptance. Thus, clinicians might ask Socratic questions like "What is the effect of focusing on this automatic thought?" or "What is the effect of changing your thinking?" or "What are the advantages and disadvantages of focusing on this thought?" Clients who consider the answers to these questions often realize that rather than accepting stressful or disappointing life circumstances, their rumination is exacerbating their emotional stress and keeping them stuck in a struggle against those circumstances. Clinicians can then help these clients adopt a present-moment focus, distancing themselves from their thoughts (i.e., cognitive defusion) and attaching less significance to them in order to achieve psychological flexibility, which allows them to live their lives according to their values even in the presence of upsetting thinking.

Socratic questioning is but one way to facilitate the evaluation of maladaptive thinking. Perhaps the most powerful tool is the *behavioral experiment*, in which clients test out, prospectively, nonjudgmentally, and usually in their own environments, the accuracy and implications of their maladaptive thinking. Consider Lisa again. If she were to take her thinking about her friend one step further, such that she predicts her friend will reject her if she reaches out to schedule another lunch date, and she accepts that prediction as truth, it is likely that Lisa will not reach out and will begin to withdraw from her friend. A behavioral experiment that she could implement in between sessions would require her to ask her friend to schedule another lunch date and then use that experience to draw a conclusion about the degree to which her thinking was accurate. Because others' reactions to clients cannot be controlled, there is always the possibility that their prediction will be realized. Thus, cognitive behavioral therapists devise a "win-win" situation, such that the results of the experiment either provide evidence that the client's thinking was inaccurate or demonstrate that the client can tolerate the distress associated with a negative result.

The techniques described thus far can be used to modify underlying beliefs in addition to situation-specific automatic thoughts. However, there exist some reappraisal strategies geared specifically toward belief modification (J. S. Beck, 2011; Persons, Davidson, & Tompkins, 2001). For example, clients can keep a positive data log, which allows them to accumulate evidence arising in daily life that supports an adaptive belief. Lisa, for example, could keep a running log of instances of friends initiating contact with her. Historical tests of beliefs provide a forum for clients to evaluate the evidence that supports the maladaptive and adaptive beliefs in discrete time periods in their lives. When they embark on a historical test of their beliefs, many clients realize that they have dismissed important life experiences that are inconsistent with the maladaptive belief that has been activated, even if they are currently experiencing many problems. Cognitive behavioral therapists also use experiential role-plays to restructure key early memories that are hypothesized to contribute to the development of a maladaptive belief. For instance, a client might play two roles, such as her current self and herself at the age in which a key negative life event occurred, and her current self would apply cognitive reappraisal tools to help her younger self interpret that life event in a more benign manner. (See chapter 22 for a discussion of additional belief modification techniques.)

## *Modifying Maladaptive Thinking*

If, after evaluating the accuracy and usefulness of their thinking, clients realize that it is problematic, then one option is to move toward modifying it. Modified automatic thoughts are often referred to as alternative responses, rational responses, adaptive responses, or balanced responses. I prefer the term "balanced response" because there are usually both negative and positive aspects to the life circumstances that clients face. Restructuring an automatic thought into a thought that is uniformly positive has the potential to be just as inaccurate as the original automatic thought. Thus, balanced responses must be believable and compelling, accounting for both the positive and negative aspects of a situation. This is why it is erroneous for cognitive restructuring to be equated with positive thinking, as the aim of cognitive reappraisal is to achieve balanced, realistic, and accepting thinking rather than positive thinking, per se.

Clinicians encourage clients to craft balanced responses on the basis of the conclusions that they drew from the guided evaluation. These balanced responses tend to be lengthier than the original automatic thought. The reason for this is that automatic thoughts tend to be quick, evaluative, and judgmental, such as Lisa's "My friend doesn't like me." Balanced responses take into account nuances, as most situations that people face in life are multifaceted. Thus, a balanced response might incorporate the highlights from the evaluation of evidence that does and does not support the automatic thought, from the reattribution exercise, from the decatastrophizing plan, or from an advantages-disadvantages analysis. As Lisa responded to her therapist's Socratic questioning, she arrived upon the following balanced response:

> It is okay to be disappointed that I was not invited to the baby shower, as I'd have liked to share this special moment with my friend. But I know that it is typical for her large family to restrict events like this to family members only. She and I recently had lunch together, and it seemed that we very much enjoyed each other's company. We even set another lunch date. What is happening here is that my belief of being undesirable has been activated, and the most adaptive course of action is to distance myself from it so that I continue to act as a good friend to her, which is important to me and which increases the likelihood that the two of us will cultivate a close friendship.

Though balanced responses are often relatively long, there are times when clients with certain clinical presentations, such as recurrent panic attacks or suicidal crisis, need a response that is relatively direct and easy to remember.

After constructing a balanced response, clients rerate the intensity of their emotional distress. They compare their ratings of emotional distress associated with the original automatic thought and with the balanced response to determine whether the cognitive restructuring exercise helped them feel better. In most cases, clinicians should not expect the ratings of emotional distress to drop to 0 or 0 percent, as clients are usually facing life circumstances that would be unpleasant or difficult for most people. However, the aim of the exercise is for the ratings to be reduced to a level that clients experience as manageable and that allows them to take skillful action. If after constructing a balanced response clients provided ratings of the degree to which they believed the original automatic thought, after they have completed the cognitive restructuring exercise they should indicate the degree to which they *now* believe the original automatic thought. From the perspective of cultivating a sense of psychological flexibility, as clients go through this process, they can also practice assuming a present-moment focus, noticing their maladaptive thinking, and taking steps to distance themselves from their thoughts. They can begin to recognize that maladaptive thoughts do not always have to be changed and that they can live a quality life even when they are present.

Similarly, maladaptive beliefs can be modified into more balanced, adaptive beliefs using the interventions described in the previous section. Clinicians encourage clients to craft an adaptive belief that is balanced, compelling, and believable (Wenzel, 2012). Recall Lisa's core belief, "I'm undesirable." If she has a history of receiving negative feedback from others, an adaptive belief like "I'm desirable" might not ring true. "I have strengths and weaknesses, just like everyone else," and "I have much to offer friends, even if I make the occasional mistake," are examples of more balanced beliefs toward which she can work.

# Tools

Cognitive reappraisal is often done verbally in the context of conversation between the client and clinician in session. In addition, clinicians often use one or more aids that help clients to organize their work and remember the fruits of their work outside of session. I describe these tools below.

## *Thought Record*

A *thought record* is a sheet of paper on which clients work through the cognitive restructuring procedure. Clients typically start with a three-column thought record, on which they record a few words about situations that increase their emotional distress, as well as accompanying cognitions and emotional experiences. As they acquire skill in identifying their thoughts, they switch to a five-column thought record, which adds two more columns—one for recording a balanced response and one to rerate the intensity of the emotional experience—to the initial three. Between sessions, clients often keep a thought record in order to work with automatic thoughts that arise in daily life. The idea behind the thought record is that it allows clients to practice the "real-time" application of cognitive restructuring so they can eventually catch and reframe unhelpful cognitions without having to write them down.

## Coping Card

A *coping card* is a reminder of the work done in session that clients can consult outside of session; typically, these reminders are written on a sheet of paper, an index card, or a business card. Coping cards are versatile and tailored to the needs of each client. For example, clients who experience recurrent automatic thoughts can work with their therapist in session to devise a compelling balanced response. Then, on the coping card, they might write the original automatic thought on one side and the balanced response on the other. Other clients prefer reminders of ways to evaluate their automatic thoughts, so they list questions on coping cards, such as "What evidence supports my thinking about this situation?" or "What evidence does not support my thinking about this situation?" Still other clients prefer to list concrete pieces of evidence to counter a recurrent automatic thought.

## Technology

In the twenty-first century, cognitive behavioral therapists are finding that many clients prefer to record their homework using technology rather than by writing it down on a sheet of paper. Microsoft Word and Excel files allow much flexibility, in that clients can use customized prompts to identify and evaluate their thinking. Other clients record their thoughts on mobile devices to catch and restructure automatic thoughts when they are on the go. Moreover, there exist many applications (i.e., apps) that provide a template for clients to record their cognitive restructuring work using smartphones or tablets. Such apps can be located by searching for "cognitive behavioral therapy" in app stores.

# Summary

Cognitive reappraisal is indicated for an array of mental health conditions, including (but not limited to) depression, anxiety disorders, obsessive-compulsive and related disorders, trauma- and stressor-related disorders, eating disorders, addictions, and adjustment to medical problems like chronic pain, cancer, and diabetes. It can even be used with clients with psychotic disorders, not necessarily to directly challenge delusional thinking but instead to help them obtain a softer perspective on the defeatist attitudes they hold about themselves and the likelihood of living a quality life (A. T. Beck, Grant, Huh, Perivoliotis, & Chang, 2013). Cognitive reappraisal is also incorporated into many CBT protocols for children with mental health disorders, whose cognitive capability is still developing (e.g., Kendall & Hedtke, 2006), and adults with traumatic brain injury, whose cognitive capabilities have been compromised (Hsieh et al., 2012). However, with these populations, it is usually implemented in a more digestible format (e.g., the development of a single coping statement, the identification and labeling of errors in thinking) than in the more sophisticated way described in this chapter.

Many clients indicate that cognitive reappraisal is a life skill that they wish they had been taught when they were younger, before there was a need to seek out a cognitive behavioral therapist. Evidence of its effectiveness lies in the degree to which clients are able to manage emotional reactivity, engage in effective problem solving, function adaptively, and achieve quality of life as a result of thinking in a more balanced manner. However, it is important to recognize that cognitive reappraisal is not indicated in all cases, and that pushing it when it is not indicated has the potential to interfere with an otherwise effective course of CBT. For example, clients who already view their situation in an accurate and realistic manner are usually helped more by interventions that promote problem solving, distress tolerance, and/or acceptance. Forcing cognitive reappraisal in these instances could be confusing or even invalidating. Moreover, as mentioned previously, some clients use cognitive reappraisal in a way that is compulsive or that reinforces an avoidance or intolerance of negative affect. Failing to recognize that these issues are exacerbated by cognitive reappraisal could increase the probability of recurrence or relapse.

Evidence is mixed, at best, regarding the degree to which cognitive reappraisal specifically affects outcome through the process of reducing the frequency or degree of belief in maladaptive cognition. The recent research of Hayes-Skelton and Graham (2013) raises the possibility that decentering accounts for its positive effect. Interestingly, data reported by Hayes-Skelton and colleagues suggest that decentering may be an important mechanism of change in a number of therapeutic approaches, such as mindfulness, acceptance-based approaches, and even applied relaxation, in addition to cognitive reappraisal (Hayes-Skelton, Calloway, Roemer, & Orsillo, 2015). It will be important for future research to identify ways to enhance cognitive reappraisal's ability to facilitate decentering. One possibility is by encouraging clients to precede cognitive reappraisal with an acceptance-based technique, as recent research indicates that cognitive reappraisal preceded by self-compassion is associated with greater reductions in depression than cognitive reappraisal alone (Diedrich, Hofmann, Cuijpers, & Berking, 2016). As cognitive behavioral therapists continue to use cognitive reappraisal with their clients, it will be important for them to do so with an eye toward facilitating decentering and increasing psychological flexibility, rather than focusing on simply changing maladaptive thoughts and beliefs.

In closing, clinicians are encouraged to take a scientist-practitioner approach to evaluating the degree to which cognitive reappraisal enhances treatment for any one client by thinking critically about the function that it serves for the client. This means that the clinician gathers observational and quantitative data from individual clients to examine not only the degree to which cognitive reappraisal reduces negative affect and improves functioning, but also the degree to which it has any unexpected, negative effects, such as the reinforcement of unhelpful beliefs about the need for certainty or the need to avoid uncomfortable affect at any cost. When cognitive reappraisal facilitates the approach toward (versus avoidance of) life problems, tolerance of uncertainty and distress, and acceptance, then it can be a powerful tool that enhances quality of life and allows clients to embrace the full array of cognitive and behavioral strategies that clinicians can offer them.

# References

Abramowitz, J. S., & Arch, J. J. (2013). Strategies for improving long-term outcomes in cognitive behavioral therapy for obsessive-compulsive disorder: Insights from learning theory. *Cognitive and Behavioral Practice, 21*(1), 20–31.

Beck, A. T., Grant, P. M., Huh, G. A., Perivoliotis, D., & Chang, N. A. (2013). Dysfunctional attitudes and expectancies in deficit syndrome schizophrenia. *Schizophrenia Bulletin, 39*(1), 43–51.

Beck, A. T., Rush, A. J., Shaw, B. F., & Emery, G. (1979). *Cognitive therapy of depression.* New York: Guilford Press.

Beck, J. S. (2011). *Cognitive behavior therapy: Basics and beyond* (2nd ed.). New York: Guilford Press.

Burns, D. D. (1980). *Feeling good: The new mood therapy.* New York: Signet.

Burns, D. D., & Spangler, D. L. (2001). Do changes in dysfunctional attitudes mediate changes in depression and anxiety in cognitive behavioral therapy? *Behavior Therapy, 32*(2), 337–369.

DeRubeis, R. J., Evans, M. D., Hollon, S. D., Garvey, M. J., Grove, W. M., & Tuason, V. B. (1990). How does cognitive therapy work? Cognitive change and symptom change in cognitive therapy and pharmacotherapy for depression. *Journal of Consulting and Clinical Psychology, 58*(6), 862–869.

Diedrich, A., Hofmann, S. G., Cuijpers, P., & Berking, M. (2016). Self-compassion enhances the efficacy of explicit cognitive reappraisal as an emotion regulation strategy in individuals with major depressive disorder. *Behaviour Research and Therapy, 82,* 1–10.

Dobson, K. S., & Dozois, D. J. A. (2010). Historical and philosophical bases of the cognitive-behavioral therapies. In K. S. Dobson (Ed.), *Handbook of cognitive-behavioral therapies* (3rd ed., pp. 3–38). New York: Guilford Press.

Gross, J. J. (1998). The emerging field of emotion regulation: An integrative review. *Review of General Psychology, 2*(3), 271–299.

Hayes, S. C., Strosahl, K. D., & Wilson, K. G. (2012). *Acceptance and commitment therapy: The process and practice of mindful change* (2nd ed.). New York: Guilford Press.

Hayes-Skelton, S. A., Calloway, A., Roemer, L., & Orsillo, S. M. (2015). Decentering as a potential common mechanism across two therapies for generalized anxiety disorder. *Journal of Consulting and Clinical Psychology, 83*(2), 395–404.

Hayes-Skelton, S., & Graham, J. (2013). Decentering as a common link among mindfulness, cognitive reappraisal, and social anxiety. *Behavioural and Cognitive Psychotherapy, 41*(3), 317–328.

Hofmann, S. G. (2004). Cognitive mediation of treatment change in social phobia. *Journal of Consulting and Clinical Psychology, 72*(3), 393–399.

Hofmann, S. G., Meuret, A. E., Rosenfield, D., Suvak, M. K., Barlow, D. H., Gorman, J. M., et al. (2007). Preliminary evidence for cognitive mediation during cognitive-behavioral therapy of panic disorder. *Journal of Consulting and Clinical Psychology, 75*(3), 374–379.

Hsieh, M. Y., Ponsford, J., Wong, D., Schönberger, M., McKay, A., & Haines, K. (2012). A cognitive behaviour therapy (CBT) programme for anxiety following moderate-severe traumatic brain injury (TBI): Two case studies. *Brain Injury, 26*(2), 126–138.

Kendall, P. C., & Hedtke, K. A. (2006). *Cognitive-behavioral therapy for anxious children: Therapist manual* (3rd ed.). Ardmore, PA: Workbook Publishing.

Persons, J. B., Davidson, J., & Tompkins, M. A. (2001). *Essential components of cognitive-behavior therapy for depression.* Washington, DC: American Psychological Association.

Smits, J. A. J., Julian, K., Rosenfield, D., & Powers, M. B. (2012). Threat reappraisal as a mediator of symptom change in cognitive-behavioral treatment of anxiety disorders: A systematic review. *Journal of Consulting and Clinical Psychology, 80*(4), 624–635.

Stice, E., Rohde, P., Seeley, J. R., & Gau, J. M. (2010). Testing mediators of intervention effects in randomized controlled trials: An evaluation of three depression prevention programs. *Journal of Consulting and Clinical Psychology, 78*(2), 273–280.

Wenzel, A. (2012). Modification of core beliefs in cognitive therapy. In I. R. de Oliveira (Ed.), *Standard and innovative strategies in cognitive behavior therapy* (pp. 17–34). Rijeka, Croatia: Intech. Available online at http://www.intechopen.com/books/standard-and-innovative-strategies-in-cognitive-behavior-therapy/modification-of-core-beliefs-in-cognitive-therapy.

# CHAPTER 22

# Modifying Core Beliefs

### Arnoud Arntz, PhD

*Department of Clinical Psychology, University of
Amsterdam; Department of Clinical Psychological
Science, Maastricht University*

## Definitions and Background

One of the most important cognitive structures conceptualized by cognitive theories of psychopathology is the *schema*. Beck (1967) introduced the schema concept in the context of cognitive therapy, stating that "a schema is a structure for screening, coding, and evaluating the stimuli that impinge on the organism" (p. 283). From an information processes point of view, it can be thought of as a generalized knowledge structure in memory that represents the world, the future, and the self. It is thought to govern such information-processing elements as attention (what to focus on), interpretation (what meaning is given to stimuli), and memory (what implicit or explicit memories are triggered by specific cues). Schemas can consist of verbal and nonverbal knowledge.

*Core beliefs* are the verbal representations of the central elements of schemas, sometimes also called central assumptions. Once a schema is activated, selective attentional processes allow much of the available information to remain unprocessed; however, a lot of meaning is added to the raw data when a schema is activated.

Because a schema steers information processing so that information that is incompatible with the schema is overlooked, distorted, or seen as irrelevant, schemas are highly resistant to change once formed. In cognitive theories, schemas bias underlying information processing.

Piaget (1923) first introduced the schema concept to psychology. He distinguished between two major ways people deal with information that is incompatible with an existing schema: accommodation versus assimilation. The default is *assimilation*: a new experience is transformed to match the existing schema. If the discrepancy is too large, however, *accommodation* might occur: an existing schema is changed to better represent reality, or a new schema is formed. A basic assumption of cognitive theories of psychopathology is that the very same phenomenon underlies the maintenance of psychopathology: people who suffer from psychopathological problems maintain their schemas by relying on assimilation instead of changing their schemas by accommodation, and it is the task of psychological treatment to help clients change their dysfunctional schemas.

Much of the research into cognitive models of psychopathology, and many therapeutic techniques of cognitive therapy, focus on biased information processes and their modification. This is somewhat surprising because the cognitive model suggests that it is better to focus on schemas rather than cognitive biases. After all, it is the schema that arguably underlies cognitive biases, and if changing cognitive biases does not result in schema alteration, change will be fragile and risk of relapse might be large. While it is true that correcting cognitive biases might lead to schema change (accommodation) if disconfirming information cannot be ignored, schema change or the formation of new schemas is difficult and thus may need to be facilitated by guided work.

Before addressing schema change, it is helpful to distinguish three layers of beliefs. At the core are *unconditional beliefs*, which represent basic assumptions about the self, others, and the world. Examples are "I am bad," "I am superior," "Others are irresponsible," "Other people are good," and "The world is a jungle." The first layer around the core consists of *conditional assumptions*, which are beliefs about conditional relationships that can be formulated in "if…, then…" terms; for example, "If I let other people discover who I really am, they will reject me"; "If I get attached to other people, they will abandon me"; "If I show weakness, others will humiliate me." So-called *instrumental beliefs*, which represent beliefs about how to act to avoid bad things and acquire good things, constitute the outer layer. Examples include "Check the hidden motives of others," "Avoid showing emotions," and "Be the boss." This ordering of beliefs not only reflects different types of beliefs, but it also distinguishes what is apparent at the surface (observable behaviors reflecting instrumental beliefs) and what is behind the surface.

Cognitive theory posits that it is necessary to change the behavioral and cognitive strategies that are governed by the outer layer of instrumental beliefs before change at the level of core beliefs is likely to occur. In large part, the strategies that follow from instrumental beliefs determine what situations clients will enter; how they will manipulate the situation, and thus how other people will behave; or what information they will pick up. Thus, without changes in strategies, information that disconfirms the existing conditional and core beliefs will not be available or processed and therefore cannot lead to schema change.

# Origins of Core Beliefs

Schemas and core beliefs start to develop very early in life, even at preverbal levels. A well-known example is attachment. Based on an inborn need for proximity to and soothing behavior from caregivers, especially at moments of stress, babies start to develop attachment representations that can have a lasting influence on later development, including that of self-esteem, emotion regulation, and intimate relationships. For instance, children who experience a secure attachment to caregivers tend to develop healthy self-worth and positive views of others, implying that they tend to trust others and equally respect their own and other people's needs. Children who experience insecure attachment tend to develop negative views about self and others. But later-formed schemas, and therefore core beliefs, can also contain nonverbal meanings. Although we can describe core beliefs in words, this does not necessarily mean they are represented in a verbal way in memory. One implication is that pure verbal ways of trying to change beliefs might fail (clients might say, "I see what you mean, but I don't feel it"), and other methods are needed.

One way schemas form is through direct (sensory) experience. Classical and operant conditioning play a role; for example, when a child is repeatedly punished when expressing negative emotions, it may result in core beliefs like "Emotions are bad" and "I am a bad person (because I experience these emotions)." A second way is through modeling: seeing how other people act offers a schematic model the child internalizes. A third way is through verbal information, such as stories, warnings, or instructions. Lastly, because people try to make sense of experiences and information, the way the individual reasons plays a role in the formation of schemas. This means that intellectual capacities and therefore all the influences on these capacities, such as developmental phase, culture, education, and so on, play a role. But this final way also implies a certain coincidence; there is a chance factor in what people make of new information that is condensed in a schematic representation.

Understanding the factors that contribute to this "making sense of experiences" is helpful in bringing about change in core beliefs. For example, when mistreated by parents, it is common for children to conclude that they themselves must be bad. Childhood and adolescence are developmental phases in which basic schemas form, but even though schema change is more difficult during adulthood, it is not impossible. Psychological therapy is a method designed to do just that.

# Discovering and Formulating Core Beliefs

In clinical practice, the therapist needs to discover and adequately formulate the core beliefs that underlie the clients' problems to adequately address them. How is this accomplished?

One way, suggested by Padesky (1994), is that the therapist can directly ask about core ideas the client might have about the self ("What does this say about you?"), others ("What does this say about others?"), and the world ("What does this say about your life/the world/how things generally go?"). To get to the real core beliefs, and to prevent avoidance, it might be important that enough affect is activated while discussing the specific problem.

Another way is to use a structured cognitive technique called the downward arrow technique. The starting point is an automatic thought or an emotion that is triggered in a concrete situation. The therapist then asks what this thought or emotion means for the client (the therapist might add "if that were true") and continues asking until detecting an unconditional basic idea that apparently lies at the root of the emotional response in the starting situation. Here's an example:

*Client:*    I was rejected for a job promotion.

*Therapist:*    What does that mean to you?

$$\downarrow$$

*Client:*    I don't meet the expectations.

*Therapist:*    [If that were true…] What does that mean to you?

$$\downarrow$$

*Client:*    I make a mess of everything.

*Therapist:*    [If that were true…] What does that mean to you?

$$\downarrow$$

*Client:*    I am a loser.

*Therapist:*    [If that were true…] What does that mean to you?

$$\downarrow$$

*Client:*    I am nothing.

Note that the therapist doesn't challenge the intermediate ideas expressed by the client but accepts them for the moment until the core belief is identified. A very similar process can be used to elicit core beliefs about other people ("What does that mean about other people?") and the world in general.

An additional approach is to ask clients to imagine the situation at the root of the present problem, and ask them what they are feeling and thinking. For example, the therapist might ask the client who was rejected for a job promotion to close his eyes and imagine again the situation in which he got the negative feelings related to learning that he was rejected for the promotion. The therapist instructs the client to imagine the situation as vividly as possible, and next focus on emotions. Then, the therapist instructs the client to let the image go but to stay with the emotion and see if any early (childhood) memory pops up spontaneously. If so, the therapist instructs the client to relive the experience by focusing on perceptual details, emotions, and thoughts. These thoughts might reveal core beliefs; if not, the therapist can ask the client what the experience means for him. Returning to the example of the client who didn't get the job promotion, he reported that he got a memory of his father ridiculing him as a child about his "stupid" interest in a specific kind of sport, giving him the feeling that he was worthless—"a nothing." A similar imagery technique can be used to focus on traumatic experiences and discover the "encapsulated beliefs" associated with these experiences.

In identifying core beliefs, it can be helpful to ask clients how they would like to view themselves, and how they would like other people and the world to be. These wishes usually form the opposite of the negative core beliefs of clients. For instance, the client who was rejected for the job promotion might say he would like to see himself as somebody with clear capacities that other people welcome and acknowledge, and that the world should be just.

Belief and schema questionnaires can also be helpful as a starting point to discuss what core beliefs played a role in elevated scores. Exploring particular items that were highly rated can give important clues as well.

It is important that core beliefs be worded in ways that make sense to the client: the therapist should work with the client to find the best formulation, asking the client to rate the believability of it (e.g., How would you rate the belief "I am nothing"?) on a scale from 0 to 100, where 100 is the highest believability. If the rating is not very high, the formulation should usually be adapted—it doesn't yet reflect a core belief. Sometimes people have dual belief systems, however, believing the core belief in certain conditions but not in others. In that case, it is important to get both believability ratings. For instance, a panic client might state that she fully believes she has a healthy heart, but when experiencing specific physical sensations she believes that she has a dangerous heart condition like angina pectoris.

# Changing Core Beliefs

Three common ways to change core beliefs are with reasoning, empirical testing, and experiential interventions.

## *Reasoning*

Using Socratic dialogues and other rational ways to stimulate clients to reflect on their core beliefs, therapists can cast doubt on these beliefs and bring about a change process. For instance, the arguments in support of and against the belief can be reviewed (pro and con technique), a reinterpretation of the original situation or situations that underlie the belief can be made, and so forth (see chapter 21 for more examples of techniques). The following three specific techniques might be especially useful in changing core beliefs.

**Investigating a (causal) relationship.** This technique can be used when clients strongly believe dysfunctional relationships (Padesky, 1994; Arntz & van Genderen, 2009). Suppose a client believes that work achievement is the only way to be liked and loved by other people. The two constructs are drawn on the whiteboard, the cause as *x*-axis (work success) and the consequence (to be loved) as *y*-axis. The client draws the line that represents his assumption: the diagonal. The therapist checks whether the client agrees that if his assumption is true, all people would cluster around the line. Next, the therapist asks the client to think of concrete people with very high work success, people with very low work success, people who are very loved, and people who are hated. After placing various people in the two-dimensional space, it may be obvious there are no data for the assumed relationship. This may help the client reevaluate the idea that success in work implies being loved, and how to achieve what he values most, if it is to have good relationships with family and friends.

**Pie chart of responsibility.** Another visual aid for changing core beliefs is the pie chart, usually employed when overresponsibility beliefs are challenged (Van Oppen & Arntz, 1994). If a client has a tendency to feel overly responsible (or guilty, etc.), the therapist can repeatedly apply this technique to specific situations. First, the therapist asks the client how responsible she feels she is, expressed as a percentage. Next, a pie chart is drawn, and all factors that played a role in bringing about a particular event are listed and given a piece of the pie that represents their percentage of responsibility. The part of the client is placed in the pie only after all other factors have been added. Often these clients have no schema for chance; they tend to believe that everything that happens is caused by intentional forces; thus, to give an appropriate part of the pie to chance factors, it is important to work on the concept. This technique often leads to vast changes in the percentage of responsibility that clients feel about situations.

**Multidimensional continuum rating.** This technique can be used when clients engage in dichotomous and/or one-dimensional reasoning to come to conclusions that are better based on a more nuanced evaluation (Padesky, 1994; Arntz & van Genderen, 2009). For instance, clients might say they are of no value to other people because of a single attribute and feel that there exist only two categories (worthless and valued). The technique starts with listing characteristics that contribute to making people worthless versus valued. Next, for each attribute a visual analogue scale (VAS) is drawn, with the anchors representing extreme positions on the attribute. The technique helps clients to realize that most conclusions should be based on nuanced evaluations of multiple aspects.

There are problems in trying to change core beliefs by reasoning: clients might have limitations in their reasoning capacities, and reasoned insight might not affect the schema. For example, clients might respond with "I see what you mean, but I don't feel it." In such situations, empirical testing and experiential methods can help bring about change on a "feeling level."

## Empirical Testing

Experiments can be used to test the tenability of beliefs. It is important to formulate clear predictions so they can be compared with the observable outcomes of the experiment. Suppose a client believes that he has a weak side that would lead to rejection if discovered by others. The client could test this by sharing with others personal feelings that he considers to reveal his weakness, and then observing how others respond. It is helpful to have clients write out old and alternative beliefs and predictions and how they can be observed before the experiment is done, and then have them write down what they observed as a result of the test. The prediction from this client's dysfunctional belief may be that others will reject him, resulting in criticism, the ending of a conversation, or the other person not wanting to see him anymore. The alternative prediction could be that others appreciate his openness and show acceptance by saying sympathetic things, sharing intimate feelings, or continuing the relationship. Special care should be taken to prevent clients from using safety behaviors that interfere with the test. If for instance the client only casually mentions a "weakness" while the focus of the conversation is on another topic, chances are high that others will ignore the statement. The client may later say that this proves that they reject him based on his weakness. A proper test would involve sharing his "weaknesses" when others are fully attuned to what he's saying.

In more severe cases, clients might not yet be able to formulate alternative and more functional beliefs. In this case, a client's core beliefs seem to be the only representation thinkable. It is best to not yet formulate alternative beliefs until existing beliefs are refuted (see Bennett-Levy et al., 2004, for an extended guide to setting up experiments for a variety of clinical problems).

Empirical tests offer powerful evidence for and against beliefs and are therefore important for belief change. Most clients will be more convinced by evidence they experience themselves than by abstract reasoning.

## Experiential Interventions

Experiential methods rely on the capacity of humans to *imagine*, bringing in new information while sensory, emotional, behavioral, and cognitive channels are activated. Experiential methods got a bad reputation in the 1960s and 1970s when they were wildly applied, but today they are fully integrated into CBT and evidence-based therapy generally. I discuss three major techniques.

**Imagery.** Research has demonstrated that imagery is more deeply connected to emotions than verbal thinking and can lead to deeper and longer lasting changes (Hackmann, Bennett-Levy, & Holmes, 2011; Holmes & Mathews, 2010). Perhaps the most important imagery technique to change core beliefs is *imagery rescripting* (Arntz & Weertman, 1999), in which one tries to identify memories of past events that lie at the root of the formation of core beliefs, which typically developed during childhood. A good way to identify such memories is to ask the client to close the eyes and imagine a recent event during which she experienced a problem. The therapist instructs the client to imagine the experience as vividly as possible, focusing on perceptions, feelings, and thoughts. Next, the therapist instructs the client to stick with the emotion but to let the image go, to see whether an image from childhood pops up (creating an affect bridge). Next, the therapist instructs the client to report how old she is, and what the situation is, and to focus on what she perceives ("What do you see, hear, smell, feel, etc., in your body?"), emotionally experiences, thinks, and needs. In other words, the therapist invites the client to experience the sequence of events from the first-person perspective, as if it is happening in the here and now.

If the client retrieves the memory, which is often of a (psychologically) traumatic nature, and emotional arousal is high enough, the therapist can—in fantasy—enter the image and intervene by stopping abuse and neglect, correcting the perpetrator(s), and taking care of the further needs of the child. In other words, the meaning of the original experience is corrected through the experiences of a different end in fantasy. Although the technique does not overwrite the original memory (there is no loss of memory or factual knowledge of what happened), there is often a dramatic change in the meaning of the original event (Arntz, 2012). In less severe cases, or later in treatment, the client can imagine entering the scene as an adult, confronting the perpetrator, and taking care of the child.

**Drama.** This technique can be used to set up almost any situation that is relevant to creating core beliefs or testing them. Three examples of the use of drama are historical role-plays, symbolic role-plays, and present-focused role-plays.

In *historical role-plays*, client and therapist play situations from the client's past (usually childhood) that contributed to the formation of core beliefs (Padesky, 1994; Arntz & van Genderen, 2009). The client describes the situation and the behavior of the other person, usually (but not necessarily) a parent. (For convenience, I describe role-plays with a child-parent interaction.) Then, the therapist plays the parent and the client the child. This usually leads to a quick activation of the beliefs and accompanying emotions. There are two options for addressing these beliefs: drama reinterpretation and drama rescripting.

With drama reinterpretation, which is used when the child might have misinterpreted the parent, roles are switched. The therapist instructs the client to play the parent and be aware of any thought, emotion, and intention from the parent's perspective. The therapist plays the client. Afterward, they discuss the client's experience in the parent role and compare it to the original interpretation. The therapist highlights discrepancies, and the client is stimulated to reinterpret the original situation. With the new interpretation, a third act follows in which the client plays the child, now realizing the new interpretation and thus behaving differently toward the parent (e.g., more assertively asking for attention, because the client realizes that his dad was unresponsive because he was embroiled in his own troubles, not because he viewed his child as worthless).

With the drama rescripting option, the drama equivalent of imagery rescripting is played out. The role-play is restarted at a good moment for intervention, and the therapist intervenes, correcting the parent (stopping abuse, bringing in safety). Note that the parent is, at that moment, not played by anyone (e.g., he or she can be seated on an empty chair). Next, the therapist takes care of the child, saying soothing things, correcting misinterpretations, and offering a healthy explanation ("It is not your fault; your father has a drinking problem and loses control over his frustrations, and that is why he beats you and says these terrible things—not because you are a bad child."). Later in therapy, or when working with healthier clients, clients can enter the play as an adult, address the parent, and take care of the child (now not played by anybody). The therapist can act as a coach for the client.

In *symbolic role-plays*, the therapist and client set up a situation that has symbolic relevance for the core belief but has never happened nor will ever happen. An example is the court play, developed to challenge core beliefs about responsibility (Van Oppen & Arntz, 1994). In this role-play a specific accusation related to the core belief is played out as if it has been brought before a court (e.g., "The defendant is guilty of the pedestrian's death because he had the intrusive thought that a pedestrian might be killed by a car the pedestrian didn't see, but he didn't act on the thought and prevent the accident"). The client and the therapist can play different roles (the public prosecutor, the defendant's advocate, the judge, the jury) and exchange arguments. Experiencing different views on the (fantasy) case helps clients to reconsider their original belief.

Lastly, core beliefs can be tested in *present-focused role-plays*. In a sense, this is a behavioral experiment done in role-play, in which clients can change roles and take different perspectives, which helps them to discover how they come across to others.

**Multiple chairs.** This technique is derived from gestalt therapy and can be applied in different ways. The basic idea is to place different perspectives on different chairs and let the client sit on these chairs and express these perspectives. For instance, the client can express a self-punitive core belief on one chair; express the impact on and needs of the self on another chair; and express a new, healthy view on still another chair. In another application, the therapist can challenge the core belief that is symbolically placed on an empty chair, while the client observes. In this way, the client can distance from the core belief and not experience the therapist's challenging as being personally criticized. The client can join the therapist in challenging the core belief, and later in treatment the client probably can do most of the challenging work alone, only needing some coaching by the therapist. In still another variation, key figures from either the past or the present are symbolically placed on the empty chairs, and the client is stimulated to express their views.

# Processes of Change

The therapeutic methods described in this chapter are known to be clinically helpful because they change core beliefs (e.g., Wild, Hackmann, & Clark, 2008). A broader focus on the kind of process-oriented research discussed in this volume will be needed to see if methods such as imagery rescripting also alter such processes as cognitive defusion (see chapter 23), self-acceptance (see chapter 24), or mindfulness (see chapter 26), but the earliest steps in that direction support the possibility (e.g., Reimer, 2014).

# Summary

Core beliefs can be addressed by many interventions, and the position taken here is that it is good to use different channels of change: reasoning, empirical testing, and experiential intervention. Clients probably differ in their sensitivity to each intervention, so it is good to have a choice of interventions and to integrate various channels. In this chapter I stressed the importance of experiencing disconfirming information, and not just trying to convince clients with verbal reasoning. The reason for this is that although the therapist and client can formulate core beliefs in words, these representations aren't always open to verbal arguments. Clients often need to experience disconfirmation on a sensory and emotional level.

The current thinking regarding the effects of psychological treatment is that old (dysfunctional) schemas and new (functional) schemas compete for retrieval (Brewin, 2006). In other words, with each encounter with a relevant cue, there is a chance that the old schema is activated and the dysfunctional core belief dominates the person. However, basic research suggests that it might be possible to change the meaning of the original knowledge representation (Arntz, 2012). If so, this will have important implications for practice, as changing the original representation is preferable to building a new representation that has to compete with the old one. For example, relapse chances are much higher when two representations have to compete than when the original representation can be changed. Future research will shed light on this issue.

# References

Arntz, A. (2012). Imagery rescripting as a therapeutic technique: Review of clinical trials, basic studies, and research agenda. *Journal of Experimental Psychopathology, 3*(2), 189–208.

Arntz, A., & van Genderen, H. (2009). *Schema therapy for borderline personality disorder.* Chichester, UK: Wiley-Blackwell.

Arntz, A., & Weertman, A. (1999). Treatment of childhood memories: Theory and practice. *Behaviour Research and Therapy, 37*(8), 715–740.

Beck, A. T. (1967). *Depression: Clinical, experimental, and theoretical aspects.* Philadelphia: University of Pennsylvania Press.

Bennett-Levy, J., Butler, G., Fennell, M., Hackmann, A., Mueller, M., & Westbrook, D. (Eds.). (2004). *Oxford guide to behavioural experiments in cognitive therapy.* Oxford: Oxford University Press.

Brewin, C. R. (2006). Understanding cognitive behaviour therapy: A retrieval competition account. *Behaviour Research and Therapy, 44*(6), 765–784.

Hackmann, A., Bennett-Levy, J., & Holmes, E. A. (Eds.). (2011). *Oxford guide to imagery in cognitive therapy.* Oxford: Oxford University Press.

Holmes, E. A., & Mathews, A. (2010). Mental imagery in emotion and emotional disorders. *Clinical Psychology Review, 30*(3), 349–362.

Padesky, C. A. (1994). Schema change processes in cognitive therapy. *Clinical Psychology and Psychotherapy, 1*(5), 267–278.

Piaget, J. (1923). *Langage et pensée chez l'enfant* (1st ed. with preface by É. Claparède). Paris: Delachaux et Niestlé.

Reimer, S. G. (2014). *Single-session imagery rescripting for social anxiety disorder: Efficacy and mechanisms.* Doctoral dissertation, University of Waterloo, Ontario. Retrieved from UWSPACE, Waterloo's Institutional Repository. (hdl.handle.net/10012/8583).

Van Oppen, P., & Arntz, A. (1994). Cognitive therapy for obsessive-compulsive disorder. *Behaviour Research and Therapy, 32*(1), 79–87.

Wild, J., Hackmann, A., & Clark, D. M. (2008). Rescripting early memories linked to negative images in social phobia: A pilot study. *Behavior Therapy, 39*(1), 47–56.

# CHAPTER 23

# Cognitive Defusion

## J. T. Blackledge, PhD
*Department of Psychology, Morehead State University*

## Definitions and Background

*Cognitive defusion* refers to the process of reducing the automatic emotional and behavioral functions of thoughts by increasing awareness of the process of thinking over and above the content or literal meaning of thought. Although the term emerged within acceptance and commitment therapy (Hayes & Strosahl, 2004), where it was originally termed deliteralization (Hayes, Strosahl, & Wilson, 1999), it is related closely to other processes, such as distancing (Beck, 1976), decentering (Fresco et al., 2007), mindfulness (Bishop et al., 2004), metacognitive awareness (Wells, 2008), and mentalization (Fonagy & Target, 1997). In this short chapter I will use the term in a broad way, deliberately including some aspects of these other concepts and methods. This broader usage seems appropriate because some studies (e.g., Arch, Wolitzky-Taylor, Eifert, & Craske, 2012) show that measures of cognitive defusion mediate the outcome of traditional cognitive behavioral methods.

Cognitive defusion techniques and strategies are designed to help psychotherapy clients take problematic thoughts less literally and to empower them to act in more effective and constructive ways when problematic thoughts are repertoire narrowing. For example, a client who believes he is unlovable because of various self-perceived shortcomings might not pursue a much desired romantic partner, or he might not self-disclose enough to a partner to build a meaningful amount of intimacy. Defusion methods could help the client put less stock in the thought "I'm unlovable," or related thoughts, and help enable him to behave in a variety of ways more conducive to building intimacy and being loved even when these thoughts are present.

Embedded in the construct of defusion and related processes is an assumption that thoughts, or words, are likely incapable of capturing the full richness and depth of direct experience. It is common for clients to view thoughts (particularly compelling ones) as the ultimate arbiters of truth, even when they fail to capture the complexities of human experience. When we are "fused" with our thoughts (i.e., when we take them literally), "thinking regulates behavior without any additional input" from our direct experiences, "overwhelm[ing] contact with the direct antecedents and consequences of behavior" (Hayes, Strosahl, & Wilson, 2012, p. 244). Human thought stands as a proxy for events, but that proxy is often, metaphorically, a two-dimensional snapshot of a three-dimensional world. More technically, "cognitive fusion is a process by which verbal events exert strong stimulus control over responding, to the exclusion of other variables" (Hayes et al., 2012, p. 69). Defusion methods are designed to increase cognitive flexibility, allowing clients to attend to other, directly experienced events, hopefully enabling more effective action.

Both defusion strategies and traditional cognitive restructuring rest on the assumption that thoughts can serve as barriers to effective action and lead to potentially problematic emotional reactions. However, more traditional cognitive perspectives (e.g., Beck, 1976) emphasize the importance of changing cognitive content in order for emotional and behavioral change to occur (see chapter 21), whereas defusion, decentering, or metacognitive awareness place greater emphasis on a person's relationship to his or her own thinking—that is, on the *context* in which thoughts are experienced.

A wide variety of contextual factors are in place when people speak in ways that their words are taken literally. A person may speak at a certain rate—not too fast (as an auctioneer speaks), and not too slow (imagine, for example, drawing out every single syllable of this sentence for several seconds). A variety of grammatical rules are followed so that adjectives, adverbs, nouns, and verbs work properly to convey intended meaning. "Correct" words need to be used to refer to the various "things" addressed by speech. In speaking an emotionally charged thought, cadence, emotional inflection, and nonverbal behavior typically match the emotion or emotions being expressed (think, for example, of how people look and sound when genuinely expressing anger, or sadness). Perhaps most importantly, when talking is being taken literally, there is a focus on the content of what's being said rather than the process of formulating and speaking those words (i.e., a listener would carefully follow a train of thought rather than focusing on the physical sensations associated with forming words or the acoustical properties of the sounds each syllable makes). If while speaking you focused too much on the process of speaking, you might quickly get derailed from your train of thought.

In other words, people have a lifelong history of being reinforced for behaving in a literal fashion when encountering verbal stimuli–literal contexts. That "context of literality" (Hayes et al., 1999, p. 64) leads those verbal and cognitive events to function in a manner consistent with their contents. The form of thoughts functions to encourage characteristic emotional, cognitive, and behavioral reactions—but only in contexts designed to produce that effect and impact (see Hayes et al., 2012, pp. 27–59, or Hayes, Barnes-Holmes, & Roche, 2003). Defusion methods deliberately change that context of literality, violating one or more of the normal conditions or language parameters discussed above, so as to disrupt the in-the-moment functions of problematic thoughts, thus enabling clients to behave in ways that are at odds with the dictates of literal thoughts.

A classic defusion method is word repetition, a method first described over one hundred years ago by Titchener (1907). Suppose a person said the word "milk" out loud once. A variety of images might show up as a result. A listener might picture a glass filled with milk, or imagine what milk tastes like or feels like when being consumed. The reader might take a moment to think of the various perceptual qualities of milk before reading the next sentence. Now, as an exercise, say the word "milk" out loud fairly quickly, over and over for about thirty seconds before continuing to the next paragraph.

You likely noticed that after about twenty seconds, the imagery and other sensations originally evoked by the word "milk" largely disappeared. All that remained were the physical sensations in your throat and mouth that repeatedly produced an odd squawking that sounded something like "MALK."

When we use language literally, we don't normally repeat the same word over and over. Doing so violates an important language parameter inherent in the context of literality and exposes that word for what it formally is: physical sensations and arbitrary sound. When spoken or thought of in a context of literality, the word functions to make psychological imagery and sensations present even when the "thing" being referred to isn't there.

The remainder of this chapter will discuss a sampling of defusion techniques that can be used in therapy, as well as a brief review of empirical literature supporting defusion and caveats regarding its use. See Blackledge (2015) for a book-length treatment of defusion and its hands-on use.

# Implementation

Because using defusion techniques involves using language in ways that depart markedly from the norm, they can strike clients as odd and be potentially off-putting. Until rapport can be built and the client begins to understand the premise behind such techniques, it is often best to use more subtle defusion strategies. Using "mind" and "thought" language conventions that identify thoughts as products of the mind and label them simply as "thoughts" (rather than indubitable reflections of reality) can be used as early as the first intake session to start reducing client fusion with troublesome thoughts. The following brief transcript demonstrates some ways these language conventions can be used:

Client:      It's just that, for most of my life, I've felt like I don't fit in anywhere—that there's something wrong with me.

Therapist:   (*Empathetically.*) "I don't fit in anywhere. There's something wrong with me." Those are some tough thoughts to have. What other thoughts show up when you think "there's something wrong with me"?

Client:      What do you mean?

Therapist:   Well, I'm guessing you might think about specific things that are wrong with you, things that you've done wrong in the past...

Client:      Oh, I see what you mean. I get too anxious about things... I'm always screwing things up.

Therapist:   How often do thoughts like that show up? Is it constant, or is it more likely to happen in certain situations?

Client:      Well, I guess it's not constant. I think it's more when I'm around other people...especially people that I like or want to make like me.

Therapist:   Yeah, when the pressure's on—that's when those scary thoughts, that anxiety, those self-doubts show up?

Client:      Exactly.

Therapist:   What other thoughts does your mind throw out at times like that?

Client:      It depends. Usually I'm worried what the other person is going to think of me. Worried that I'll say something stupid and they won't like me.

Therapist:   I think I understand. It sounds like you have a lot of pessimistic thoughts about doing things wrong—a lot of thoughts about how things aren't going to turn out well.

These "thought" and "mind" conventions are actually common in many forms of therapy, and they may help explain some of the early benefits that clients experience in these therapies. Such conventions can be readily integrated into assessment (and later sessions), allowing clinicians to simultaneously gather pertinent information about the client and help her start to see her problematic thoughts from a different perspective. While the use of such language typically doesn't have a profound effect on its own over time, it is not uncommon for clients to more readily disclose distressing thoughts and for those thoughts to be somewhat less emotionally provocative when it is used. Of equal importance, using these conventions helps shape the client to more consistently recognize thoughts as thoughts, aiding the use of more robust defusion techniques later on.

# Changing Other Literal Language Parameters

A client's "context of literality" can be undermined in a variety of ways that are more robust than using the simple language conventions from the last section. I'll discuss several here. It must be emphasized that to avoid invalidating the client, the more-invasive defusion techniques typically should not be used until the therapist has demonstrated good empathy with the client. Toward the same end, the client should understand that it is not his individual narrative per se that is being questioned, but rather that therapist and client are working together to expose how language and thoughts in general are suspect and that our minds claim to know a lot more than they actually know. Finally, rather than being used in a preplanned, structured fashion, such techniques are typically best used as a flexible, natural response to times when a client is struggling with an issue and appears to be relatively fused with the content of his narrative.

**The word repetition exercise.** The word repetition, or "milk," exercise introduced earlier in this chapter can be used as a relatively invasive defusion exercise. One way to explore its use is to approach it as a kind of experiment:

*Therapist:* I'd like to look at what you're struggling with from a little different perspective, to see if something different might happen. I don't know how to eliminate some of these difficult and well-practiced thoughts, but I do know how to do something that might help us look at them differently. The exercise may not seem initially to have much to do with what we're talking about, but would you be willing to try something different as a kind of experiment? We'll then roll it back around so that we can see if it is useful.

After introducing the notion of an experiment, the "milk" exercise is conducted much as it was just presented a few pages ago. The therapist then asks the client to condense a core distressing thought to one or two words (e.g., a person who thinks she is a bad person might have that thought condensed down to "I'm bad"). As in the milk example, the therapist might ask the client to say that word or phrase out loud once, and to notice the various feelings, thoughts, and sensations that show up. Then, the client repeats the words out loud, fast, for about thirty seconds, and again the therapist asks the client to notice what experiences and sensations show up. Thirty seconds is common because research has shown that benefits reach an asymptote after that amount of time (Masuda, Hayes, Sackett, & Twohig, 2004). Typically, clients will have a significantly different experience with the word or phrase by the end of this time period. The intensity of the affect associated with it may diminish somewhat, and they may take the thought less seriously, or at least see how odd or suspect the word is, and so on. A good way to finish the exercise is by saying something along these lines:

*Therapist:* I wonder if "I'm bad" is maybe a lot like "milk": Your mind is very good at convincing you it's true when you think it. It's very good at convincing you that "badness" is in the room, just like it's very good at convincing you that "milk" is in the room—even when it really isn't. What if that's simply what words do? Try to convince us that they've captured the complete Truth of things when in fact they're just sounds and sensations?

**"Having" thoughts.** The "thought" language convention discussed above can be made more explicit. When a client is fused with a distressing or counterproductive narrative, asking her to speak the phrase "I'm having the thought that…" in advance of each thought in that narrative can often help her defuse from those thoughts. This technique may likely facilitate defusion for at least two reasons. First, it explicitly labels each thought as a "thought," something not done when a person takes language literally. Second, the somewhat laborious repetition of the phrase before every thought in the narrative slows things down, reducing the relatively quick train of thoughts—a hallmark of the context of literality—to a more awkward, halting pace that typically changes how those thoughts are experienced. An exchange between therapist and client using this technique might play out as follows:

*Client:* It's been like this for almost twenty years. I just can't pull myself up out of it. I've tried everything I can think of, but I can't make it work. I'm hopeless, and I'll always be hopeless. It's just senseless. There's no point in trying to improve myself, because I just can't do it.

*Therapist:* I hear you. It's been like this for a long, long time. I'm wondering if maybe we can slow this down a bit. You look trapped by all those thoughts. Would you be willing to look at them from a little different perspective, so that maybe we can make some room?

*Client:* I guess so. What perspective?

*Therapist:* Well, there can be a danger in taking every one of our thoughts at face value. If you're willing, I'd like you to continue telling me about the situation you're in. But this time, I'd like you to say "I'm having the thought that" before each sentence you speak.

*Client:* I don't see how that's going to get me out of this. I've been thinking this way for a long time.

*Therapist:* I hear you. And it probably won't change those thoughts. But it might change how you look at them. Are you willing to give it a try?

*Client:* Okay.

*Therapist:* Good. So, you were talking about how things feel hopeless, about how you can't make things in your life work.

*Client:* I can't. I mean, I was telling you earlier about how much I messed up that talk with my wife. I…

*Therapist:* Okay, and let me interrupt you. Can you say, "I'm having the thought that I really messed up that talk with my wife"?

*Client:* I'm having the thought that I really messed up that talk with my wife.

*Therapist:* And if you could preface the next thought with "I'm having the thought that…"

*Client:* But I really did… I mean, I'm having the thought that I really did mess things up with my wife. I shouldn't have been so hard…

*Therapist:* And that thought too.

*Client:* I'm having the thought that I shouldn't have been so hard on her.

*Therapist:* And the next one?

*Client:* I'm having the thought that I always do this… I'm having the thought that I don't understand why she's still with me.

*Therapist:*    Good.

*Client:*    I'm having the thought that I'm not good enough for her... I'm having the thought that I'm not good enough for anything.

*Therapist:*    Okay.

**Slow speech, singing, and silly voices.** Dramatically altering rate of speech (Hayes et al., 1999) or expressing thoughts in ways markedly inconsistent with their content can result in defusion. With regard to altering rate of speech, it is simpler to get a client to speak at a reliably slow versus sufficiently fast rate. Rationales similar to those listed in the transcripts above can be used to introduce the endeavor. The rate of speech should be very slow—counting quickly to five per syllable (about two seconds) seems to be an effective pace when using this technique. Speaking more quickly than that tends to retain too much of the words' meanings.

There are a variety of ways to help a client express thoughts in ways that differ greatly from the way he "should" express them if he were accurately conveying the emotions that underlay them. There are a variety of apps available for smartphones that transform the audio qualities of spoken thoughts. These apps temporarily record whatever you say and then play it back in an altered voice. One advantage of such apps is that the client can easily use them, as needed, between sessions. Many have multiple preset options (e.g., "chipmunk," "robot," and "helium" voices) that often dramatically change the tone and pitch of a recorded voice. An app store search will reveal dozens of apps, though it should be noted that many do not markedly change voices enough to facilitate defusion. It is advisable to first test any app you recommend for a client, and even help the client find the voice settings within the chosen app that seem to produce higher degrees of defusion.

The therapist could ask the client directly to "change his tone." If the client is willing, the therapist could ask him to speak a troublesome thought in the voice of one of his favorite cartoon characters or superheroes (or any TV or movie character with a highly idiosyncratic tone). The tone and overall "feel" of the voice must be at least significantly inconsistent with the original emotive tone of the thought. For example, speaking anxious or insecure thoughts in Christian Bale's Batman voice, or sadness-laden thoughts in a Mickey Mouse voice, could readily facilitate defusion. Alternatively, the client could sing the distressing thoughts to the tune of an upbeat song, in an operatic or otherwise exaggerated or emotively inconsistent voice, or in any way inconsistent with the literal functions of the thoughts. Such invasive defusion techniques must be predicated on a good, empathic therapeutic relationship and the client's clear understanding that his narrative is not being ridiculed, but rather viewed from a different perspective.

**Thoughts on cards.** Writing down the client's distressing thoughts and emotions, one by one, and laying them out in front of her on a table or desk can facilitate defusion. This strategy may likely work best when each thought is written on a separate index card or piece of paper (rather than continuously on a single page), to spatially break up the narrative and to visually highlight each thought as separate. Even thoughts that are reactions to or commentaries on the exercise should be written down, to emphasize that *all* thoughts are just thoughts and to build a more consistent context of defusion. As with the "I'm having the thought that..." language convention, typically the therapist should be careful to write down every thought the client discloses. This helps counter the natural social and therapeutic pull to discuss what the client is saying at a literal level.

Once multiple (perhaps even dozens of) cards are generated, they can be used in multiple ways. Simply having the client look at the assortment of separate thoughts as they are written down and placed on the table can serve a potent defusive function. If the client is willing, she can fold up and carry the cards in her pocket as she engages in important activities likely to produce similar thoughts and feeling. They serve as a reminder and extension of the original experience's lesson, and as a metaphorical lesson that troublesome thoughts can simply be carried along as she engages life.

Another in vivo exercise has the therapist attempt to throw each index card on the client's lap while she remains seated, doing whatever she can to avoid contacting her various thoughts. Have the client reflect on what the experience was like, which typically involves noting how frenetic it was and how she still ended up contacting most of her unwanted thoughts. Then repeat the exercise and ask the client to simply allow the "thoughts" to land in her lap. Typically, clients realize that they can simply allow troublesome thoughts to be there as thoughts, and that they don't need to engage in tiresome and fruitless efforts to keep them away.

# Empirical Support

The effects of cognitive defusion interventions have been assessed several dozen times in published research, therapy outcome studies, mediational studies, and analogue laboratory experiments (e.g., see Blackledge, 2015, for a recent summary). New measures of cognitive defusion have been developed that work in theoretically coherent ways (e.g., Gillanders et al., 2014). A recent meta-analysis (Levin,

Hildebrandt, Lillis, & Hayes, 2012) shows that defusion methods have a consistently positive effect on the believability of difficult thoughts and distress.

# Caveats

Most defusion techniques have the potential to make a client feel invalidated if there is not a strong therapeutic alliance or the treatment rationale is not clear (see Blackledge, 2015). When using defusion methods with other methods, two additional caveats apply.

**Mixing defusion and thought change strategies.** Using defusion techniques alongside techniques that imply a client must come to think differently about her experiences can lead to confusion for both client and therapist. Therapists who elect to use defusion techniques in therapy should think carefully about the assumptions behind other techniques they are using to see if there are any direct or implied contradictions that could create confusion. If the therapist decides to use techniques with potentially contradictory assumptions together, that in and of itself requires a coherent rationale. For example, the therapist may ask the client to consider that learning to think about thoughts differently can be helpful in providing new emotional or behavioral alternatives. If cognitive change strategies are helpful, then use them; if learning how to view thoughts simply as thoughts works better, then use *those* strategies.

**Using defusion in isolation.** Within the context of modern process-oriented cognitive behavioral therapy, cognitive defusion is one psychological process among many that can be used to help the client "unhook" from counterproductive thoughts and facilitate greater psychological flexibility in the presence of psychological distress. Analogue component defusion studies have so far suggested that defusion can decrease psychological distress at least over the short term, and therapy outcome studies have repeatedly shown that defusion leads to reduced distress over time. However, in both cases, defusion is explicitly and consistently used as a way to experience a more fulfilling and vital life *even when* psychological distress is present. With some clients defusion can raise issues of the proper role of judgment and meaning, and clients can become confused about when to use defusion. Using defusion alongside values-driven treatment strategies (see chapter 25) can help answer these questions, namely that defusion is a tool that can promote the client's own pursuit of values and meaning when automatic thoughts get in the way.

# References

Arch, J. J., Wolitzky-Taylor, K. B., Eifert, G. H., & Craske, M. G. (2012). Longitudinal treatment mediation of traditional cognitive behavioral therapy and acceptance and commitment therapy for anxiety disorders. *Behaviour Research and Therapy, 50*(7–8), 469–478.

Beck, A. T. (1976). *Cognitive therapy and the emotional disorders.* New York: International Universities Press.

Bishop, S. R., Lau, M., Shapiro, S., Carlson, L., Anderson, N. D., Carmody, J., et al. (2004). Mindfulness: A proposed operational definition. *Clinical Psychology: Science and Practice, 11*(3), 230–241.

Blackledge, J. T. (2015). *Cognitive defusion in practice: A clinician's guide to assessing, observing, and supporting change in your client.* Oakland, CA: New Harbinger Publications.

Fonagy, P., & Target, M. (1997). Attachment and reflective function: Their role in self-organization. *Development and Psychopathology, 9*(4), 679–700.

Fresco, D. M., Moore, M. T., van Dulmen, M. H. M., Segal, Z. V., Ma, S. H., Teasdale, J. D., et al. (2007). Initial psychometric properties of the experiences questionnaire: Validation of a self-report measure of decentering. *Behavior Therapy, 38*(3), 234–246.

Gillanders, D. T., Bolderston, H., Bond, F. W., Dempster, M., Flaxman, P. E., Campbell, L., et al. (2014). The development and initial validation of the cognitive fusion questionnaire. *Behavior Therapy, 45*(1), 83–101.

Hayes, S. C., Barnes-Holmes, D., & Roche, B. (2003). *Relational frame theory: A post-Skinnerian account of human language and cognition.* New York: Kluwer Academic/Plenum Publishers.

Hayes, S. C., & Strosahl, K. (2004). *A practical guide to acceptance and commitment therapy.* New York: Springer.

Hayes, S. C., Strosahl, K. D., & Wilson, K. G. (1999). *Acceptance and commitment therapy: An experiential approach to behavior change.* New York: Guilford Press.

Hayes, S. C., Strosahl, K. D., & Wilson, K. G. (2012). *Acceptance and commitment therapy: The process and practice of mindful change* (2nd ed.). New York: Guilford Press.

Levin, M. E., Hildebrandt, M. J., Lillis, J., & Hayes, S. C. (2012). The impact of treatment components suggested by the psychological flexibility model: A meta-analysis of laboratory-based component studies. *Behavior Therapy, 43*(4), 741–756.

Masuda, A., Hayes, S. C., Sackett, C. F., & Twohig, M. P. (2004). Cognitive defusion and self-relevant negative thoughts: Examining the impact of a ninety year old technique. *Behaviour Research and Therapy, 42*(2), 477–485.

Titchener, E. B. (1907). *An outline of psychology.* New York: Macmillan.

Wells, A. (2008). Metacognitive therapy: Cognition applied to regulating cognition. *Behavioural and Cognitive Psychotherapy, 36*(6), 651–658.

# CHAPTER 24

# Cultivating Psychological Acceptance

John P. Forsyth, PhD
Timothy R. Ritzert, MA

*Department of Psychology, University at Albany,
State University of New York*

## Definitions and Background

The idea of acceptance is quite old. It appears in religious traditions, Eastern contemplative practices, and most psychotherapy approaches when discussing therapeutic alliance and process. More recently it entered into evidence-based psychotherapy as a core process, both of psychopathology and of therapeutic change. Psychological *acceptance*, as we frame it here, is "the voluntary adoption of an intentionally open, receptive, flexible, and nonjudgmental posture with respect to moment-to-moment experience" (Hayes, Strosahl, & Wilson, 2012, p. 272). Such an experience includes *internal* events (e.g., thoughts, emotions, memories, physical sensations, urges/impulses) and closely related *contextual* situations that evoke them. Thought of in this way, psychological acceptance is opening up to what life is offering, just as it is. Acceptance is a skill, not merely a set of techniques. It is also a process, and not simply an outcome.

*Acceptance* as a term can be readily misunderstood. It is not giving up, tolerating, or passively resigning. It is rather a behavior and a choice. It involves approaching (often distressing) psychological events and related situations, without unnecessarily trying to change, avoid, suppress, escape from, or prolong them. Choosing to approach and open up to difficult psychological experiences is, paradoxically, doing something new.

Acceptance entails a change in *how* one approaches psychological events (Cordova, 2001), responding to them with openness, flexibility, and compassion. Thus, a key component of this work is altering a client's relationship with the experiences he is having anyway. Metaphorically the posture of acceptance can be demonstrated experientially with the simple gesture of standing up, with eyes wide open and somewhat playful, and stretching both arms as wide as one can. This receptive posture is contrasted with closing the arms and wrapping them around the torso as tightly as one can, standing rigidly with eyes tightly closed.

Acceptance is not about wallowing in distress, nor adopting a clever tactic to control difficult private content. Rather, acceptance is a process designed to help clients let go of needless struggle, live in the moment, make choices guided by personal values, and take actions that matter to them and stand to increase quality of life. When difficult psychological experiences show up, acceptance asks, "Are you willing to have that stuff, fully and without defense, just as it is, and carry it forward, if that meant you could do what truly matters to you?"

Research suggests that acceptance-based interventions work not by directly altering thoughts and emotions, but by reducing their unhelpful *influence* over behavior (Levin, Luoma, & Haeger, 2015). In the process, new possibilities open up, and change efforts can be guided more by self-regulation focused on vitality, joy, meaning, and purpose.

## Why Acceptance Is Often Needed

Neuroscience teaches us that human beings are historical—our nervous systems are additive, not subtractive. What goes in stays in, short of brain insult or injury. Viewed this way, the difficulties our clients experience now are simply a product of everything that has come before.

As historical creatures, we come into this world much like empty vessels, differing in genetic predispositions but basically conscious containers for our experience. Like a chef creating a soup, life experience adds various ingredients to our vessels and continues to do so. Some ingredients are clearly discernable—the trauma, the fiftieth birthday party—and each ingredient has its unique taste, some sweet, others sour, others bitter. More subtle flavors emerge from whatever happens to be in the mix at any moment. There's no healthy way to *remove* ingredients and flavors once they are added. New ingredients can be added, but these do not subtract from what is already present.

Language and cognition (see chapter 7) increase our ability to access our history. No verbally able human escapes the possibility of pain, because it can be brought to mind anytime, anywhere via language and cognition. Ironically, even though psychological pain is a normal part of the human experience (Eifert & Forsyth, 2005; Hayes et al., 2012), when experience is deemed unacceptable, pain is likely to increase because it leads to experiential avoidance (EA). *EA* is an unwillingness to experience psychological events even when efforts to escape or avoid such events have caused behavioral harm (Hayes, Wilson, Gifford, Follette, & Strosahl, 1996). EA appears to underpin many forms of psychological suffering precisely because when applied *rigidly* and *inflexibly*, it tends to increase pain and suffering and interfere with meaningful action (e.g., Chawla & Ostafin, 2007; Eifert & Forsyth, 2005). A large body of evidence suggests that EA is costly, effortful, and ineffective in the long term (e.g., Gross, 2002; Wenzlaff, & Wegner, 2000).

While control strategies work well outside the skin, they are often misapplied inside the skin, where thoughts, memories, and emotions cannot be readily controlled or eliminated. In short, if you don't want it, you've got it. What one *can* do is alter one's relationship with thoughts and feelings. This is where acceptance can make a real difference.

# Cultivating Psychological Acceptance

Cultivating acceptance involves creating a new context in which to experience thoughts and emotions. The remainder of this chapter offers practical guidance about how to cultivate acceptance.

## *Confront the Unworkability of Control*

An important precursor to acceptance work is helping clients recognize which aspects of experience they cannot control, and to open up to doing something new. Normally, this can be done in the first or second session and then be revisited as needed. Two simple questions are central to this process:

What have you tried so far to solve the problem(s)?

In your experience, how has that worked? In the short term? Long term?

When explored with compassion and gentleness, these questions begin to expose the unworkability and costs of the struggle itself. The client's own experience often reveals that control works in the short term, mainly in terms of offering psychological relief. However, these brief honeymoons from pain are costly—emotionally, physically, and in terms of moments away from doing something important. In this very brief clinical dialogue, with a twenty-seven-year-old female client who has long-standing struggles with social anxiety, the therapist begins to draw this out.

*Therapist:*   What's it like for you when anxiety shows up?

*Client:*    Well, I get a sinking feeling in my stomach, tense up, and don't feel like doing anything. I just sit alone watching TV.

*Therapist:*    So, if I hear you right, one of the things you do when anxiety shows up is sit alone in front of your TV? In your experience, how has that worked in taking care of the anxiety?

*Client:*    (*Confused.*) Honestly, it only works for a bit. Really, I just sit there feeling badly about myself, and how everyone else is out there, having fun, living their lives—and I'm not.

*Therapist:*    So, doing nothing and watching TV doesn't seem to be helping and may even make you feel worse. And, your mind is telling you that you're missing out. What else have you tried?

Eventually the therapist can simply reflect back what the client is saying (e.g., "It sounds like your experience is telling you that what appear to be sensible strategies end up not working in the long run. Does that sound about right?"). The intention is not to make the client feel bad, but rather to reveal the costs of the struggle itself and to help the client to consider the possibility that her own experience is valid, regardless of what her mind is saying.

Well-placed metaphors or exercises can draw out the costs of needless control efforts and orient the client toward new, more hopeful directions. Acceptance and commitment therapy contains numerous metaphors that can be readily used for this purpose (see Hayes et al., 2012; Stoddard & Afari, 2014). For example, a client might be given a short length of rope, and the tug-of-war with emotion can be acted out in therapy. The therapist's dialogue can orient the client toward the seeming need to win this tug-of-war with internal "monsters" (emotions) even though the fight puts off the ability to do more useful things (e.g., as both therapist and the client tug on their ends of the rope).

*Therapist:*    Your mind is telling you that you need to beat me before you can move on. What's showing up for you now?

*Client:*    I need to pull harder!

*Therapist:*    And isn't that like what you've actually been doing? Does it sometimes feel like this?

*Client:*    Just like this.

*Therapist:*    (*Continuing to pull.*) Have you ever won this tug-of-war once and for all? And notice also that you are not going to the dance you want to go to.

This kind of dialogue continues in the interaction (see Eifert & Forsyth, 2005; Hayes et al., 2012) until the client eventually sees an alternative: to let go of the rope. That action then becomes a physical metaphor for acceptance, and for the tricks of mind that keep it from being used.

It can be useful to have clients use an initial worksheet, recording (a) difficult situations, thoughts, and feelings that show up; (b) what they do in response to them (including times when they "picked up the rope"); and (c) short- and long-term consequences (i.e., what they have given up or missed out on when they got caught in a tug-of-war with their monsters).

## Teach Perspective-Taking Skills

One cannot truly accept what one does not know or see. This is why acceptance pivots on *perspective-taking skills*, or learning how to observe psychological experiences just as they are. Defusion skills (learning to look *at* thoughts and emotions, rather than *from* them; see chapter 23) can facilitate healthy perspective-taking and acceptance.

A variety of experiential exercises build perspective-taking skills, including formal and informal mindfulness exercises (see chapter 26). Traditional breath-focused meditation and other concrete mindfulness exercises (Kabat-Zinn, 2005) foster the ability to notice thoughts and feelings with openness. Therapists can also foster perspective taking by encouraging clients to speak as an observer of their experience in session (e.g., "I am noticing that I am experiencing an urge to shut down and withdraw."). Therapists can model and shape perspective taking linked to emotional openness in their own talk (for instance, "I notice I am feeling a sense of urgency inside me…as if I need to quickly do something to be useful to you.").

## Nurture Self-Kindness and Compassion

Many clients are incredibly hard on themselves and relate to their history and difficult psychological and emotional content with resistance, anger, and self-blame, adding more suffering to their pain. Acceptance work is not about asking clients to *like* what they think and feel. Instead, we are inviting clients to change the quality of their relationship with the experiences they are having anyway. Instead of turning away, acceptance asks the client to soften, to open up, and to meet difficult content with kindness, friendliness, gentleness, and, dare we say, love.

*Self-compassion* and *self-kindness* are not feelings—they are actions to be practiced, both in and out of session. They involve expanded awareness that (a) pain in life is inevitable, and (b) all human beings confront obstacles, problems, and pain (Neff, 2003).

We often use the metaphor of a parent dealing with a difficult child as we begin this work:

> When their child is upset or does something wrong, parents learn that yelling or telling the child to stop crying is sometimes ineffective and escalates the situation. Sometimes, parents opt for a softer approach. They don't resort to fighting or punishing behavior simply because their child is behaving badly. They see through that first impulse (to react with negative energy), and instead wish for their child to know kindness and love, and so they respond in a caring way that shows that. I wonder if approaching yourself and your history in the same way might be helpful. Isn't it true that self-blame has only escalated the situation? Isn't it time for something new?

You might even ask clients to hold their painful content as if it were a young infant, cradling it close to their heart with compassion and kindness. Guided meditation exercises, such as "holding anxiety gently," can be used to cultivate compassionate responses (see Forsyth & Eifert, 2016). After bringing the client into a state of eyes-closed open awareness, invite the person to do the following:

> *Take both of your hands and cup them to make the shape of a bowl, palms facing up. Allow them to rest softly in your lap. Notice the quality of those hands and the shape they are in. They are open and ready to hold something. As you get in touch with that, become aware that those very hands have been used by you in many ways. They have been used for work, for love, to touch and be touched [continue with half a dozen similar things]. Allow yourself to sink into the goodness contained in your hands.*
>
> *From that place of goodness, see if you can allow, even if just for a moment, a small, tiny piece of your [name emotional concern here; e.g., anxiety] to settle there. Like a feather floating down, imagine that piece of it gently comes to rest in the middle of your kind and loving hands.*
>
> *Take a moment to sink into that—this piece of [emotional concern] is now resting within the goodness of your hands. What is it like to hold it in this way? Simply notice, breathe, and sense the warmth and goodness of your hands. There's nothing else to do here.*

## Foster Willingness and Mindful Acceptance

*Willingness* is a choice to be open to whatever the mind and history offer. It is a kind of leap of faith—a dive into the future, open but without truly knowing what will happen. Thus, when we ask clients if they are willing to experience what shows up, we invite them to exercise control in terms of their choices and behavior, not knowing what they may experience as they step into the unknown.

The goal is for them to be willing to have a mindful, compassionate stance toward their experiences as they show up. Learning this posture is fostered by starting small, focusing on developing acceptance skills, and then expanding to more difficult content. Mindfulness practices (Brach, 2004; see also chapter 26) provide a useful structure to learn how to apply willingness. For example, guided meditations that direct attention, one domain and area at a time, toward emotions, bodily sensations, thoughts, and the like (e.g., the "acceptance of thoughts and feelings exercise" from Forsyth & Eifert, 2016) can be used in session to practice mindful acceptance. For instance, a difficult memory can be dismantled into a series of thoughts, images, physical sensations, and/or urges, and each piece can then be explored and contacted willingly, mindfully, and compassionately (see the "tin can monster" exercise in Hayes et al., 2012). Such exercises are, in essence, a kind of exposure exercise, done in the context of willingness and self-compassion.

## Frame Acceptance in the Context of Client Values

It helps to motivate acceptance by linking it to client *values*—chosen qualities of being and doing (see chapter 25) and other forms of positive motivation (see chapter 27). Doing so helps prevent acceptance from being a new form of avoidance or self-soothing.

Framing acceptance work in the context of client values is particularly important when doing exposure-based work. The aim is to help the client learn to change his *relationship* with unpleasant aspects of his history, while expanding the range of behavioral options. A brief dialogue with the socially anxious client mentioned earlier shows how the therapist began to draw this out.

*Therapist:*   Last time, we talked about seeing what it might be like for you to go out dancing with some of your friends this coming weekend. I just wanted to check in with you to see where you are with that.

*Client:*   I dunno… I've been thinking about it all week, and I'm really anxious about it.

*Therapist:*   (*Senses that the difficult content is showing up in the room and sees this as an opportunity to do some exposure-like acceptance work.*) What's showing up for you right now? Like, where do you feel it in your body?

*Client:*        (*Points to her stomach.*)

*Therapist:*   What sensations are there?

*Client:*        It's like butterflies… I feel queasy, like I might get sick, and then I'll make a fool of myself.

*Therapist:*   Okay, so let's notice that. You're sensing something in your body. And, your mind is protesting and jumping in as it does…telling you that this is unacceptable and you're not okay. Let's take a moment to notice that…thoughts showing up…and see if we can allow them to be here. Now, I'd like to invite you to do something, if you're willing.

*Client:*        Okay… But you're not going to try to get me to grab that rope again, are you? (*Smiling.*)

*Therapist:*   No, no rope this time. Instead, I'd like us to take a moment to see what's really there. I'd like to invite you to close your eyes and get in touch with your breath like we've done many times before. When you start feeling connected to your breath, your safe refuge, I'd like you to notice that one sensation in your belly. Simply notice it, and with each breath see if you can make more space for the sensation within you to just be there. (*Pausing for about thirty seconds or so.*) As you soften to it, look again and see if this sensation is really your enemy. Can you soften to it and hold it gently, and with some kindness, as you see yourself out with your friends, dancing and enjoying the freedom in that? Take a few moments, and when you've noticed some space and tenderness, come back to just being here, and slowly open your eyes when you're ready.

The therapist then explored other sensations, urges, and thoughts with the client—one at a time, with qualities of mindful awareness and gentle allowing. The therapist repeatedly checked in with the client to assess her willingness, and also what was new or different in her experience, as she explored difficult content, or barriers, that had gotten in the way of her going out and connecting with friends while dancing.

The client, in turn, felt encouraged to practice willingness and mindful acceptance at home, first dancing alone and eventually taking a step in a valued direction by going out and dancing with her friends. When the anxiety monster showed up on the dance floor, she did not "pick up the rope" but instead treated it with kindness and compassion. In session the following week, the client even joked that she danced "with her anxiety monsters at the club," and she felt empowered and alive doing so.

# Recommendations, Common Traps, and Clinical Errors

Acceptance work can be challenging for therapists. Below we outline some suggestions and some common traps and errors you may experience along the way.

**The therapeutic stance and your own personal work.** Acceptance work asks the therapist to go into difficult places with clients while modeling an open, receptive, and compassionate stance. That can be challenging, which is why *therapist* experiential avoidance predicts a failure to use exposure strategies (e.g., Scherr, Herbert, & Forman, 2015). For acceptance to be instigated, modeled, and supported, therapists need to practice acceptance with their own difficult psychological events. It is not necessary to be masters of acceptance, because coping models are actually more effective. When we, as therapists, are working to approach our own history and imperfections with kindness, compassion, and patience, it becomes easier to support client efforts to so the same.

**Resist the temptation to offer easy explanations or quick fixes.** Though in therapy the tendency to jump in and offer solutions, explanations, or promises about thinking and feeling better is great, doing so can backfire in the context of acceptance work. It is more important to focus on aligning with clients and their experiences as they are, and to move toward changes from that foundation of openness. This does not mean condoning what has not worked in the client's experience, approving of unhealthy client behaviors, or "accepting" unhealthy environments or situations. It means starting with the validity of client experience, and allowing client experience to guide therapy toward what works.

**Make it experiential.** Experiential exercises are more effective than mere instructions about how to accept thoughts and feelings (McMullen et al., 2008). Intellectual conversations *about* acceptance are rarely helpful in therapeutic contexts. Acceptance is more like riding a bicycle: it is learned through direct experience. If you ever find yourself explaining acceptance, or trying to convince the client to accept, just stop, and say something like "Did you notice what just happened? Both of our minds really got going there." Then return to something experiential.

**Lay the groundwork, and avoid using acceptance in a control context.** Acceptance with the goal of eliminating difficult private events is unlikely to be helpful in the long run. Going directly to acceptance without exploring the costs of needless control can backfire because clients see acceptance as a clever new way to "win the tug-of-war" rather than to do what is in the etymology of the word "acceptance": to receive the gift that is inside difficult experiences. A stance that embodies kindness, curiosity, compassion, and openness is necessary before that gift is likely to be received.

**Acceptance is a process, not a "one and done" technique.** Often the temptation is great to focus on the techniques of acceptance, perhaps even doing them in a linear way, while missing that acceptance is a functional process. As a process, acceptance often unfolds gradually and is revisited again and again in various ways over the course of therapy and a lifetime. Many evidence-based methods (exposure, mindfulness, behavioral activation) contain the opportunity to learn acceptance as a process. Therapists who have a process focus will be more likely to work successfully with clients to cultivate acceptance.

**Frame acceptance in the context of client values.** Values dignify the hard work of therapy, particularly acceptance-based work. Without a positive life focus, acceptance can feel like wallowing in the muck, without a direction. The purpose is not to open up to pain for its own sake. The purpose is to foster what the client truly cares about. Thus, it is important to link this work to what matters to the client and to let the work of acceptance be about that.

# Applications and Contraindications

Generally speaking, acceptance is most applicable to experiences *inside the skin*, whereas direct change efforts are often most applicable to the world *outside the skin*. Acceptance is not indicated when the client can effectively change something about the environment or behavior that would produce an increased quality of life. For instance, if a client is being subjected to racial discrimination in the workplace, it would not be helpful to accept this state of affairs. Rather, one might work with this client to help her accept the anxiety that comes with contacting a human resources department to report the discrimination. The same applies to some experiences within the skin, although here we need to be careful. If a client has a headache and experience and data suggest that aspirin would alleviate it without harm, there is no reason for him to not take the aspirin. Conversely, a person with chronic pain syndrome may need to learn to carry pain with her because, for example, the long-term impact of opiates is unhelpful.

To make this discrimination, it can be useful to think functionally by considering questions such as these:

- Is this a problem that is old, a part of the client's history, and/or one for which reasonable control and change efforts have largely failed (think long term)?

- Is the outcome of control and change efforts one of expansion and increased vitality and range of functioning, or not?

- Based on the client's experience with the problem, would doing more of the same offer any hope?

- If the client no longer pursued the struggle and control agenda, would that open up new opportunities that are seemingly unavailable now?

It appears from the evidence that acceptance is much more broadly applicable than clients and clinicians initially suppose. That said, it is important to develop a context for acceptance-based work and skills and to be open to alternatives. Once a client has nurtured acceptance skills as a new and potentially more vital alternative to the typical change agenda, life itself can help the client learn when it is the best approach and when it is not.

# Conclusions

Psychological acceptance is a radically empowering form of clinical change. Instead of changing first before being open to what is present, acceptance focuses on whether it is possible to be a functional, whole, and complete human being now. Though many clients enter therapy seemingly trapped in a cage of suffering and despair, desperate to find a way out, acceptance illuminates the door that has been open all along. There is enormous freedom in that. A growing evidence base shows that acceptance skills are central to psychological well-being and help guide and explain the impact of psychotherapy with many forms of human suffering.

# References

Brach, T. (2004). *Radical acceptance: Embracing your life with the heart of a Buddha*. New York: Bantam Books.

Chawla, N., & Ostafin, B. (2007). Experiential avoidance as a functional dimensional approach to psychopathology: An empirical review. *Journal of Clinical Psychology, 63*(9), 871–890.

Cordova, J. V. (2001). Acceptance in behavior therapy: Understanding the process of change. *Behavior Analyst, 24*(2), 213–226.

Eifert, G. H., & Forsyth, J. P. (2005). *Acceptance and commitment therapy for anxiety disorders: A practitioner's treatment guide to using mindfulness, acceptance, and values-based behavior change strategies.* Oakland, CA: New Harbinger Publications.

Forsyth, J. P., & Eifert, G. H. (2016). *The mindfulness and acceptance workbook for anxiety: A guide to breaking free from anxiety, phobias, and worry using acceptance and commitment therapy* (2nd ed.). Oakland, CA: New Harbinger Publications.

Gross, J. J. (2002). Emotion regulation: Affective, cognitive, and social consequences. *Psychophysiology, 39*(3), 281–291.

Hayes, S. C., Strosahl, K. D., & Wilson, K. G. (2012). *Acceptance and commitment therapy: The process and practice of mindful change* (2nd ed.). New York: Guilford Press.

Hayes, S. C., Wilson, K. G., Gifford, E. V., Follette, V. M., & Strosahl, K. D. (1996). Experiential avoidance and behavioral disorders: A functional dimensional approach to diagnosis and treatment. *Journal of Consulting and Clinical Psychology, 64*(6), 1152–1168.

Kabat-Zinn, J. (2005). *Wherever you go, there you are: Mindfulness meditation in everyday life* (10th anniversary ed.). New York: Hachette Books.

Levin, M. E., Luoma, J. B., & Haeger, J. A. (2015). Decoupling as a mechanism of change in mindfulness and acceptance: A literature review. *Behavior Modification, 39*(6), 870–911.

McMullen, J., Barnes-Holmes, D., Barnes-Holmes, Y., Stewart, I., Luciano, M. C., & Cochrane, A. (2008). Acceptance versus distraction: Brief instructions, metaphors and exercises in increasing tolerance for self-delivered electric shocks. *Behaviour Research and Therapy, 46*(1), 122–129.

Neff, K. (2003). Self-compassion: An alternative conceptualization of a healthy attitude toward oneself. *Self and Identity, 2*(2), 85–101.

Scherr, S. R., Herbert, J. D., & Forman, E. M. (2015). The role of therapist experiential avoidance in predicting therapist preference for exposure treatment for OCD. *Journal of Contextual Behavioral Science, 4*(1), 21–29.

Stoddard, J. A., & Afari, N. (2014). *The big book of ACT metaphors: A practitioner's guide to experiential exercises and metaphors in acceptance and commitment therapy.* Oakland, CA: New Harbinger Publications.

Wenzlaff, R. M., & Wegner, D. M. (2000). Thought suppression. *Annual Review of Psychology, 51,* 59–91.

# CHAPTER 25

# Values Choice and Clarification

Tobias Lundgren, PhD
Andreas Larsson, PhD

*Department of Clinical Neuroscience, Center for Psychiatry Research, Karolinska Institute; Stockholm Health Care Services*

## Definitions and Background

Clients often come into therapy stuck in a difficult life situation with troublesome emotions, thoughts, memories, and physical pains. In their struggles, it is not uncommon for them to have lost contact with what gives life meaning and purpose. Cognitive and behavioral treatments have increasingly been willing to address this deficit by reorienting them toward their values choices.

Values and discussions of valued choices are a core part of acceptance and commitment therapy (Hayes, Strosahl, & Wilson, 1999, 2011), behavioral activation (see chapter 19), motivational interviewing (see chapter 27), and a wide variety of other evidence-based methods. Historically speaking, values work in psychotherapy was the province of humanistic psychotherapies. Viktor Frankl wrote extensively on the drive for *meaning*, drawing on his experience in a Nazi concentration camp during World War II, and applied these ideas in logotherapy (Frankl, 1984). Carl Rogers, another famous humanist, thought the pursuit of values to be essential in self-actualization and ultimately psychological health. Using a card-sorting task comparing a client's self-perception to an ideal self before and after therapy, he developed data supporting his person-centered approach (Rogers, 1995). Rogers's ideas were brought into evidence-based therapy by motivational interviewing, in particular (Miller & Rollnick, 2002).

*Values* in the cognitive behavioral literature have been defined in multiple ways (Dahl, Plumb, Stewart, & Lundgren, 2009; Hayes et al., 2011), but for the purposes of this chapter we will adopt the definition of "freely chosen, verbally constructed consequences of ongoing, dynamic, evolving patterns of activity, which establish predominant reinforcers for that activity that are intrinsic in engagement in the valued behavioral pattern itself" (Wilson & DuFrene, 2009, p. 64). It seems worthwhile to unpack this definition to see how it may guide us in working with values.

**Values are freely chosen.** "Freely chosen" means they are chosen in a context free from aversive control. As much as possible, a reduction in aversive control is almost a prerequisite for choosing values. People formulate and choose values that are *theirs*, and therapists need to be cautious about suggesting that their own values are preferable over client choices.

**Values are verbally constructed consequences of ongoing, dynamic, evolving patterns of activity.** Values are not just the direct consequences of action—they are constructed as important consequences through speaking and symbolic thought (see chapter 7). Values are part of the context of action systems and cannot be separated from action. They are not some kind of entity out there to be discovered or held onto.

**Values establish predominant reinforcers for that activity that are intrinsic in engagement in the valued behavioral pattern itself.** Values are about what is important and sought after. Values are an inseparable part of the behavior they reinforce, in the moment when the behavior occurs.

For example, imagine you are at home with your child and there is a lot of work to get through that you left undone at the office. Now in this moment, seeing that your child needs your attention, you put down your laptop and choose to fully engage in conversation and play with your child. If this moment of connection with the importance of active parenting makes it more likely that you will do the same the next time, we can say that being an active parent is a value of yours.

Values work can function in therapy as a motivator for change, as a metric for the effectiveness of actions, and as a guide in the development of new behavioral repertoires. Values work can be done at any point in the therapeutic process. Values interventions are used to help clients stop vicious, negative life cycles and get in contact with more effective behavior patterns.

# Implementation

We will give an extended example of values work using the Bull's-Eye Values Survey (BEVS). During the last decade, the BEVS has also been developed and investigated as an outcome and mediator measure in research. Changes in valued living as measured by the BEVS are associated with higher quality of life and lower depression, anxiety, and stress (Lundgren, Luoma, Dahl, Strosahl, & Melin, 2012). BEVS scores mediate changes in behavioral health (Lundgren, Dahl, & Hayes, 2008) and mental health areas (Hayes, Orsillo, & Roemer, 2010). The aim of the BEVS is to (1) help clients clarify their values, (2) measure how well they are living in accordance with their values, (3) operationalize obstacles for valued living and measure their perceived effect, and (4) create a bold but reasonable valued action plan that challenges expressed obstacles. In the following section, a client-therapist interaction will demonstrate all four parts of the BEVS.

This clinical example is based on the case of Erik, a forty-year-old carpenter. Erik suffers from depression and anxiety symptoms and has been rehabilitating a back injury that has left him with chronic pain. He has two children and a wife who works in the children's day-care system.

When Erik came into the office he looked tired. He answered questions but was not particularly responsive with eye contact or in his body language. After two sessions creating rapport and collecting information, the therapist decided to help Erik clarify his deeply held values so as to increase the likelihood of new action paths in his life.

*Therapist:* Erik, I would like to understand what you have lost during your fight with depression, anxiety, and pain.

*Erik:* I have lost everything, my life…

*Therapist:* (*Pauses a couple of moments.*) Tell me more about the life you have lost…

*Erik:* I have lost contact with my kids, my wife, lost my friends, my love for sports…lost taking care of myself. It awakens memories of how things were before. (*Looking at the therapist.*) I remember playing sports with my kids, talking about life with my wife, and just hanging out with friends playing basketball and laughing. I really miss that.

*Therapist:* Okay, it seems to me that there is something really important here. Is it okay for you to look more closely at this?

*Erik:* Sure, if it can help me get better, I am open to anything.

Erik has lost a lot in his struggle with depression and anxiety. In the next section, we'll illustrate how the BEVS can be used to explore that issue: clarifying values and investigating values consistency.

The bull's-eye dartboard, used in the BEVS, is a visual representation of the four areas of living that are important in people's lives: work/education, leisure, relationships, and personal growth/health. It is okay to use these areas as they are defined here, and to go through all of them with a client; it's also fine to not have the domains predefined, and to instead define them with your client. The following descriptions of these four areas should clarify what we mean by "values" and should stimulate thinking around values:

1. *Work/education* refers to career aims, values about improving education and knowledge, and generally feeling of use to those close to you or in your community (i.e., volunteering, overseeing your household, etc.).

2. *Leisure* refers to how you play in life, how you enjoy yourself, hobbies, or other activities that you spend free time doing (e.g., gardening, sewing, coaching a children's soccer team, fishing, playing sports).

3. *Relationships* refers to intimacy in life—relationships with children, family of origin, friends, and social contacts in the community.

4. *Personal growth/health* refers to your spiritual life, either in organized religion or personal expressions of spirituality; exercise; nutrition; and addressing health risk factors such as drinking, drug use, smoking, and weight.

## Clarify Your Values

Start your work with the BEVS by asking the client to describe her values within each of the four values areas. The therapist invites the client to think about each area in terms of her dreams, as if she had the possibility to get her wishes completely fulfilled. What are the qualities that she would like to get out of each area, and what are her expectations from these areas of life? Her values should reflect how she would like to live life over time rather than a specific goal. For example, getting married might be a *goal* that reflects the *value* of being an affectionate, honest, and loving partner. To accompany her son to a baseball game might be a *goal*; to be an involved and interested parent might be the *value*.

## Suggestions to Deepen Values Work

**Expand on experiences.** Was there a time in the past when your client had a life worth living? Ask your client to close her eyes, take a couple of breaths, and connect with situations in the past, when life was good and really worth living.

Help her see herself in one of those situations. Deepen the experience by asking for emotions and images. How was that life, and how was your client acting back then? What can she see? Are there other people involved in those memories? How did she act, and how were the interactions for her? Try to get the client to really connect with the past experience of having a life worth living.

**Take your time.** If your client is open, willing, and able to connect with past experiences of having a life with purpose and meaning, don't rush the work. Help your client to stay inside the values context. You want to help your client to be able to do this outside the therapy room, and you start the process in therapy. Explore that value, feel it, and stimulate further exploration of it.

**You find values in suffering.** Values are often found inside suffering. For example, a client would rarely be afraid of other people or of being rejected if relationships were not important. This means that values themselves, and values talk, may also evoke suffering. Take it slow, and acknowledge that suffering and values often go hand in hand.

**Go beyond goals.** Often clients can start describing goals instead of values. Try to help clients go *beyond* the goals. If a client states that he would like to start working out three times a week, ask why doing so is important to him. Why is taking care of the body by working out important? How does he want to approach the workouts? What are the important qualities in your client's actions that will make working out a good experience? How are they related to a meaningful life?

**Balance pushing and choosing.** Be aware that sometimes values work is not the best way to move forward. If the suffering is too overwhelming, questions about values may fall flat. If you have pushed for values and doing so has not worked, be ready to change your approach. You may need to do other therapeutic interventions first and come back to values later. However, sometimes it can be effective to push on. The art of psychotherapy is to be present with your client and to continuously keep your functional analysis in mind. You need to figure out how you need to act in order to be of service to your client.

In the following conversation, Erik and his therapist deepened their values work.

*Therapist:* In this exercise, I want us to look more closely at your values. Is there a life domain that you would like to start with?

*Erik:* The most important thing for me is the contact with my kids. My wife too, of course, but I would say kids first.

Therapist:    Okay, let's start there then. Can you contact an experience, a moment in the past when you were how you want to be with your kids? When you had the contact and relationship you want with them? Take your time.

Erik:    Yeah. (Smiles.) I remember when we were playing soccer in the garden. We had fun and laughed together; I didn't think of possible pain, or ruminate. We were just there together, hanging out. Thinking of that also makes me a bit sad. I miss that contact.

Therapist:    Mixed feelings here, both joy and sadness. What does that contact mean to you?

Erik:    It meant and means the world to me! I can really sense our relationship, the connection, the happiness in my body and my love for them.

Therapist:    If we could strive to get that relationship back into your life, would you be willing to work for that?

Erik:    Absolutely, I would do anything!

Therapist:    Take a couple of moments and write down a brief description of the relationship you would like to have with your kids. What's in that experience you contacted? How were you acting with them at that time?

Erik then wrote this values statement in relation to his kids:

I want to be a present dad. I want to play with my kids, see them, and be there for them not only when we have fun but also when they have a hard time. I want to be active, listen, and show them that I care for them. Even if I physically can't be the person I used to be, I love my kids and need and want to find a way to be with them. I want them to know that I love them very much.

Erik and the therapist always could have reinvestigated values as therapy proceeded, but at that point in therapy the therapist used Erik's statement for the BEVS work. They had established a value to guide therapy and to help motivate Erik to break vicious action patterns and establish new ones. For the purposes of this chapter, we will not go through all the areas of the BEVS. Instead, we will use Erik's relationship with his kids as an example of how values clarification work can be done and explain the different functions of the values work.

Erik and his therapist then investigated how Erik's actions coincided with his value.

*Therapist:*  Now, look at this dartboard we developed. We'll use the relationship area. The middle of the dartboard, the bull's-eye, represents being a present and active dad: the dad you want to be with and for your kids. Now, mark an X on the dartboard that best represents how well you have acted in line with those values during the last two weeks. An X in the bull's-eye means that you have been living completely in line with how you want to be as a dad. An X far from the bull's-eye means that you have not been living as you want in relation to your kids.

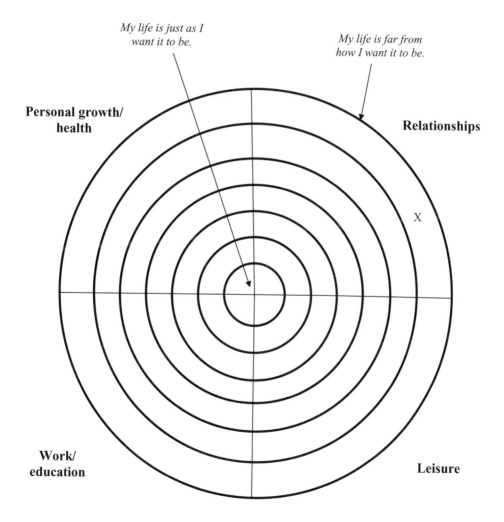

FIGURE 1. Erik placed his X far from the bull's-eye.

Erik and his therapist then went on to talk about the discrepancy between how Erik wanted to be with his kids and how he actually had acted during the previous two weeks. His actions did not coincide with his value, and this discrepancy became a motivator for change.

*Therapist:* In our previous talks, you told me that your actions lately have been about avoiding shame and guilt around not being a good enough father. What does looking at the dartboard tell you?

*Erik:* It tells me that I am far from being the dad I want… It makes me sad on the one hand but also eager. I want something else. I want to be in the bull's-eye. I have not thought about the dad I want to be or those moments we have had together in a long time. I have been so filled up by anxiety and thoughts about not being good enough. When I think of the dad I am today, it is far from the one I want to be. I want to make a change.

*Therapist:* That sounds really important and also painful—to see what you are missing.

Seeing the discrepancy between Erik's values and his actions created a space that he was eager to fill with meaning and valued actions. Hopefully this work can establish a verbal operant to motivate choices in line with his values.

The therapist and Erik then examined obstacles for change.

*Therapist:* Erik, I want you again to contact the obstacles that pop up for you when thinking about being the dad you want to be. Take your time and really connect with that.

*Erik:* (Tearing up.) I feel ashamed that I haven't done better… I feel tired…hopelessness…fear that if I start to be active it will increase my pain, and also that they will reject me.

*Therapist:* Feelings and thoughts, intertwined around fear of not being the dad you had imagined you would be… Can I ask you a question? When these thoughts and feelings emerge in situations around your kids, how often are they controlling what you do? (The therapist gives Erik a sheet of paper with a horizontal line of numbers, with the 1 representing little control of feelings, and 7 representing complete control. The therapist instructs him to circle the number that best represents how often his feelings and thoughts prevent him from being the dad he wants to be.)

| 1 | 2 | 3 | 4 | 5 | (6) | 7 |
|---|---|---|---|---|-----|---|

Doesn't prevent me at all                                    Prevents me completely

In situations with his children, and when Erik thought about his role as a dad, obstacles emerged and Erik began to avoid rather than to act in line with his values. Avoidance reduces fear and pain in the short term, but in the long run it may reduce life quality. His actions narrowed his life path. It is important to note that as therapists we need to work with these obstacles using all our knowledge of cognitive and behavioral treatments. Values work supplements and supports this work.

The final step in the BEVS is to create a valued action plan. The therapist asked Erik to formulate actions he could take in daily life that would tell him that he was zeroing in on the bull's-eye in the area of being the dad he wanted to be. These actions could be small steps toward a particular goal, or they could just be actions that reflect how he wanted to be as a dad. Usually, taking a valued step includes being willing to encounter the obstacle or obstacles the client identified earlier, and to take the action anyway. The therapist asked Erik to identify at least one value-based action he was willing to take in the area of being the dad he wanted to be.

*Therapist:* Erik, what would be a step that you would be willing to take that would move you in the direction of being the present, active dad you want to be even in the face of emotional difficulties and obstructing thoughts? It doesn't need to be a big step, but most often the step means that you will challenge your fears a little.

*Erik:* One thing that I have thought about is to ask my eldest son to go to a hockey game. We did that before, but now I have been afraid that I would be tired and need to cancel, so I haven't even asked. Both Ludwig, my son, and I really liked going to games, and I am pretty sure that he would like to do that again.

*Therapist:* Great. I can see that means something for you. So, when is there a game you could go to? And when can you ask him?

*Erik:* There is a game at home this weekend, and I could ask him tonight because we probably need to get tickets right away.

*Therapist:* Okay, so you will ask him tonight and get tickets together. How is it for you to plan reconnecting with your son?

*Erik:*       It feels great doing that, and also a bit scary. What if I get anxious, and what if he says no?

*Therapist:*  Your fears will probably pop up now and then in this process. Can you let them come along when you reconnect with Ludwig?

*Erik:*       Sure. For my son, absolutely!

## Summary of Working with the BEVS

Erik was occupied with troublesome thoughts and emotions, and the BEVS work helped him to both clarify his values and what his actions had led to in the short and the long runs. Prior to Erik's contact with the therapist, his values had been put on hold. Through their work together, the therapist and Erik brought his values forth into attention again, stimulating new behaviors. This was not the end of the therapeutic journey for Erik—values work usually sets the stage for interventions designed to handle the obstacles that emerge once values are put into action. Those methods are covered elsewhere in this volume.

# Clinical Pitfalls

**Words are tricky.** Be aware of how your clients talk about their values. Statements like "I really *need* to be a better dad" or "I *must* do this or that" can indicate that values are entangled with avoidance and suffering.

**Outcomes can dominate over process.** Values work is not about forcing behavioral outcomes. Often therapists suggest goals or actions, and when an action occurs, they assume therapy has been successful. It is important to focus on how valued actions occur, because when they truly are valued, they tend to become a natural part of the client's behavioral repertoire.

**Just do it!** Done incorrectly, values work can sound like "Ignore your pain and move forward no matter what." That kind of stoic, teeth-clenched change is not what we want as therapists. We want clients to develop new skills, and by doing so live a meaningful and psychologically healthy life.

**Goals vs. values.** This is a place where therapists often get stuck, especially beginner therapists. If a client answers values questions with concrete goals, try to move up in the hierarchy to qualities of being and doing.

**Morals vs. values.** It is easy to get stuck in what is right and wrong when it comes to values. With values work we want to help our clients to formulate statements that function to motivate actions in line with living a personally good life. If your client states values that you are not willing to support, you should consider referring the client to another therapist. This doesn't happen often, but if it does try to see what's best for your client.

**Clients are not stating values as I know values!** We are looking to develop values statements, closely connected to client experiences, that motivate action in helpful directions. The topography of words is not interesting in and of itself. If you find yourself wrestling your client into stating the "right" words, pause, reflect, and ask the client to tell you more about what he cares about, what he misses in life, and what matters to him. Don't push clients to formulate certain values words. Doing so will not be as effective as trying to understand and take the perspective of your client. Be curious and learn to understand the words your client is using to express his values.

**Client barriers becoming therapy barriers.** If you start to think *This person needs X before she can move in a valued direction*, you are likely encountering a barrier, oftentimes a barrier the client is also experiencing. Often this means you are stuck in thinking that the client's expressions of obstacles are literal truths. They are not; they are expressions of suffering and inflexibility in that moment that you need to treat functionally. Try to work with the barrier using your normal therapeutic interventions, and investigate to see if you can find a way to help your client, allowing values and expressed barriers to coexist.

**Fused values becoming new ways to punish oneself.** If values statements become rigid and aversive, they are no longer values as we mean them. Particularly for people who are highly prone to self-shame or have a performance-based self-esteem, values can become a way to punish themselves. Often that itself becomes a barrier to moving in valued directions.

# Applications

Values work can be an important part of any treatment. Even if not explicitly addressed, therapists should generally include some values work in their analysis of client behavior and its functions. Values are often useful when setting more traditional treatment goals. Here are some common clinical examples, broken down by problem areas.

**Work-site stress.** It's difficult to overestimate the pressure that a well-crafted organization can place on an individual. This does not mean organizations are evil, just that when building an organization, certain functional properties are put in place to make people productive. This may lead some people to create rules basing their self-worth on productivity. If, for one reason or another, they produce less, this may impact their sense of self-worth.

**Eating disorders.** Eating disorders, bulimia, and anorexia nervosa are characterized by individuals trying to control internal experiences through food intake, most often in order to fulfill an idealized appearance. This is virtually an inverse of values. Because of the heavy dominance of aversive control, and how long the disorders have been present with people—meaning they have a lot of practice being aversively controlled—eating-disorders work often requires building a values repertoire.

**Behavior medicine.** In behavior medicine, values work can be especially important with chronic conditions, such as pain, diabetes, or epilepsy. Values are often put on hold when dealing with medical conditions. It is important to bring values back into an individual's context to help the person find motivation for growth and change, even if the medical condition persists.

**Addiction.** In addiction work, it is common for past failures in valued domains (e.g., parenting) due to an addiction to dominate over engaging in the opportunities that arise in the moment (e.g., taking care of your child who is in front of you now). The importance of valued actions is especially clear during relapses. When people struggling to step out of addiction veer off a valued path, it is common to think *I've broken the rule, so I might as well do a good job of it!* By returning to the values conversation, it becomes possible for the person to see that the real choice is between a pattern of quit/relapse/quit and quit/relapse/fail. If the values behind abstaining, sobriety, or moderation have remained in place, that choice is clearer (Wilson, Schnetzer, Flynn, & Kurtz, 2012).

**Depression.** Lack of access to values-congruent reinforcement seems to be a key ingredient to maintaining depression. Values work is used to link behavior change to immediately reinforcing properties. It appears that doing more things that are meaningful is helpful in depression, and it is best for the clients to do these meaningful things not because they want to get out of the depression, but because these things matter deeply to them and move them in valued directions that lead to a more healthy, fulfilling, and meaningful life.

**Anxiety problems.** For anxiety, values and exposure work can go hand in hand. Values work lessens aversive control. If, as a therapist, you perform exposure based on values rather than symptom reduction, you are not just supporting nonavoidant behavior, you may be helping to reduce aversive control more globally, building out the "freely chosen" part of the definition of values given earlier.

# Summary

Values work can empower most forms of evidence-based therapy by linking behavior change to meaning and purpose. Choosing and clarifying values appears to be a key process with wide applicability across problem types and treatment methods.

# References

Dahl, J., Plumb, J. C., Stewart, I., & Lundgren, T. (2009). *The art and science of valuing in psychotherapy: Helping clients discover, explore, and commit to valued action using acceptance and commitment therapy.* Oakland, CA: New Harbinger Publications.

Frankl, V. E. (1984). *Man's search for meaning: An introduction to logotherapy* (Rev. and updated). New York: Pocket Books.

Hayes, S. A., Orsillo, S. M., & Roemer, L. (2010). Changes in proposed mechanisms of action during an acceptance-based behavior therapy for generalized anxiety disorder. *Behaviour Research and Therapy, 48*(3), 238–245.

Hayes, S. C., Strosahl, K. D., & Wilson, K. G. (1999). *Acceptance and commitment therapy: An experiential approach to behavior change.* New York: Guilford Press.

Hayes, S. C., Strosahl, K. D., & Wilson, K. G. (2011). *Acceptance and commitment therapy: The process and practice of mindful change* (2nd ed.). New York: Guilford Press.

Lundgren, T., Dahl, J., & Hayes, S. C. (2008). Evaluation of mediators of change in the treatment of epilepsy with acceptance and commitment therapy. *Journal of Behavioral Medicine, 31*(3), 225–235.

Lundgren, T., Luoma, J. B., Dahl, J., Strosahl, K., Melin, L. (2012). The Bull's-Eye Values Survey: A psychometric evaluation. *Cognitive and Behavioral Practice, 19*(4), 518–526.

Miller, W. R., & Rollnick, S. (2002). *Motivational interviewing: Helping people change.* New York: Guilford Press.

Rogers, C. R. (1995). *On becoming a person: A therapist's view of psychotherapy.* New York: Houghton Mifflin.

Wilson, K. G., & DuFrene, T. (2009). *Mindfulness for two: An acceptance and commitment therapy approach to mindfulness in psychotherapy.* Oakland, CA: New Harbinger Publications.

Wilson, K. G., Schnetzer, L. W., Flynn, M. K., & Kurtz, S. (2012). Acceptance and commitment therapy for addiction. In S. C. Hayes & M. E. Levin (Eds.), *Mindfulness and acceptance for addictive behaviors: Applying contextual CBT to substance abuse and behavioral addictions* (pp. 27–68). Oakland, CA: New Harbinger Publications.

# CHAPTER 26

# Mindfulness Practice

Ruth Baer, PhD

*Department of Psychology, University of Kentucky*

## Definitions and Background

In the psychological literature, *mindfulness* is often described as a form of nonjudgmental attention to present-moment experiences; these include internal phenomena, such as sensations, cognitions, emotions, and urges, as well as environmental stimuli, such as sights, sounds, and scents. Mindfulness also includes awareness of current activity and is often contrasted with behaving automatically or mechanically with attention focused elsewhere. Establishing a consensus about a more precise definition of mindfulness has been difficult, in part because the term is used in a variety of interventions, each with its own theoretical foundations. The Buddhist roots of several current mindfulness-based methods, and attempts to describe contemporary mindfulness in ways consistent with foundational Buddhist teachings, have also contributed to lack of consensus about a definition; this problem is complicated by the variety of ways in which mindfulness is described within Buddhist texts (Dreyfus, 2011). Despite these difficulties, a perusal of contemporary psychological descriptions of mindfulness shows that many include two general elements that can be loosely characterized as *what one does* and *how one does it*. The examples of this shown in table 1 suggest that mindfulness is generally agreed to be a type of attention or awareness that is open, curious, accepting, friendly, nonjudgmental, compassionate, and kind.

# Table 1. Contemporary psychological descriptions of mindfulness: what and how

| AUTHOR | WHAT | HOW |
|---|---|---|
| Kabat-Zinn, 1994, 2003 | Paying attention, or the awareness that arises through paying attention... | ...on purpose, in the present moment, and nonjudgmentally.<br><br>...with an affectionate, compassionate quality, a sense of openhearted, friendly presence and interest. |
| Marlatt & Kristeller, 1999 | Bringing one's complete attention to present experiences... | ...on a moment-to-moment basis, with an attitude of acceptance and loving-kindness. |
| Bishop et al., 2004 | Self-regulation of attention so that it is maintained on the immediate experience... | ...with an orientation characterized by curiosity, openness, and acceptance. |
| Germer, Siegel, & Fulton, 2005 | Awareness of present experience... | ...with acceptance: an extension of nonjudgment that adds a measure of kindness or friendliness. |
| Linehan, 2015 | The act of focusing the mind in the present moment... | ...without judgment or attachment, with openness to the fluidity of each moment. |

A more technical and theory-based definition is found in acceptance and commitment therapy (ACT; Hayes, Strosahl, & Wilson, 2012), which conceptualizes mindfulness as having four elements: contact with the present moment, acceptance, defusion, and self-as-context; each of these is defined in terms of ACT and relational frame theory (Fletcher & Hayes, 2005; see chapters 23 and 24 in this volume). Though conceptually rigorous, this approach to defining mindfulness is roughly consistent with the framework of *what* and *how*. Present-moment experiences, particularly thoughts and feelings, are observed in a particular way: with willingness to experience them as they are, recognition that they need not control behavior, and the understanding that they do not define the person who is experiencing them. Similar formulations are central to other mindfulness-based interventions (Segal, Williams, & Teasdale, 2013)

Many authors agree that both the what and the how are essential to a clear understanding of mindfulness. For example, a person in a sad mood might be intensely aware of feeling sad but might respond to the sadness by judging the sad mood as ridiculous; criticizing the self as weak and foolish for feeling sad; ruminating about how the sad mood arose and how to get rid of it; or attempting to suppress, avoid, or escape the sad feelings in harmful ways. These responses to sadness are inconsistent with mindfulness and increase the risk of a downward spiral into depression (Segal et al., 2013).

Mindfulness of sadness includes closely observing the associated sensations, including where in the body they are felt and whether they are changing over time. The mindful observer of sadness brings an attitude of openness, friendly interest, and compassion to the experience while allowing the sadness to be present. When ruminative thought patterns arise, the mindful observer gently redirects attention to the present-moment sensations. The purpose of mindfulness of sadness is to encourage wise choices about potentially adaptive responses: taking constructive steps to address a problem, engaging in an activity to lift mood, or simply allowing sadness to run its natural course without reacting to it in ways that cause harm or are inconsistent with longer-term values and goals.

# Implementation

Mindfulness-based interventions (MBIs) have a growing body of support (for a recent meta-analysis, see Khoury et al., 2013). The MBIs with the strongest evidence base are ACT and its close cousin acceptance-based behavior therapy (Roemer, Orsillo, & Salters-Pednault, 2008); dialectical behavior therapy (DBT; Linehan, 1993, 2015); and mindfulness-based cognitive therapy (MBCT; Segal et al., 2013) and the closely related methods of mindfulness-based stress reduction (MBSR; Kabat-Zinn, 1982) and mindfulness-based relapse prevention (Bowen, Chawla, & Marlatt, 2011). Loving-kindness meditation and compassion-focused methods (Gilbert, 2014; Hofmann, Grossman, & Hinton, 2011) also have promising support. Each of these programs includes a variety of exercises and practices to cultivate mindfulness skills. Some involve formal meditation, while others encourage mindful awareness of routine daily activities.

## *Meditative Practices*

Sitting meditation is a commonly used practice with strong roots in meditation traditions. In a posture that is comfortable and relaxed, yet awake and alert, participants direct their attention to a series of internal or external foci, often beginning with the sensations and movements of breathing. Without trying to control the breath, they simply observe as it enters and leaves the body at its own pace and rhythm. Before long, attention is likely to wander. When this happens, participants are encouraged to recognize that the mind has wandered, note briefly where it went (e.g., planning, remembering, daydreaming), and gently return their attention to breathing while letting go of judgments and criticisms about the wandering mind. As the practice continues, the focus of attention typically shifts sequentially to other present-moment experiences, including bodily sensations, sounds, thoughts, and emotions. These experiences are observed with gentle interest, acceptance, and compassion as they come and go, whether they are pleasant, unpleasant, or neutral. Brief, silent labeling of observed experience is sometimes encouraged. For example, participants might say "aching," "self-critical thoughts are here," or "a feeling of anger is arising" as they notice these phenomena.

The body scan is another widely used meditative practice. Participants sit or lie comfortably with their eyes closed and focus their attention sequentially on many parts of the body, noticing sensations with friendly interest. When their minds wander, which is described as inevitable, they notice this and gently return attention to the body while letting go of judgment and self-criticism. If pain arises, they observe its qualities as best they can. Urges to move are observed nonjudgmentally. If participants choose to act on an urge, they are invited to notice with friendly curiosity the intention to act, the actions themselves, and any aftereffects or consequences. The body scan cultivates several essential mindfulness skills, including directing attention in particular ways; noticing when it has wandered; returning it kindly to the present moment; and being nonjudgmental, curious, and accepting about observed experience, whether it is pleasant or unpleasant.

## Movement-Based Practices

Several MBIs use gentle yoga and mindful walking to cultivate mindful awareness while moving or stretching the body. Participants are invited to observe their bodily sensations with compassionate awareness, to notice when their minds wander, and to gently return their attention to sensations. The goal is not to strengthen muscles, improve flexibility or balance, or increase physical fitness, although such changes may occur with consistent practice. The only goal is to practice mindful awareness and acceptance of the body and mind as they are in the moment.

## Mindfulness of Routine Activities

Many MBIs invite participants to bring moment-to-moment, nonjudgmental awareness to daily activities, such as eating, driving, or washing dishes. As with the other practices, participants gently return attention to the activity when the mind wanders away and bring an attitude of acceptance, allowing, openness, curiosity, kindness, and friendliness to all observed experiences, even those that are unwanted or unpleasant. Mindfulness of breathing in daily life is another way to encourage ongoing present-moment awareness. The breath is a useful target of mindful observation because it creates continuous observable sensations and movements. Breathing does not require voluntary control and therefore provides individuals an opportunity to allow the observed experience to be as it is, without trying to change it. Moreover, qualities of breathing (pace, depth, rhythm) shift with emotional and bodily states. By observing these patterns, people can become more aware of the constant fluctuations of emotion and sensation they experience in daily life.

With children or developmentally delayed or cognitively impaired populations, other attentional anchors, such as the soles of the feet, are sometimes used (Singh, Wahler, Adkins, & Myers, 2003). This target can help participants learn to regulate disruptive behavior because they can pay attention to their feet on the playground or during social interactions.

## Breathing Spaces

The breathing space, which originated in MBCT, is a three-step practice designed to encourage participants to apply mindfulness skills in daily life, especially in stressful situations. First, they bring attention to the inner landscape of thoughts, emotions, and sensations; they gently note these experiences and allow them to be as they are, as if they were weather patterns in the mind and body. Then they narrow attention to focus only on breathing, and then widen it again to include the whole body. The breathing space is taught as a three-minute exercise but can be practiced more quickly or slowly depending on situational demands. It is not an escape or distraction strategy but rather an opportunity to step out of automatic patterns, see more clearly what the present moment holds, and make wise choices about what to do next.

## Other Mindfulness Exercises

Several interventions have developed other creative exercises designed to cultivate mindfulness skills. In DBT, for example, each person in a group might be given an object, such as a lemon or a pencil. After a few moments of closely observing its shape, size, color, texture, and markings, all objects are returned to the group leader, who then shuffles them, sets them in the middle of a table, and asks participants to see if they can find the one they just examined. Participants might also be invited to sing a song or play a game mindfully. A short and somewhat more meditative practice is the conveyor belt exercise from DBT. With eyes closed, participants are invited to imagine that the mind is like a conveyor belt that brings thoughts, emotions, and sensations into awareness. Each is observed nonjudgmentally as it appears, including negative thoughts (*This is a waste of time.*) and mind wandering. ACT includes a similar exercise known as cubby-holing. Participants briefly consider a list of categories, such as sensation, thought, memory, emotion, and urge; then they close their eyes for a few minutes and observe the experiences that arise, noting with a single word the category that each represents.

## Loving-Kindness and Compassion Meditation

Loving-kindness meditation and compassion meditation are closely related to mindfulness and sometimes are included in MBIs. Typically, participants practice them while sitting still, often with the eyes closed. Participants extend goodwill toward themselves and a sequence of others by silently repeating short phrases, such as "May he [I, she, they] be safe," "May he be healthy," "May he be happy," "May he be peaceful." A recent review (Hofmann et al., 2011) concludes that such practices, though less extensively studied than mindfulness practices, may be useful in the treatment of a wide range of problems and disorders.

# Empirical Support

In mental health contexts, mindfulness is not practiced purely for its own sake but because mindfulness skills appear to have beneficial effects on psychological symptoms and well-being. Indeed, systematic reviews of mediation studies (Gu, Strauss, Bond, & Cavanagh, 2015; Van der Velden et al., 2015) report that there is consistent evidence that MBSR and MBCT lead to significant increases in self-reported mindfulness skills and that the acquisition of these skills is strongly associated with improvements in mental health. The specific psychological processes through which mindfulness skills exert these benefits are less clear. Several theoretical models and summaries of relevant literature propose lists of potential mechanisms (Brown, Ryan, & Creswell, 2007; Hölzel et al., 2011; Shapiro, Carlson, Astin, & Freedman, 2006; Vago & Silbersweig, 2012). These include forms of awareness (body awareness or general self-awareness), forms of self-regulation (attention regulation, emotion regulation), and perspectives on the self and internal experience (meta-awareness, decentering, reperceiving). The remainder of this chapter discusses mechanisms with empirical support from mediation analyses in outcome studies of MBIs (see Ciarrochi, Bilich, & Godsell, 2010; Gu et al., 2015; and Van der Velden et al., 2015, for reviews). The mechanisms with the best support include changes in cognitive and emotional reactivity, repetitive negative thought (rumination and worry), self-compassion, decentering (also known as metacognitive awareness or meta-awareness), and psychological flexibility. A few studies have also examined the role of positive affect. These processes have been defined and operationalized within a variety of theoretical and empirical contexts, and several of them appear to overlap conceptually and functionally. They are summarized in the following sections.

## Cognitive Reactivity

As originally defined, *cognitive reactivity* is the extent to which a mild dysphoric state activates dysfunctional thinking patterns (Sher, Ingram, & Segal, 2005). It is typically studied with a laboratory task, in which the experimenter induces a temporary dysphoric state by asking participants to dwell on a sad experience while listening to gloomy music, or similar procedures. Participants complete a measure of dysfunctional attitudes (e.g., happiness requires success in all endeavors, asking for help is a sign of weakness, personal worth depends on others' opinions) before and after the mood induction. Cognitive reactivity is shown by increases in dysfunctional attitudes immediately following the induction. People with a history of depressive episodes show higher cognitive reactivity to the induced mood, even if they are in remission when tested. Higher scores for cognitive reactivity are also associated with greater susceptibility to future depressive episodes (Segal et al., 2013).

Cognitive reactivity can also be assessed with the Leiden Index of Depression Sensitivity–Revised (LEIDS-R; Van der Does, 2002), a questionnaire that defines the construct more broadly as the tendency to show several maladaptive reactions to low mood, including rumination, avoidance of difficulties (neglecting tasks), aggressive behavior (sarcasm, temper outbursts), and perfectionism. LEIDS-R scores are consistently higher in previously depressed adults than in those who have never been depressed; scores also predict the amount of change in dysfunctional thinking following a negative mood induction. A recent study of a community sample found that MBCT led to significant decreases in reactivity, as assessed by the LEIDS-R, and that this effect was mediated by the extent to which participants had learned mindfulness skills during the intervention (Raes, Dewulf, van Heeringen, & Williams, 2009).

## Emotional Reactivity

Several studies have shown relationships between mindfulness and reduced emotional reactivity to stress, specifically in recovery time following a negative mood induction or other unpleasant experience (see Britton, Shahar, Szepsenwol, & Jacobs, 2012, for a summary). In a randomized trial comparing MBCT to a wait-list control in adults with partially remitted depression, Britton and colleagues (2012) studied emotional reactivity with the Trier Social Stress Test (Kirschbaum, Pirke, & Hellhammer, 1993), administered before and after treatment. In the presence of a camera and judges, this test requires participants to make a five-minute speech and then to perform a difficult mental arithmetic task aloud. Emotional reactivity was measured with self-ratings of distress pretask, during the task, immediately following the task, and at forty and ninety minutes posttask.

Following the eight-week course, MBCT participants' distress before and during the task were unchanged from before treatment. However, significant reductions in emotional reactivity were seen at the posttask, forty-minute, and ninety-minute assessment points, suggesting that after mindfulness training the task continued to elicit distress, but that participants recovered from it more quickly. Wait-list participants showed no change over the eight-week period, except that their pretask scores increased, suggesting that anticipatory anxiety was worse for their second experience with the task.

Although the study did not examine what treatment participants were doing during the posttask phase, MBCT teaches friendly acceptance of sensations and emotions while decentering from the content of thoughts and disengaging from ruminative thought patterns. It therefore seems plausible that after mindfulness training, participants were better able to refrain from several forms of reactivity to the stress associated with the task.

## Repetitive Negative Thought

Several studies have examined the role rumination and worry may play in accounting for the therapeutic effects of MBIs on psychological symptoms, such as depression, anxiety, and stress. In their systematic review, Gu and colleagues (2015) found consistent evidence that reductions in repetitive negative thinking significantly mediate the effects of mindfulness-based treatment on outcomes. Van der Velden and colleagues (2015) report that evidence for rumination and worry as mediators of change in MBCT for depression is mixed. However, they note that while the frequency of rumination may not always decrease following treatment, the relationship between rumination and later relapse may change if participants develop skills for decentering from the content of negative thoughts.

## Self-Compassion

According to Neff (2003), *self-compassion* has three components: self-kindness in the face of suffering, seeing one's difficulties as part of a larger human experience, and "holding one's painful thoughts and feelings in balanced awareness rather than over-identifying with them" (p. 223). Gu and colleagues (2015) found three studies of self-compassion as a mediator of the effects of MBIs, and results were conflicting. Two of the studies used nonclinical samples and found that MBSR led to significant increases in self-compassion, but that these increases did not mediate effects on anger expression or anxiety. However, the strongest of the three studies (Kuyken et al., 2010) compared MBCT with antidepressant medication for clients with recurrent depression and found that increases in self-compassion over the eight-week course of MBCT mediated reductions in the likelihood of a depressive episode over the next fifteen months.

Kuyken and colleagues (2010) also included in the study the cognitive reactivity task described earlier, finding that cognitive reactivity was unexpectedly higher in the MBCT group than the medication group at the end of the eight-week treatment. However, in the medication group, cognitive reactivity post-treatment predicted the likelihood of relapse over the following fifteen months, whereas in the MBCT group reactivity post-treatment was unrelated to later relapse. Self-compassion moderated this pattern, such that the toxic relationship between cognitive reactivity post-treatment and depressive relapse over the next fifteen months was absent for those who showed greater improvements in self-compassion. This finding suggests that a kind and nonjudgmental response to dysfunctional thoughts, when they arise, may weaken the link between such thoughts and the later onset of depressive episodes.

## Decentering

Decentering is also known as meta-awareness or metacognitive awareness and is similar to defusion as defined in the ACT literature. Hölzel and colleagues (2011) describe a similar construct as a change in perspective in which the contents of consciousness are recognized as constantly fluctuating and transient experiences. *Decentering* is the term used in the MBCT literature, in which it refers to a perspective from which thoughts and feelings are recognized as temporary phenomena rather than as true or important reflections of reality or as essential aspects of oneself. A decentered perspective allows people to take their thoughts and feelings less literally and to be less driven by them. Decentering has been shown to mediate the effects of MBCT for depression (Van der Velden et al., 2015) and MBSR for generalized anxiety disorder (Hoge et al., 2015).

## Psychological Flexibility

Psychological flexibility is the central theoretical construct in ACT and includes six components. Four of these, as noted earlier, are conceptualized as elements of mindfulness (contact with the present moment, acceptance, defusion, and self-as-context). The other two components (values and committed action) are behavior change processes. *Psychological flexibility*, therefore, is the ability to be mindfully aware of the present moment and to behave in values-consistent ways, even when difficult thoughts and feelings are present. ACT includes many exercises and practices designed to cultivate the components of mindfulness, as well as strategies for helping participants to identify their values and engage in values-consistent behavior. A large body of literature shows that increases in psychological flexibility mediate the beneficial effects of ACT in a wide range of adult samples, including people with anxiety and mood disorders, chronic pain, self-harming behavior, and health-related goals such as smoking cessation and weight management (Ciarrochi et al., 2010).

## Positive Affect

A few studies suggest that mindfulness training increases daily experiences of positive affect, and that this may be an important mediator of the effect of MBCT on depressive symptoms and risk of relapse (Geschwind, Peeters, Drukker, van Os, & Wichers, 2011; Batink, Peeters, Geschwind, van Os, & Wichers, 2013). Although the processes through which this occurs are not well studied, a newly articulated mindfulness-to-meaning theory (Garland, Farb, Goldin, & Fredrickson, 2015) suggests that mindfulness leads to decentering from thoughts and emotions, which facilitates the reappraisal of adversity and the savoring of positive experiences, which in turn increases purposeful engagement with life. Additional study of this promising theory is needed.

## Summary of Mindfulness Processes

As noted earlier, the literature on the mechanisms of mindfulness includes a variety of conceptual and theoretical perspectives, each with its own terms and constructs that are used in somewhat overlapping ways. In general, the literature suggests that the practice of mindfulness teaches participants to adopt a new perspective on, or relationship to, their own internal experiences (sensations, cognitions, emotions, urges). This perspective includes decentering or defusion; acceptance or allowing; friendly curiosity, kindness and compassion; and the understanding that thoughts and feelings are not facts, don't have to control behavior, and don't define the person who is having them. Adopting this perspective appears to reduce unhelpful reactions to stressful events and the uncomfortable thoughts and feelings associated with them. For example, mindful awareness of difficult experiences may prevent the onset of dysfunctional attitudes and rumination; alternatively, if these cognitive patterns arise, the person may be able to decenter or defuse from them more readily, with an attitude of kindness and compassion. This may facilitate quicker recovery from stress and pain, increased positive affect and savoring, clearer recognition of values and goals, and increases in values-consistent behavior. Figure 1 summarizes the current literature's conclusions about how mindfulness may influence mental health.

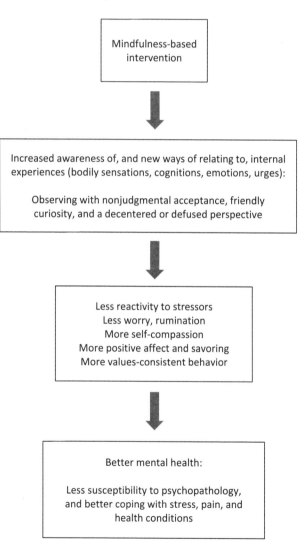

FIGURE 1. A model summarizing the current empirical literature's conclusions about the mechanisms of mindfulness training.

# Conclusions

For many years, cognitive and behavioral therapies focused primarily on methods of change. A large body of literature supports the efficacy of strategies for changing behavior, cognitions, emotions, and aspects of the environment. Until recently, fewer strategies have been available for managing painful realities that can't readily be changed, or difficult thoughts and feelings that paradoxically intensify when attempts are made to change them. The introduction of mindfulness to the cognitive and behavioral therapies provides a set of principles and practices that help people develop the skills to manage such experiences. For this reason, mindfulness training is often described as an acceptance-based approach, but it does not promote passivity or helplessness. It cultivates the ability to see what is happening in the present moment and to make wise choices about how to respond.

Mindful awareness, therefore, may provide a foundation for the effective use of the skills and methods discussed in this volume. Mindfulness training seems to help clients recognize and acknowledge their internal experiences (thoughts, emotions, sensations, urges) and choose constructive ways to respond to them. In some circumstances, helpful responses might include change-based strategies, such as arousal reduction, cognitive restructuring, behavioral activation, problem solving, or interpersonal skills use. In other circumstances, defusion and acceptance skills may be more helpful. Responses that are self-compassionate and consistent with personal values and goals are likely to promote flourishing and well-being. Mindfulness, therefore, may be critical to a broad perspective on how to alleviate problems and help people thrive.

# References

Batink, T., Peeters, F., Geschwind, N., van Os, J., & Wichers, M. (2013). How does MBCT for depression work? Studying cognitive and affective mediation pathways. *PLoS One, 23*(8), e72778.

Bishop, S., Lau, M., Shapiro, S., Carlson, L., Anderson, N. D., Carmody, J., et al. (2004). Mindfulness: A proposed operational definition. *Clinical Psychology: Science and Practice, 11*(3), 230–241.

Bowen, S., Chawla, N., & Marlatt, G. A. (2011). *Mindfulness-based relapse prevention for addictive behaviors: A clinician's guide.* New York: Guilford Press.

Britton, W. B., Shahar, B., Szepsenwol, O., & Jacobs, W. J. (2012). Mindfulness-based cognitive therapy improves emotional reactivity to social stress: Results from a randomized controlled trial. *Behavior Therapy, 43*(2), 365–380.

Brown, K. W., Ryan, R. M., & Creswell, J. D. (2007). Mindfulness: Theoretical foundations and evidence for its salutary effects. *Psychological Inquiry, 18*(4), 211–237.

Ciarrochi, J., Bilich, L., & Godsell, C. (2010). Psychological flexibility as a mechanism of change in acceptance and commitment therapy. In R. A. Baer (Ed.), *Assessing mindfulness and acceptance processes in clients: Illuminating the theory and practice of change* (pp. 51–76). Oakland, CA: New Harbinger Publications.

Dreyfus, G. (2011). Is mindfulness present-centred and nonjudgmental? A discussion of the cognitive dimensions of mindfulness. *Contemporary Buddhism, 12*(1), 41–54.

Fletcher, L., & Hayes, S. C. (2005). Relational frame theory, acceptance and commitment therapy, and a functional analytic definition of mindfulness. *Journal of Rational-Emotive and Cognitive-Behavioral Therapy, 23*(4), 315–336.

Garland, E. L., Farb, N. A., Goldin, P. R., & Fredrickson, B. L. (2015). Mindfulness broadens awareness and builds eudaimonic meaning: A process model of mindful positive emotion regulation. *Psychological Inquiry, 26*(4), 293–314.

Germer, C. K., Siegel, R. D., & Fulton, P. R. (Eds.). (2005). *Mindfulness and psychotherapy.* New York: Guilford Press.

Geschwind, N., Peeters, F., Drukker, M., van Os, J., & Wichers, M. (2011). Mindfulness training increases momentary positive emotions and reward experience in adults vulnerable to depression: A randomized controlled trial. *Journal of Consulting and Clinical Psychology, 79*(5), 618–628.

Gilbert, P. (2014). The origins and nature of compassion focused therapy. *British Journal of Clinical Psychology, 53*(1), 6–41.

Gu, J., Strauss, C., Bond, R., & Cavanagh, K. (2015). How do mindfulness-based cognitive therapy and mindfulness-based stress reduction improve mental health and wellbeing? A systematic review and meta-analysis of mediation studies. *Clinical Psychology Review, 37,* 1–12.

Hayes, S. C., Strosahl, K. D., & Wilson, K. G. (2012). *Acceptance and commitment therapy: The process and practice of mindful change* (2nd ed.). New York: Guilford Press.

Hofmann, S. G., Grossman, P., & Hinton, D. E. (2011). Loving-kindness and compassion meditation: Potential for psychological interventions. *Clinical Psychology Review, 31*(7), 1126–1132.

Hoge, E. A., Bui, E., Goetter, E., Robinaugh, D. J., Ojserkis, R., Fresco, D. M., et al. (2015). Change in decentering mediates improvement in anxiety in mindfulness-based stress reduction for generalized anxiety disorder. *Cognitive Therapy and Research, 39*(2), 228–235.

Hölzel, B. K., Lazar, S. W., Gard, T., Schuman-Olivier, Z., Vago, D. R., & Ott, U. (2011). How does mindfulness meditation work? Proposing mechanisms of action from a conceptual and neural perspective. *Perspectives on Psychological Science, 6*(6), 537–559.

Kabat-Zinn, J. (1982). An outpatient program in behavioral medicine for chronic pain patients based on the practice of mindfulness meditation: Theoretical considerations and preliminary results. *General Hospital Psychiatry, 4*(1), 33–47.

Kabat-Zinn, J. (1994). *Wherever you go, there you are: Mindfulness meditation in everyday life.* New York: Hyperion.

Kabat-Zinn, J. (2003). Mindfulness-based interventions in context: Past, present and future. *Clinical Psychology: Science and Practice, 10*(2), 144–156.

Khoury, B., Lecomte, T., Fortin, G., Masse, M., Therien, P., Bouchard, V., et al. (2013). Mindfulness-based therapy: A comprehensive meta-analysis. *Clinical Psychology Review, 33*(6), 763–771.

Kirschbaum, C., Pirke, K. M., & Hellhammer, D. H. (1993). The "Trier Social Stress Test": A tool for investigating psychobiological stress response in a laboratory setting. *Neuropsychobiology, 28*(1–2), 76–81.

Kuyken, W., Watkins, E., Holden, E., White, K., Taylor, R. S., Byford, S., et al. (2010). How does mindfulness-based cognitive therapy work? *Behaviour Research and Therapy, 48*(11), 1105–1112.

Linehan, M. M. (1993). *Cognitive-behavioral treatment of borderline personality disorder.* New York: Guilford Press.

Linehan, M. M. (2015). *DBT skills training manual* (2nd ed.). New York: Guilford Press.

Marlatt, G. A., & Kristeller, J. L. (1999). Mindfulness and meditation. In W. R. Miller (Ed.), *Integrating spirituality into treatment: Resources for practitioners* (pp. 67–84). Washington, DC: American Psychological Association.

Neff, K., (2003). The development and validation of a scale to measure self-compassion. *Self and Identity, 2,* 223–250.

Raes, F., Dewulf, D., van Heeringen, C., & Williams, J. M. G. (2009). Mindfulness and reduced cognitive reactivity to sad mood: Evidence from a correlational study and a non-randomized waiting list controlled study. *Behaviour Research and Therapy, 47*(7), 623–627.

Roemer, L., Orsillo, S. M., & Salters-Pednault, K. (2008). Efficacy of an acceptance-based behavior therapy for generalized anxiety disorder: Evaluation in a randomized controlled trial. *Journal of Consulting and Clinical Psychology, 76*(6), 1083–1089.

Segal, Z. V., Williams, J. M. G., & Teasdale, J. D. (2013). *Mindfulness-based cognitive therapy for depression* (2nd ed.). New York: Guilford Press.

Shapiro, S. L., Carlson, L. E., Astin, J. A., & Freedman, B. (2006). Mechanisms of mindfulness. *Journal of Clinical Psychology, 62*(3), 373–386.

Sher, C. D., Ingram, R. E., & Segal, Z. V. (2005). Cognitive reactivity and vulnerability: Empirical evaluation of construct activation and cognitive diatheses in unipolar depression. *Clinical Psychology Review, 25*(4), 487–510.

Singh, N. N., Wahler, R. G., Adkins, A. D., & Myers, R. E. (2003). Soles of the feet: A mindfulness-based self-control intervention for aggression by an individual with mild mental retardation and mental illness. *Research in Developmental Disabilities, 24*(3), 158–169.

Vago, D. R., & Silbersweig, D. A. (2012). Self-awareness, self-regulation, and self-transcendence (S-ART): A framework for understanding the neurobiological mechanisms of mindfulness. *Frontiers in Human Neuroscience, 6*(Article 296), 1–30.

Van der Does, A. (2002). Cognitive reactivity to sad mood: Structure and validity of a new measure. *Behaviour Research and Therapy, 40*(1), 105–120.

Van der Velden, A. M., Kuyken, W., Wattar, U., Crane, C., Pallesen, K. J., Dahlgaard, J., et al. (2015). A systematic review of mechanisms of change in mindfulness-based cognitive therapy in the treatment of recurrent major depressive disorder. *Clinical Psychology Review, 37,* 26–39.

402

# CHAPTER 27

# Enhancing Motivation

## James MacKillop, PhD

*Peter Boris Centre for Addictions Research, Department
of Psychiatry and Behavioural Neurosciences,
McMaster University; Homewood Research Institute,
Homewood Health Centre*

## Lauren VanderBroek-Stice, MS

*Department of Psychology, University of Georgia*

## Catharine Munn, MD, MSc

*Peter Boris Centre for Addictions Research, Department of
Psychiatry and Behavioural Neurosciences, McMaster
University; Student Wellness Centre, McMaster University*

## Background

An ostensible truism for a person seeking psychological treatment is that he or she wants to get better. In turn, a corollary of this assumption is that when a mental health professional provides a way to understand the problem, and, particularly in behavioral and cognitive therapies, lays out a plan of action for addressing it, the client will vigorously embrace those steps needed to alleviate the existing distress. The reality, however, is that the course of psychological treatment is often far less simple and linear. Clients avoid prescribed intersession activities, do not complete

This work was partially supported by a grant from the Ontario Ministry of Training, Colleges, and Universities Mental Health Innovation Fund (James MacKillop and Catharine Munn). Dr. MacKillop is the holder of the Peter Boris Chair in Addictions Research, which partially supported his role.

homework, miss sessions, or voluntarily lapse into the distressing behaviors that were the impetus for treatment.

One reason for suboptimal outcomes is that, fundamentally, behavior change is not easy. This is in part because seemingly dysfunctional behaviors are serving a function, typically keeping an experience that is even more undesirable than the manifest symptoms at bay. In other words, maladaptive behaviors often serve as transient, short-term solutions to problems that are ultimately exacerbated in a vicious cycle. Thus, an unhealthy behavioral homeostasis is achieved, and these functional/dysfunctional behaviors gain a persistent momentum that is challenging to change. This is compounded by the fact that clients may not commit to treatment out of ambivalence about addressing the presenting problem. Importantly, it is not ambivalence in the sense that they are indifferent to the outcome. Clients are ambivalent in the literal sense of being pulled in two directions: by a desire for change and by the inertia of existing behavioral patterns. The earliest forms of psychological treatment, starting with Freud, recognized the "neurotic paradox" that such ambivalence creates. Behavior therapists likewise recognized it as a challenge to the rational assumptions of learned behavior (Mowrer, 1948). Fundamentally, it is the question of why, if a maladaptive behavior leads to distress and the desire for change, does actual behavior change not naturally follow.

In the contemporary context, this inability to change can be understood as a problem of motivation. At a superficial level, client motivation is often assumed to be self-evident from the fact that treatment is being sought. Therapists inaccurately assume it to be a stable, unwavering trait. Instead, motivation for change is increasingly understood as a dynamic and fluctuating process, with a waxing and waning periodicity. Actively considering and cultivating motivation for change in psychological treatment is the focus of this chapter, which draws on the extensive body of work on motivational interviewing (MI; Miller & Rollnick, 2002, 2013), a therapeutic method for facilitating a client's intrinsic motivation to change behavior. Regardless of treatment modality or form of psychopathology, motivation is a sine qua non of successful behavior change, and MI has been found to be a powerful intervention, both on its own and as a platform for other psychological interventions.

MI was originally developed in the treatment of addiction, for which ambivalence is arguably a hallmark of the disorder, but its reach far exceeds addictive disorders. This chapter will introduce some of the language and concepts of MI, but it should not be considered the equivalent of formal training. As Miller and Rollnick (2009) wisely and concisely noted, "MI is simple, but not easy" (p. 135), and there is evidence that learning MI requires more than superficial training

(Barwick, Bennett, Johnson, McGowan, & Moore, 2012; Madson, Loignon, & Lane, 2009; Miller, Yahne, Moyers, Martinez, & Pirritano, 2004).

Motivational interviewing has its roots in William Miller's research on alcohol-use disorders in the early 1980s, when it was found that clinician empathy was more predictive of treatment outcome than the active effects of behavioral treatment (Miller, Taylor, & West, 1980). This serendipitous finding led to subsequent explorations of how interpersonal processes and clinician style promote behavior change, and an initial description of motivational interviewing as an approach emphasizing empathetic, person-centered therapy that focuses on evoking and strengthening the client's own arguments for change (Miller, 1983). Included in this approach was a deeper theoretical grounding that emphasized two major elements. The first was Rogers's (1959) humanistic emphasis on the value of a positive and empathetic environment, in which clients can express feelings and explore issues without fear of judgment. The second included both Festinger's (1957) idea that cognitive dissonance occurs when individuals perform an action that conflicts with a core belief or value and leads to motivation to restore consistency of actions and beliefs; and Bem's (1967) self-perception theory that proposed people become more attached to attitudes that they verbalize and hear themselves defend. Reflecting these ideas, MI cultivates a strong client-clinician relationship characterized by high levels of empathy, and it draws attention to discrepancies between clients' current circumstances and their values using a Socratic style that elicits the discrepancy from the clients in their own words (evoking, not telling). More concretely, MI combines an empathic therapeutic style with intentional selective reinforcement of client language that favors change (Miller & Rose, 2009).

This perspective differed dramatically from the dominant models of addiction treatment at the time. In the 1980s, the prevailing view of individuals with substance-use disorders was that many were in "denial" of their problems, an attribution that unfortunately persists and for which there is little evidence (Chiauzzi & Liljegren, 1993; MacKillop & Gray, 2014). Clinicians commonly sought to persuade clients to change and to argue against their resistance, often inadvertently provoking clients to defend the status quo. The MI perspective was qualitatively different, assuming instead that many afflicted individuals were aware of the need for change and possessed some degree of internal motivation to do so, an assumption that is robustly supported by client reports on motivation for change.

It helped that MI emerged contemporaneously to the transtheoretical model of change (Prochaska & Di Clemente, 1982), although MI is distinct. The transtheoretical framework emphasizes motivation for change as a continuum and the importance of meeting clients at their own motivational level across the stages of precontemplation, contemplation, preparation, action, and maintenance (and potentially relapse, returning a person to an earlier stage). MI is highly compatible with this perspective, to the extent that it is suited for working with clients who are less motivated and can be understood as a strategy for moving them forward in terms of stages of change (Miller & Rollnick, 2013).

# Processes and Principles

MI is less a therapeutic technique than a method of interacting with clients. To capture the "MI spirit" (Miller & Rollnick, 2013), there are four core principles. The client-clinician relationship is seen as a *partnership*, an active collaboration between experts: the clinician, who possesses professional expertise, and the client, who is an expert on himself. The MI spirit emphasizes *acceptance*, defined as actively trying to respect the client's autonomy, understand the client's perspective, and recognize the client's strengths and efforts (see chapter 24). Importantly, acceptance does not imply that the clinician must agree with or endorse the client's beliefs and actions. Another principle is *compassion*, which involves a genuine effort to prioritize the client's needs, goals, and values, albeit with an orientation toward behavior change and healthy outcomes. Finally, the principle of *evocation* refers to the assumption that the client already possesses all of the qualities and wisdom needed to change, and that the clinician serves as a guide who can help the client call forth her own motivation and strengths in order to achieve goals.

Several interactional elements are critical in client-clinician communication, denoted by the acronym OARS (Miller & Rollnick, 2013), which refers to asking "open" questions, "affirming," using "reflective" listening, and "summarizing." An interactional style characterized by the four elements of OARS is the foundation upon which the clinician develops discrepancies between the client's current situation and his or her priorities and values. Understanding what people value and how their current behaviors are in conflict with those values is key to resolving the conflict and moving the client in the direction of change (see chapter 25). This can take place via open-ended questions (e.g., "What do you hope your life will look like in one year? What about in ten years?"), or via specific techniques discussed below.

In addition to considering what one says as a clinician, it is also critical to be aware of what one hears from a client. MI is somewhat unique because the client's speech provides immediate feedback that can inform the clinician's approach to an issue. *Change talk* is any client language that suggests the client is considering the possibility of positively changing a particular behavior. In contrast, *sustain talk* is any language that favors the status quo.

Increasing change talk is a key process that fosters MI effects (Amrhein, Miller, Yahne, Palmer, & Fulcher, 2003; Moyers et al., 2007). Apodaca and Longabaugh (2009) investigated MI change mechanisms for substance-use treatment and found that both in-session client utterances in favor of change and experiences of a behavior-value discrepancy were related to better outcomes, whereas MI-inconsistent behaviors (e.g., confronting, directing, warning) on the part of the clinician were associated with poorer outcomes.

It appears that change talk requires a certain level of cognitive facility in order to be effective. A recent study of MI for cocaine use (Carpenter et al., 2016) found a relationship between in-session client change talk and positive clinical outcomes, but only among participants who—in an experimental "relational frame" task (see chapter 7)—could learn to derive symbolic relations between cocaine-related stimuli, nonsense words, and the consequences of cocaine use.

Some clients believe that change is important but lack confidence in their ability to change. Additionally, a client's confidence may decrease following apparent setbacks and roadblocks along the way. Therefore, a secondary goal of MI is to support client self-efficacy throughout the change process. The process for evoking client *confidence talk*, or ability language, is similar to evoking change talk more broadly. The clinician listens for and reflects statements that include words like "can," "possible," and "able." The clinician also asks open questions to elicit information about a past instance when the client successfully made positive life changes, ideas the client has for how to go about making changes, and obstacles the client might encounter and how they could be dealt with.

Learning to recognize these different forms of talk in session is aptly described as "detecting a signal within noise. It is not necessary to eliminate…the noise, just follow the signal" (Miller & Rollnick, 2013, p. 178). Clinicians need to notice language that expresses a desire or intention to change, optimism about the client's ability to change, reasons for or benefits of change, and the need to change or problems with continuing the way things are (Rosengren, 2009). Sustain talk may appear in the form of defending a position or behavior, interrupting the clinician, or disengaging from the conversation (e.g., ignoring the clinician or appearing distracted). An increase in sustain talk should signal to the clinician the need to "roll with resistance" by slowing down, reevaluating the conversation, or including the client in the problem-solving process (Miller & Rollnick, 2013). It may be appropriate for the clinician to apologize for misunderstanding the client, to affirm the client's point of view in order to diminish defensiveness, or to shift the conversation away from the touchy topic rather than intensifying it. Being aware of these verbal patterns is important because clinician style affects the ratio of change talk to sustain talk (e.g., Glynn & Moyers, 2010), especially in substance-use populations. (e.g., Apodaca, Magill, Longabaugh, Jackson, & Monti, 2013;

Vader, Walters, Prabhu, Houck, & Field, 2010). Beyond client treatment engagement, as measured by attendance and treatment completion, it is still unclear which specific processes contribute to positive MI outcomes in other areas of clinical work, such as mood and anxiety disorders, psychosis, and comorbid conditions (Romano & Peters, 2015).

If MI is working as anticipated, the conversation will shift from whether the client wants to change to how change can be accomplished, sometimes referred to as the choice point or decision point. To know if the time is right, the clinician should look for increased change talk (and decreased sustain talk), stronger commitment language, greater apparent personal resolve, questions about change, or signs that the client has taken concrete steps to experiment with change. When the client appears sufficiently ready, the clinician should test the water by directly asking him if he's ready to start planning for change, either by summarizing his motivations for change or by posing a key question (e.g., "So, what do you think you'll do?" or "Where do you want to go from here?").

# Empirical Support

With regard to efficacy, early studies sought to determine the factors that influence client motivation for initiating formal, extended alcohol treatment (Miller, Benefield, & Tonigan, 1993; Miller, Sovereign, & Krege, 1988). These studies involved a single-session intervention that combined MI with feedback from a personal assessment of the individual's drinking relative to norms and recommendations (i.e., "Drinker's Check-up"; Miller et al., 1988). While the results did not show that the MI intervention provoked high rates of engagement in subsequent formal treatment, participants exhibited a significant, self-directed reduction in drinking at follow-up in general. A review of similar studies found that the effectiveness of brief MI interventions was comparable with more intensive treatments for reducing problematic drinking (Bien, Miller, & Tonigan, 1993). Given these promising findings, research on MI was expanded to evaluate its independent usefulness in different capacities and with various populations and conditions.

Since these initial findings, literally hundreds of studies have evaluated the efficacy of MI. The evidence is strongest for substance-use disorders, including the use of alcohol, marijuana, tobacco, and other drugs (Heckman, Egleston, & Hofmann, 2010; Hettema, Steele, & Miller, 2005). In a large multisite clinical trial, a four-session MI intervention generated equivalent outcomes to eight sessions of either cognitive behavioral treatment or twelve-step facilitation (Project MATCH Research Group, 1997, 1998). In addition, across an ever-expanding range of problem behaviors, MI has demonstrated significant positive effects on behavioral outcomes, including reducing risky behaviors (e.g., unprotected sex, sharing needles), promoting healthy behaviors (e.g., exercise, better eating habits), and increasing treatment engagement (for a review of four meta-analyses, see Lundahl & Burke, 2009). Across all problem behaviors studied, MI is significantly more effective than standard controls, and it is equally effective as other active treatments, though MI takes less time to implement (Lundahl, Kunz, Brownell, Tollefson, & Burke, 2010).

Regarding treatment format, MI can be implemented as a brief, stand-alone intervention, but the effect of MI is greatest when combined with another active treatment, such as cognitive behavioral therapy (Burke, Arkowitz, & Menchola, 2003). When used in conjunction with another intervention, MI is helpful as a precursor for increasing initial client engagement and as a strategy for maintaining motivation throughout treatment (Arkowitz, Miller, & Rollnick, 2015). MI has demonstrated positive results for clients regardless of their problem's severity, gender, age, and ethnicity, although its supportive, nonconfrontational tone may be selectively more effective for some ethnic groups, such as Native Americans who rely on similar communication patterns (Hettema et al., 2005). MI may also be more effective than cognitive behavioral therapy for clients with alcohol-use disorder who report higher levels of trait-level anger and dependence (Project MATCH Research Group, 1997).

# Tools

With regard to in-session tools, perhaps the most versatile and efficient measures are motivational "rulers" or "ladders" (Boudreaux et al., 2012; Miller & Rollnick, 2013). These are single-item questions that assess readiness to change, importance of change, and/or confidence in the ability to change (on a scale from 0 to 10). They can be administered verbally, on paper, or via computer and serve two main functions. First, these measures quantify the client's motivation in a short and face-valid way. Second, these measures allow the discussion to ramify around the reported number. For example, self-efficacy can be explored by asking what makes the client's rating of confidence 8 out of 10 or why the client's rating of importance is 9 out of 10. Importantly, asking what makes these values as high as they are elicits pro-change statements (e.g., what makes them feel ready or gives them confidence). However, the opposite is also true: asking clients why their ratings are not higher will elicit reasons to not change and thus should be avoided.

Another strategy for implementing MI is to collaboratively complete a decisional balance exercise or change plan. These are relatively short procedures that formalize either the costs and benefits of the problematic behavior or the steps that will be taken following the session. The decisional balance exercise involves collaboratively completing a two-by-two matrix that crosses costs and benefits with the status quo versus making a change. It is a simple and straightforward way for the client and clinician to articulate and formalize the impelling and countervailing motivational forces at hand. However, an embedded risk within this tool is that the fully crossed matrix includes a focus on reasons not to change and costs of changing. Thus, it can have the unintended consequence of evoking sustain talk if used unskillfully.

A change plan is a worksheet the client completes while in discussion with the clinician. Common sections include the changes the individual wants to make, the most important reasons for doing so, the steps that are already being taken, potential impediments, people who can help, and benchmarks for success. A benefit of the change plan is that it provides the clinician with an oblique angle from which to encourage the client to describe objective goals. If the desired change is too nebulous, the goal is undermined because it is unclear whether a person is succeeding or failing, except in gross terms. For example, "It's time to get my drinking under control" is an excellent example of change talk, but it is largely undefined. Conversely, "I really need to not drink at all during the week and no more than four drinks on Friday and Saturday night" reflects both change talk and clear objective goals that can be targeted and achieved.

These two tools can be thought of as bookends to the choice points that naturally emerge in treatment; the decisional balance exercise reflects the critical process of cultivating maximum motivation to change, and the change plan provides a format for identifying objective goals and plans, after the client and clinician have agreed that change is a priority. The clinician often gives these worksheets to the client, and they can serve as powerful reminder stimuli between sessions.

A lengthier strategy is a structured card-sorting exercise regarding values (see chapter 25). For this activity, the client categorizes up to one hundred pregenerated and client-generated values in piles based on how important the listed values are to him. The clinician follows up the activity by asking open-ended questions that lead the client to explore why the selected values are important and how they are expressed (or not expressed) in the client's life. This can then be followed up with questions about how the presenting problem is incongruent with the client's personal values. The activity can take a full session, and it provides a powerful way for a person to operationalize personal values and consider the effects of the presenting problem in direct juxtaposition to those values.

Two additional implementation recommendations may also be useful. First, a microtechnique that can be very powerful is integrating direct invitations to clients over the course of the therapeutic dialogue. For example, this might happen when a clinician transitions from unstructured dialogue to a more structured aspect of the session, such as offering objective feedback about performance on specific assessments (e.g., drinking levels, symptom severity): "Next, I'd like to give you some objective feedback about how your drinking compares with other students here. Would you like to see that?" (or "Are you interested?" or "How does that sound?") These invitations typically elicit an affirmative response (and are highly informative when they do not) and implicitly emphasize client autonomy and agency, communicating to clients that proceeding is their choice. Including direct invitations intermittently is a small way of communicating respect for the client and fostering a collaborative partnership.

Second, an implementation strategy that helps orient the clinician is to consider the function of therapeutic in-session behavior in terms of the MI components: expressing empathy, developing discrepancy, rolling with resistance, and supporting self-efficacy (Miller & Rollnick, 2002). For example, developing a change plan and problem solving specific behavior-change strategies clearly support self-efficacy. Explicitly considering how an activity or dialogue fits into a domain of MI can be especially useful for novice clinicians.

A variety of additional tools and measures are available to support MI work (see http://www.motivationalinterviewing.org), but a comprehensive review is beyond the scope of this chapter. Nonetheless, given the large and rich array of resources, it is recommended that clinicians leverage them as much as possible.

# Conclusions

Motivation to change is a key issue in all forms of clinical intervention. MI is a framework for thinking about how clinicians can help clients help themselves; it is a mind-set that recognizes the fluctuating nature of motivation and its essential importance in behavior change.

# References

Amrhein, P. C., Miller, W. R., Yahne, C. E., Palmer, M., & Fulcher, L. (2003). Client commitment language during motivational interviewing predicts drug use outcomes. *Journal of Consulting and Clinical Psychology, 71*(5), 862–878.

Apodaca, T. R., & Longabaugh, R. (2009). Mechanisms of change in motivational interviewing: A review and preliminary evaluation of the evidence. *Addiction, 104*(5), 705–715.

Apodaca, T. R., Magill, M., Longabaugh, R., Jackson, K. M., & Monti, P. M. (2013). Effect of a significant other on client change talk in motivational interviewing. *Journal of Consulting and Clinical Psychology, 81*(1), 35–46.

Arkowitz, H., Miller, W. R., & Rollnick, S. (Eds.). (2015). *Motivational interviewing in the treatment of psychological problems* (2nd ed.). New York: Guilford Press.

Barwick, M., Bennett, L. M., Johnson, S. N., McGowan, J., & Moore, J. E. (2012). Training health and mental health professionals in motivational interviewing: A systematic review. *Children and Youth Services Review, 34*(9), 1786–1795.

Bem, D. J. (1967). Self-perception: An alternative interpretation of cognitive dissonance phenomena. *Psychological Review, 74*(3), 183–200.

Bien, T. H., Miller, W. R., & Tonigan, J. S. (1993). Brief interventions for alcohol problems: A review. *Addiction, 88*(3), 315–335.

Boudreaux, E. D., Sullivan, A., Abar, B., Bernstein, S. L., Ginde, A. A., & Camargo Jr., C. A. (2012). Motivation rulers for smoking cessation: A prospective observational examination of construct and predictive validity. *Addiction Science and Clinical Practice, 7*(1), 8.

Burke, B. L., Arkowitz, H., & Menchola, M. (2003). The efficacy of motivational interviewing: A meta-analysis of controlled clinical trials. *Journal of Consulting and Clinical Psychology, 71*(5), 843–861.

Carpenter, K. M., Amrhein, P. C., Bold, K. W., Mishlen, K., Levin, F. R., Raby, W. N., et al. (2016). Derived relations moderate the association between changes in the strength of commitment language and cocaine treatment response. *Experimental and Clinical Psychopharmacology, 24*(2), 77–89.

Chiauzzi, E. J., & Liljegren, S. (1993). Taboo topics in addiction treatment: An empirical review of clinical folklore. *Journal of Substance Abuse Treatment, 10*(3), 303–316.

Festinger, L. (1957). *A theory of cognitive dissonance.* Stanford, CA: Stanford University Press.

Glynn, L. H., & Moyers, T. B. (2010). Chasing change talk: The clinician's role in evoking client language about change. *Journal of Substance Abuse Treatment, 39*(1), 65–70.

Heckman, C. J., Egleston, B. L., & Hofmann, M. T. (2010). Efficacy of motivational interviewing for smoking cessation: A systematic review and meta-analysis. *Tobacco Control, 19*(5), 410–416.

Hettema, J., Steele, J., & Miller, W. R. (2005). Motivational interviewing. *Annual Review of Clinical Psychology, 1*, 91–111.

Lundahl, B., & Burke, B. L. (2009). The effectiveness and applicability of motivational interviewing: A practice-friendly review of four meta-analyses. *Journal of Clinical Psychology, 65*(11), 1232–1245.

Lundahl, B. W., Kunz, C., Brownell, C., Tollefson, D., & Burke, B. L. (2010). A meta-analysis of motivational interviewing: Twenty-five years of empirical studies. *Research on Social Work Practice, 20*(2), 137–160.

MacKillop, J., & Gray, J. C. (2014). Controversial treatments for alcohol use disorders. In S. O. Lilienfeld, S. J. Lynn, & J. M. Lohr (Eds.), *Science and pseudoscience in clinical psychology* (2nd ed., pp. 322–363). New York: Guilford Press.

Madson, M. B., Loignon, A. C., & Lane, C. (2009). Training in motivational interviewing: A systematic review. *Journal of Substance Abuse Treatment, 36*(1), 101–109.

Miller, W. R. (1983). Motivational interviewing with problem drinkers. *Behavioural Psychotherapy, 11*(2), 147–172.

Miller, W. R., Benefield, R. G., & Tonigan, J. S. (1993). Enhancing motivation for change in problem drinking: A controlled comparison of two therapist styles. *Journal of Consulting and Clinical Psychology, 61*(3), 455–461.

Miller, W. R., & Rollnick, S. (2002). *Motivational interviewing: Preparing people for change* (2nd ed.). New York: Guilford Press.

Miller, W. R., & Rollnick, S. (2009). Ten things that motivational interviewing is not. *Behavioural and Cognitive Psychotherapy, 37*(2), 129–140.

Miller, W. R., & Rollnick, S. (2013). *Motivational interviewing: Helping people change* (3rd ed.). New York: Guilford Press.

412

Miller, W. R., & Rose, G. S. (2009). Toward a theory of motivational interviewing. *American Psychologist, 64*(6), 527–537.

Miller, W. R., Sovereign, R. G., & Krege, B. (1988). Motivational interviewing with problem drinkers: II. The Drinker's Check-up as a preventive intervention. *Behavioural Psychotherapy, 16*(4), 251–268.

Miller, W. R., Taylor, C. A., & West, J. C. (1980). Focused versus broad-spectrum behavior therapy for problem drinkers. *Journal of Consulting and Clinical Psychology, 48*(5), 590–601.

Miller, W. R., Yahne, C. E., Moyers, T. B., Martinez, J., & Pirritano, M. (2004). A randomized trial of methods to help clinicians learn motivational interviewing. *Journal of Consulting and Clinical Psychology, 72*(6), 1050–1062.

Mowrer, O. H. (1948). Learning theory and the neurotic paradox. *American Journal of Orthopsychiatry, 18*(4), 571–610.

Moyers, T. B., Martin, T., Christopher, P. J., Houck, J. M., Tonigan, J. S., & Amrhein, P. C. (2007). Client language as a mediator of motivational interviewing efficacy: Where is the evidence? *Alcoholism: Clinical and Experimental Research, 31*(s3), 40s–47s.

Prochaska, J. O., & Di Clemente, C. C. (1982). Transtheoretical therapy: Toward a more integrative model of change. *Psychotherapy: Theory, Research, and Practice, 19*(3), 276–288.

Project MATCH Research Group. (1997). Project MATCH secondary a priori hypotheses. *Addiction, 92*(12), 1671–1698.

Project MATCH Research Group. (1998). Matching alcoholism treatments to client heterogeneity: Project MATCH three-year drinking outcomes. *Alcoholism: Clinical and Experimental Research, 22*(6), 1300–1311.

Rogers, C. R. (1959). A theory of therapy, personality, and interpersonal relationships, as developed in the client-centered framework. In S. Koch (Ed.), *Psychology: A study of a science* (Vol. 3, pp. 184–256). New York: McGraw-Hill.

Romano, M., & Peters, L. (2015). Evaluating the mechanisms of change in motivational interviewing in the treatment of mental health problems: A review and meta-analysis. *Clinical Psychology Review, 38*, 1–12.

Rosengren, D. B. (2009). *Building motivational interviewing skills: A practitioner workbook.* New York: Guilford Press.

Vader, A. M., Walters, S. T., Prabhu, G. C., Houck, J. M., & Field, C. A. (2010). The language of motivational interviewing and feedback: Counselor language, client language, and client drinking outcomes. *Psychology of Addictive Behaviors, 24*(2), 190–197.

# CHAPTER 28

# Crisis Management and Treating Suicidality from a Behavioral Perspective

Katherine Anne Comtois, PhD, MPH

*Department of Psychiatry and Behavioral Sciences,
University of Washington*

Sara J. Landes, PhD

*Department of Psychiatry, University of Arkansas for Medical
Sciences, and Central Arkansas Veterans Healthcare System*

## Background

When suicidality arises in therapy, there are two paths to follow: management of suicide risk and treatment of controlling variables to resolve the suicidality. Management includes the steps one takes to minimize the acute risk of suicide and self-harm, including the management of lethal means, development of a safety plan, and generation of hope. Though the management of risk is important, therapists often mistake it for suicide prevention treatment. Treatment is a collaborative and often reasonably long-term process between therapist and client to change the controlling variables for suicide, self-harm, and the factors that make life not worth living, such as pain, isolation, or lack of meaning.

This confusion between the management and treatment of suicidality often arises because therapists see suicide and self-harm only as symptoms of or tangents from the disorder or problem they are treating. They expect that suicidality will resolve as the disorder or problem resolves, and that it does not require treatment per se. ·

A more powerful alternative is to target suicidality directly with both management and treatment. This method may help resolve immediate symptoms/problems, and those that persist after suicidality has been resolved can be targeted without concern that the client might attempt or die by suicide before they are resolved.

The principles and guidelines in this chapter are based on principles and protocols of dialectical behavior therapy (DBT; Linehan, 1993, 2015a, 2015b) and the Linehan Risk Assessment and Management Protocol, or LRAMP, formerly the University of Washington Risk Assessment and Management Protocol, or UWRAMP (Linehan, Comtois, & Ward-Ciesielski, 2012; Linehan Institute, Behavioral Tech, n.d.; Linehan, 2014). This brief chapter is meant to provide general guidance for the behavioral management and treatment of suicidality, but additional formal training in DBT and LRAMP methods is recommended.

# Managing Suicide Risk

Managing suicide risk includes a number of tasks: suicide risk assessment, suicide risk decision making, safety or crisis response planning, and means safety. Each of these are described in detail below.

## Suicide Risk Assessment

Suicide risk management starts with coming to a shared understanding with clients of what led to past suicidal behavior and current suicidal thinking. The target includes their behavior and that of others, as well as the emotions, cognitions, bodily sensations, and urges associated with suicidality. It can be useful to gather data using an assessment, such as the Scale for Suicidal Ideation (Beck, Brown, & Steer, 1997; Beck, Kovacs, & Weissman, 1979) in the interview or questionnaire form. This measure rates key areas, including desire for life and death, history of attempts, fear of death and other barriers to suicide, as well as efforts to prepare for suicide, and it has been shown to predict death by suicide among mental health outpatients (Beck, Brown, Steer, Dahlsgaard, & Grisham, 1999). The assessment can be administered both for current suicidal ideation as well as for ideation at its worst point, the latter being a stronger predictor of subsequent suicide (Beck et al., 1999).

It is critical to gather a history of all suicide attempts and nonsuicidal self-injuries (NSSI). Two measures can be considered. The Suicide Attempt Self-Injury interview (SASII; Linehan, Comtois, Brown, Heard, & Wagner, 2006) is a structured interview that is essentially a functional analysis reformulated as a series of questions about the method, precipitants, consequences, and functions of self-injury. The Lifetime Suicide Attempt Self-Injury Count (L-SASI; Comtois & Linehan, 1999; Linehan & Comtois, 1996), a briefer version of the SASII, examines the range of suicidal behavior over a lifetime (or a recent time period) using the SASII rating scales. The L-SASI is an efficient initial assessment that can be completed in three to twenty minutes (depending on the number of suicidal behaviors). It begins with a few questions about the first, most recent, and most severe self-injuries and then efficiently gathers a total count of suicide attempts and NSSI by method, lethality, and medical treatment. A combination of the L-SASI with a full SASII on the most recent and worst suicide attempts provides a comprehensive history of behavior on which to base management decisions.

In addition to gathering history, it is important to observe any patterns of which the client may be unaware. The client's environment may operantly reinforce suicidality, NSSI, or suicide communications. For instance, parents may have a large reaction and/or provide needed help when their adolescent harms herself, but when the adolescent is not self-harming the parents may orient their attention elsewhere. They may overlook or even punish attempts to ask for help and fail to attend to their adolescent until suicidal communications or actions occur. Thus, there is limited reinforcement for adaptive behavior, punishment for normative expressions of pain and requests for help, and reinforcement of suicidal behaviors. Another example is a client who functions at a high level until he feels overwhelmed and then attempts suicide. The spouse was likely unaware of the ways in which her husband felt himself a burden or needed assistance (as is often the case in situations like this) until after the suicidal behavior occurred. Attempts to then provide support or to remove overwhelming tasks are inadvertently timed with suicidal behavior, so they reinforce it in the future. These patterns generally develop without the conscious intent of the client or others—a fact that needs to be clear to the client and others. However, to prevent suicide it is equally critical that these contingencies are not ignored or missed, but rather that they are understood and changed.

## Suicide Risk Decision Making

Once the risk and protective factors are known, the next step is to determine the level of risk and the immediate treatment response. Clear empirical support suggests that outpatient psychosocial treatments are the most efficacious at reducing suicide ideation, attempts, and deaths (Brown & Green, 2014; Comtois & Linehan, 2006; Hawton et al., 2000). Rigorous studies have not been conducted comparing inpatient with outpatient mental health treatment. Only a single randomized controlled study of inpatient hospitalization has been conducted (Waterhouse & Platt, 1990), and it did not find a difference in subsequent suicide attempts. However, the study was flawed in that only those at low risk of suicide were included and the inpatient intervention was minimal. Thus, there is little empirical evidence on which to base clinical decision making regarding hospitalization. Predicting individual risk is essentially impossible given the low base rate of suicide attempts and suicide.

Evidence-based treatments for suicidality recommend basing clinical decision making regarding suicide risk on not only epidemiological risk and protective factors but also the controlling variables for the individual's suicide risk and his or her commitment to an outpatient treatment plan. Those at high and imminent risk of suicide who are willing and able to take action to reduce their immediate risk in the short term may be managed in an outpatient setting, whereas individuals at lower risk but who are uninterested in or unable to engage in outpatient treatment may require referral to emergency or inpatient services. Knowledge of the controlling variables for suicidal behavior is therefore key to decision making. For each controlling variable, it is critical to evaluate the individual's capacity and motivation for change. If individuals are capable of changing the controlling variable themselves or with the help of family, other support, or social services, then outpatient treatment is more feasible. This ability to change controlling variables is why the teaching of skills and coping strategies is central to behavioral psychotherapies that work with suicidal individuals. However, capability without the motivation to change is of limited value. Based on the assessment of an individual's capability and commitment to change and sense of what constitutes a life worth living, the clinician and client can determine what the initial treatment response should be.

There is no formula that can tell a clinician whether a particular client will make a suicide attempt if treated in an outpatient setting. This is a matter of clinical judgment that is based on the best-quality assessment possible. Therapists benefit most from making these decisions in consultation with a clinical team or, at a minimum, a colleague familiar with the client. What clinicians, family, and friends need most when a client commits suicide is the conviction that the clinicians working with the client did all they could (for management guidance for this situation, see Sung, 2016). The clinician best achieves this conviction by consulting with others when making decisions, laying out the controlling variables and assessment of the client's ability and commitment to change so others can offer their perspective, asking further assessment questions, and concuring with or helping edit the treatment plan. This thinking is then documented in the medical record. The risk of negligence (i.e., the basis of legal action against the therapist) is reduced when the decision-making process is clear and multiple clinicians concur on the plan, both of which increase the confidence of all concerned and buffer the self-doubt and/or blame that can follow a suicide.

It may seem that going through the effort to have a plan thoroughly evaluated will prevent its development, but the opposite is the case. Behavioral principles apply to the clinician as much as the client, and the future review of the clinical record, let alone suicide attempt or death by suicide, is too rare of an event to function directly as a consequence. A sense of relief or reassurance can be a powerful reinforcer, but a plan will function as a reinforcer only if it has been thoroughly evaluated and confirmed by those who might review it—such as the malpractice insurer, attorney, risk management office of a particular agency, organizational leadership, suicide prevention expert, and so forth—in the case of a negative outcome. Taking the time to develop the plan and paperwork and have them reviewed and endorsed by the relevant players can go a long way toward offering the clinician reassurance and relief, which increases the likelihood that this consultation and paperwork will be done for all subsequent clients. If the plan survives a negative outcome, and the result is what the plan is designed for and is not traumatizing for the clinician, the relief the clinician will feel for having followed the plan also increases.

Simultaneously, the aversiveness of completing extra paperwork must be addressed. If guidelines or a plan are put in place that are burdensome, especially for a rare outcome like suicidal behavior, the clinician will inevitably be reinforced for avoiding or minimizing it. Developing templates—either paper forms or those maintained in electronic health records—is a strategy that can improve the quality of documentation and the likelihood that a clinician will complete it correctly. Examples include the Suicide Status Form (Jobes, 2006; Jobes, Kahn-Greene, Greene, & Goeke-Morey, 2009), the Linehan Suicide Safety Net (Linehan et al., 2012; Linehan Institute, Behavioral Tech, n.d.), therapeutic risk management (Homaifar, Matarazzo, & Wortzel, 2013; Wortzel, Matarazzo, & Homaifar, 2013), and the Department of Veterans Affairs' electronic health record templates for suicide risk assessment and safety plans. Templates have a number of advantages. For example, they contain prompts for all key content areas (e.g., suicide risk or protective factors), so the clinician does not need to be concerned about missing important components. Furthermore, many items involved in suicide decision making are fairly standard and lend themselves to templates, allowing clinicians to select from prepared text options (e.g., "Conducted assessment of risk and protective factors," "Completed safety plan with client," etc.) or combinations of prepared text and fields for open text (e.g., "Considered both hospitalization and continuing the outpatient treatment plan and decided not to hospitalize because..." or "Risk and protective factors remain the same as at the last assessment except..."). These options spare clinicians from substantial typing while also conveying a lot of information.

## Safety or Crisis Response Planning

Making a public commitment to life can be therapeutic (Rudd, Mandrusiak, & Joiner Jr., 2006), and clients can do this without having to make a contractual promise not to harm themselves. A safety or crisis response plan is a more effective and useful method. These plans include two components: what the individuals can do themselves and how to effectively reach out for help. For example, in the safety plan developed by Greg Brown, Barbara Stanley, and colleagues (Kayman, Goldstein, Dixon, & Goodman, 2015; B. Stanley et al., 2015), the clinician and client identify (a) warning signs that suicidality may reappear so action can be taken at the earliest point, (b) coping strategies the individual can use, and (c) people and places the client can utilize for distraction until the suicidal moment passes. These strategies are designed to promote action on the part of clients and teach them how to self-manage their suicidality. The safety plan also includes social support the client can call on for help, including professional help.

For several reasons clinicians should strongly consider having suicidal individuals use crisis lines instead of the emergency room (ER). First, unless the ER has a psychiatric emergency service or mental health expert on call, its medical/surgical staff has less suicide prevention expertise than mental health clinicians and may have little to offer beyond temporarily securing the patient. A combination of volunteers and supervisors staff crisis lines, and assessing and responding to suicidal risk is their area of expertise. Crisis lines affiliated with the National Suicide Prevention Lifeline, funded by the Substance Abuse and Mental Health Services Administration, have specific standards and regular evaluations to ensure they use evidence-based suicide care (e.g., Gould et al., 2016; Gould, Munfakh, Kleinman, & Lake, 2012; Joiner et al., 2007). Second, a visit to the ER is both time consuming and expensive for the client and often involves coercive means, such as physical or chemical restraint, that may be distressing or traumatic. A crisis line is free and results in immediate help without coercive means. The crisis line has relationships with police and emergency services, so if its risk assessment indicates an immediate rescue is needed—voluntary or involuntary—it can ensure this is done swiftly and efficiently. Third, referring clients to the ER can have iatrogenic consequences. For example, the client may think the referral means the therapist is unable to help her, or the client may even view it as abandonment. Unless the therapist is indeed unable to help, referral to the ER should be avoided.

Crisis lines can also provide ongoing support to clients that supplements the therapist's availability. This support reduces the amount of time the therapist must spend working with an acutely suicidal client, as well as the emotional demands, freeing up time and emotional energy for psychotherapy sessions and for out-of-session contact the therapist provides within his or her personal and professional limits. This, in turn, helps the therapist stay with a client who becomes suicidal until the suicidality can be treated and resolved. Thus, an intervention such as a crisis line that provides additional support to suicidal individuals and allows them to remain with their therapist is ideal.

## Means Safety

A safety plan also includes a strategy for means safety, formerly termed means restriction, which has been abandoned due to its negative, counterproductive connotation (Anglemyer, Horvath, & Rutherford, 2014; I. H. Stanley, Hom, Rogers, Anestis, & Joiner, 2016; Yip et al., 2012). In outpatient psychosocial treatment, it is critically important for clients to make their environment free of the means for them to impulsively take their life. There are several guidelines for means safety that clinicians can consult to facilitate this discussion with clients (Harvard T. H. Chan School of Public Health, n.d.; Suicide Prevention Resource Center, n.d.). Removing access to lethal means is the ideal scenario. However, when the client is unwilling or reluctant to do so, the clinician faces the dilemma of whether to move assertively to reduce the client's access to means and risk losing access to the client (e.g., the client leaves treatment or lies to the clinician).

As with suicide decision making in general, there is no rule to follow when making decisions about means safety. Again, the most effective strategy is to find consensus with other clinicians, who consider alternatives and agree that the therapist's strategy is the most effective given the limitations of the situation. The clinician should collaborate with the client in session to make an initial decision. Except in rare cases of imminent risk, there is ample opportunity in the hours and days following the session to consult with other clinicians and, if it's recommended, change the plan either by calling the client or as part of a subsequent session. Whatever decisions are made, the decision making and who is consulted should be clear in the medical record. In the case of a tragic outcome, the ability to review documentation that shows the thinking and information available at the time is critical, both for the therapist—in order to feel reassured about his work with the client—and others reviewing the records.

# Treating Suicidality

There are two primary behavioral interventions for suicidal behavior with replicated randomized trials: DBT (Linehan, 1993; Linehan, Comtois, Murray et al., 2006; Stoffers et al., 2012) and cognitive behavioral therapy (CBT) for suicide

421

prevention (Brown et al., 2005; Rudd et al., 2015; Wenzel, Brown, & Beck, 2009). Both interventions have several common areas that clinicians can bring to their work: a focus on suicide rather than diagnosis; a focus on active engagement and retention in treatment; a functional assessment of the precipitants and controlling variables of suicidal behavior; problem solving; an active and directive stance toward helping clients develop alternative ways of thinking and behaving during periods of acute emotional distress instead of engaging in suicidal behavior; and generating hope for the future.

The first commonality is a focus on suicide as the primary target of treatment. This means that while depression, substance use, or other diagnoses are addressed in treatment, suicidality is not considered a symptom or a complication of the diagnosis that will necessarily be resolved as the diagnostic condition improves. Instead, it is considered not only an independent issue but a primary issue of treatment that remains the focus until it resolves.

Making treatment about preventing suicide and resolving a client's desire to die requires the client to be engaged and committed to this target as well. Engaging the client is therefore also a focus. Both DBT and CBT have explicit strategies for engaging the client in treatment, preventing dropout, and troubleshooting and overcoming barriers to care. The DBT framework prioritizes clients taking action for themselves, whereas CBT includes an active case-management arm; however, both anticipate clients having problems attending treatment and view the responsibility to remain in treatment as shared between therapist and client. DBT also includes well-defined, active commitment strategies for linking treatment to the client's goals as well as to preventing suicide. CBT enhances commitment by providing clients the opportunity to share their suicide narrative, with active validation from the therapist, as well as through psychoeducation.

A core element of behavioral interventions for suicide prevention is a functional assessment of suicidal thinking and behavior to determine the controlling variables, as discussed in detail above. The goal is to have an idiographic understanding that will lead to idiographic solutions. Once problems are identified, problem solving is a prominent therapy strategy to resolve controlling variables that are solvable. Simultaneously, the therapist teaches strategies for tolerating what cannot be solved or for coping until problems are solved. The goal is to collaborate with clients to find the most effective solutions for the problems that drive suicidal thinking and to get them to practice those solutions—even when emotions are high and perspective is limited, as is the case in moments of suicide risk.

Finally, a critical aspect of therapy for suicide prevention is creating a vision of and hope for the future. This will guide the person toward a life worth living instead of suicide and will obviate the need for suicidal coping. A central tenet of

DBT treatment is to achieve a life worth living and of sufficient quality so that suicide is no longer an issue. In this way, DBT is a longer treatment. Suicidal coping is generally replaced by skillful coping in the first one to four months of DBT, which is typical of CBT and other behavioral interventions. The rest of therapy (six months, one year, or longer) focuses on resolving quality of life–interfering behaviors that prevent the client from achieving a life worth living. Therapy-interfering behavior—which is addressed early on and throughout treatment to increase a client's skillful engagement in therapy and prevent dropout— falls between the primary target of suicidal and crisis behavior and the target of quality of life.

By contrast, CBT approaches to suicidality are much briefer—sixteen sessions or fewer—with a focus on resolving the suicidal coping and preventing relapse. Clients can pursue further therapy elsewhere for general quality of life. Thus, in these shorter therapies, the focus is on hope rather than achieving a life worth living. A key strategy in CBT is the "hope kit," a box or other container that holds items and mementos, such as photographs and letters, that serve as reminders of reasons to live. The hope kit serves as a powerful and personal reminder of a client's connection to life that can be used when suicidal feelings arise. Clients often find the process of constructing a hope kit very rewarding, as it leads them to discover or rediscover reasons to live.

# References

Anglemyer, A., Horvath, T., & Rutherford, G. (2014). The accessibility of firearms and risk for suicide and homicide victimization among household members: A systematic review and meta-analysis. *Annals of Internal Medicine, 160*(2), 101–110.

Beck, A. T., Brown, G. K., & Steer, R. A. (1997). Psychometric characteristics of the Scale for Suicide Ideation with psychiatric outpatients. *Behaviour Research and Therapy, 35*(11), 1039–1046.

Beck, A. T., Brown, G. K., Steer, R. A., Dahlsgaard, K. K., & Grisham, J. R. (1999). Suicide ideation at its worst point: A predictor of eventual suicide in psychiatric outpatients. *Suicide and Life-Threatening Behavior, 29*(1), 1–9.

Beck, A. T., Kovacs, M., & Weissman, A. (1979). Assessment of suicidal intention: The Scale for Suicide Ideation. *Journal of Consulting and Clinical Psychology, 47*(2), 343–352.

Brown, G. K., & Green, K. L. (2014). A review of evidence-based follow-up care for suicide prevention: Where do we go from here? *American Journal of Preventive Medicine, 47*(3, Supplement 2), S209–S215.

Brown, G. K., Ten Have, T., Henriques, G. R., Xie, S. X., Hollander, J. E., & Beck, A. T. (2005). Cognitive therapy for the prevention of suicide attempts: A randomized controlled trial. *JAMA, 294*(5), 563–570.

Comtois, K. A., & Linehan, M. M. (1999). *Lifetime parasuicide count: Description and psychometrics.* Paper presented at the 9th Annual Conference of the American Association of Suicidology, Houston, TX.

Comtois, K. A., & Linehan, M. M. (2006). Psychosocial treatments of suicidal behaviors: A practice-friendly review. *Journal of Clinical Psychology, 62*(2), 161–170.

Gould, M. S., Lake, A. M., Munfakh, J. L., Galfalvy, H., Kleinman, M., Williams, C., et al. (2016). Helping callers to the National Suicide Prevention Lifeline who are at imminent risk of suicide: Evaluation of caller risk profiles and interventions implemented. *Suicide and Life-Threatening Behavior, 46*(2), 172–190.

Gould, M. S., Munfakh, J. L. H., Kleinman, M., & Lake, A. M. (2012). National Suicide Prevention Lifeline: Enhancing mental health care for suicidal individuals and other people in crisis. *Suicide and Life-Threatening Behavior, 42*(1), 22–35.

Harvard T. H. Chan School of Public Health. (n.d.). Lethal means counseling. https://www.hsph.harvard.edu/means-matter/lethal-means-counseling/.

Hawton, K., Townsend, E., Arensman, E., Gunnell, D., Hazell, P., House, A., et al. (2000). Psychosocial versus pharmacological treatments for deliberate self harm. *Cochrane Database of Systematic Reviews, 2*(CD001764).

Homaifar, B., Matarazzo, B., & Wortzel, H. S. (2013). Therapeutic risk management of the suicidal patient: Augmenting clinical suicide risk assessment with structured instruments. *Journal of Psychiatric Practice, 19*(5), 406–409.

Jobes, D. A. (2006). *Managing suicidal risk: A collaborative approach.* New York: Guilford Press.

Jobes, D. A., Kahn-Greene, E., Greene, J. A., & Goeke-Morey, M. (2009). Clinical improvements of suicidal outpatients: Examining Suicide Status Form responses as predictors and moderators. *Archives of Suicide Research, 13*(2), 147–159.

Joiner, T., Kalafat, J., Draper, J., Stokes, H., Knudson, M., Berman, A. L., et al. (2007). Establishing standards for the assessment of suicide risk among callers to the National Suicide Prevention Lifeline. *Suicide and Life-Threatening Behavior, 37*(3), 353–365.

Kayman, D. J., Goldstein, M. F., Dixon, L., & Goodman, M. (2015). Perspectives of suicidal veterans on safety planning: Findings from a pilot study. *Crisis: The Journal of Crisis Intervention and Suicide Prevention, 36*(5), 371–383.

Linehan, M. M. (1993). *Cognitive behavioral treatment of borderline personality disorder.* New York: Guilford Press.

Linehan, M. M. (2014). Linehan Risk Assessment and Management Protocol (LRAMP). Seattle: Behavioral Research and Therapy Clinics. Retrieved from http://blogs.uw.edu/brtc/files/2014/01/SSN-LRAMP-updated-9–19_2013.pdf.

Linehan, M. M. (2015a). *DBT skills training handouts and worksheets* (2nd ed.). New York: Guilford Press.

Linehan, M. M. (2015b). *DBT skills training manual* (2nd ed.). New York: Guilford Press.

Linehan, M. M., & Comtois, K. A. (1996). Lifetime Suicide Attempt and Self-Injury Count (L-SASI). (Formerly Lifetime Parasuicide History, SASI-Count). Seattle: University of Washington. Retrieved from http://depts.washington.edu/uwbrtc/resources/assessment-instruments/.

Linehan, M. M., Comtois, K. A., Brown, M. Z., Heard, H. L., & Wagner, A. (2006). Suicide Attempt Self-Injury Interview (SASII): Development, reliability, and validity of a scale to assess suicide attempts and intentional self-injury. *Psychological Assessment, 18*(3), 303–312.

Linehan, M. M., Comtois, K. A., Murray, A. M., Brown, M. Z., Gallop, R. J., Heard, H. L., et al. (2006). Two-year randomized controlled trial and follow-up of dialectical behavior therapy vs. therapy by experts for suicidal behaviors and borderline personality disorder. *Archives of General Psychiatry, 63*(7), 757–766.

Linehan, M. M., Comtois, K. A., & Ward-Ciesielski, E. F. (2012). Assessing and managing risk with suicidal individuals. *Cognitive and Behavioral Practice, 19*(2), 218–232.

Linehan Institute, Behavioral Tech (n.d.). Linehan Suicide Safety Net. Retrieved from http://behavioraltech.org/products/lssn.cfm.

Rudd, M. D., Bryan, C. J., Wertenberger, E. G., Peterson, A. L., Young-McCaughan, S., Mintz, J., et al. (2015). Brief cognitive-behavioral therapy effects on post-treatment suicide attempts in a military sample: Results of a randomized clinical trial with 2-year follow-up. *American Journal of Psychiatry, 172*(5), 441–449.

Rudd, M. D., Mandrusiak, M., & Joiner Jr., T. E. (2006). The case against no-suicide contracts: The commitment to treatment statement as a practice alternative. *Journal of Clinical Psychology, 62*(2), 243–251.

Stanley, B., Brown, G. K., Currier, G. W., Lyons, C., Chesin, M., & Knox, K. L. (2015). Brief intervention and follow-up for suicidal patients with repeat emergency department visits enhances treatment engagement. *American Journal of Public Health, 105*(8), 1570–1572.

Stanley, I. H., Hom, M. A., Rogers, M. L., Anestis, M. D., & Joiner, T. E. (2016). Discussing firearm ownership and access as part of suicide risk assessment and prevention: "Means safety" versus "means restriction." *Archives of Suicide Research, 13*, 1–17.

Stoffers, J. M., Völlm, B. A., Rücker, G., Timmer, A., Huband, N., & Lieb, K. (2012). Psychological therapies for people with borderline personality disorder. *Cochrane Database of Systematic Reviews, 8*(CD005652).

Suicide Prevention Resource Center. (n.d.). CALM: Counseling on Access to Lethal Means. http://www.sprc.org/resources-programs/calm-counseling-access-lethal-means.

Sung, J. C. (2016). Sample individual practitioner practices for responding to client suicide. March 21. http://www.intheforefront.org/sites/default/files/Sample%20Individual%20Practices%20-%20SPRC%20BPR%20-%20March%202016.pdf.

Waterhouse, J., & Platt, S. (1990). General hospital admission in the management of parasuicide: A randomised controlled trial. *British Journal of Psychiatry, 156*(2), 236–242.

Wenzel, A., Brown, G. K., & Beck, A. T. (2009). *Cognitive therapy for suicidal patients: Scientific and clinical applications.* Washington, DC: American Psychological Association.

Wortzel, H. S., Matarazzo, B., & Homaifar, B. (2013). A model for therapeutic risk management of the suicidal patient. *Journal of Psychiatric Practice, 19*(4), 323–326.

Yip, P. S., Caine, E., Yousuf, S., Chang, S.-S., Wu, K. C.-C., & Chen, Y.-Y. (2012). Means restriction for suicide prevention. *Lancet, 379*(9834), 2393–2399.

425

# CHAPTER 29

# Future Directions in CBT and Evidence-Based Therapy

Steven C. Hayes, PhD

*Department of Psychology, University of Nevada, Reno*

Stefan G. Hofmann, PhD

*Department of Psychological and Brain Sciences,
Boston University*

In the early days of the behavior therapy movement, the late Gordon Paul, then just a few years past his PhD, wrote one of the most quoted questions about the proper goal of a science of evidence-based interventions (1969, p. 44): "What treatment, by whom, is most effective for this individual with that specific problem, under which set of circumstances, and how does it come about?" We included this quote in chapter 1 because it opened the door to a scientific approach to therapeutic intervention that links contextually specific evidence-based procedures to evidence-based processes that solve the problems and promote the prosperity of particular people. This approach did not quite go far enough, however, because in the early days of behavior therapy there was far too much trust that learning principles and theories was an adequate basis for clinical procedures. Indeed, that may explain why two years earlier Paul (1967) hadn't included the phrase "and how does it come about" in the original formulation of this question, instead focusing entirely on contextually specific evidence-based procedures. Processes of change were an afterthought.

A truly process-based approach gives high priority to evidence-based processes and to evidence-based procedures as they are linked to these processes. At this point in the volume, we are finally in a position to put a fine point on the foundational question the field of clinical change needs to focus on in order to make a priority choice. The central question in modern psychotherapy and intervention science now is "What core biopsychosocial processes should be targeted with this client given this goal in this situation, and how can they most efficiently and effectively be changed?" Answering these questions is the goal of any form of *process-based empirical therapy*, but we argue that it is now, most especially, becoming the goal of processes-based cognitive behavioral therapy (CBT).

Relieving human suffering is a challenging goal in every way. It requires powerful conceptual tools that will parse human complexity into a manageable number of issues. It requires clinical creativity that will lead to the successful targeting of key domains and dimensions of human functioning. It depends on methodological tools that permit the development of generalizable knowledge from detailed experience with myriad individuals.

In the early days, learning principles and an artful approach to functional analysis were the bulk of what was available to take this approach, and they simply were not enough. The principles and procedures were too limited, and linking principles and procedures with individuals—a task in itself—needed more bolstering from science. In the decades that followed, the behavioral movement expanded its conceptual and procedural armamentarium, becoming CBT as a result. That was a step forward, although as we explored in section 2 of this book, the field is still learning how best to develop and use a more catholic set of principles and to organize them into pragmatically useful forms; and, as we showed in section 3, many modern procedures are only now coming into their own, scientifically speaking.

Government agencies also wanted to see the development of evidence-based therapy (EBT), but they had their own ideas about how to do so, driven largely by ideas from the psychiatric establishment. After the third version of the American Psychiatric Association's *Diagnostic and Statistical Manual of Mental Disorders* was developed in 1980, the US National Institute of Mental Health (NIMH) decided to pour resources into funding randomized trials of specific protocols targeting psychiatric syndromes. This combination had an enormous impact on the field of CBT, and on EBT more generally, bringing prestige and attention to psychotherapy developers but also inadvertently narrowing their vision.

In the grand arc of history, these developments did a lot of good for the field. The study of protocols for syndromes captured *some* of the essence of Paul's agenda, and there was an enormous increase in the amount of data available about psychotherapy and other psychosocial interventions, the impact of psychiatric medications, the development of psychopathology, and other key issues. Among other things, the concerns raised by Eysenck (1952) about whether evidence-based psychotherapy could be shown to be better than doing nothing at all were answered once and for all. CBT was a prime beneficiary of this growth of evidence, leading to its current position as the best-supported intervention approach.

428

The biomedicalization of human suffering that underlay these developments, however, left behind several key features of Paul's clinical question. The new question—"What protocol is best for the symptoms of this syndrome?"—intervention scientists were answering failed to capture adequately the needs of the individual, the context of interventions, the specificity of procedures, the specificity of problems, and the link to processes of change. In other words, protocol- and syndrome-based empirical therapy left behind a number of the defining features of a process-based empirical therapy approach.

The field is still dealing with the practical and intellectual challenges that resulted. Theory suffered as a more purely technological approach blossomed. How important are processes and principles if they are just used as a vague setup for technologies and are not formally tested as moderators and mediators of intervention? The inability to develop robust theories of behavior change should be expected if theory development is merely an untested ritual engaged in before the real action of protocol development linked to syndromes occurs.

As the new research program unfolded in the thirty-year period between 1980 and 2010, it was extremely discouraging, scientifically speaking, that a focus on syndromes never seemed to lead to conclusive evidence on etiology, course, and response to treatment. Said in another way, a syndromes approach never led to the discovery of diseases, which is the ultimate purpose of syndromal classification. Comorbidity and client heterogeneity was so great within syndromal groups that traditional diagnosis felt more like an empty ritual than a vitally important and progressive process. After 2010 the NIMH began withdrawing its interest—in effect, abandoning the very approach it had taken on board as its developmental strategy thirty years earlier, bringing CBT researchers along for the ride. The DSM-5 was released in 2013 with a notable lack of enthusiasm in almost every corner of the field.

CBT has gone through changes as well. In this book we avoided the language of the "third wave" because it can feel offensive to some in the field, and our entire goal is to try to bring the different wings and traditions together under a more process-based approach. Still, it is worth looking beyond reactions to that specific label for the new generation of work that was emerging within CBT (Hayes, 2004); the key features that these developments emphasized are ways to possibly improve understanding and outcomes. An original, italicized statement summarizing third-wave ideas emphasized that what was emerging was an "empirical, principle-focused approach…[that] is particularly sensitive to the context and functions of psychological phenomena…and reformulates and synthesizes previous generations of behavioral and cognitive therapy and carries them forward into questions, issues, and domains previously addressed primarily by other traditions" (Hayes, 2004, p. 658). Stated another way, CBT had arrived at a point where a

429

process-based empirical approach could be used to open up the tradition to the full range of issues that can be examined in EBT.

The present volume attempts to step forward in that way. A process-based approach reflects to some degree the pressures that have led the NIMH to focus on the framework of the Research Domain Criteria Initiative instead of the DSM as a way forward (Insel et al., 2010), but it does so by taking intervention science in a process-based direction. We organized the book around the recent consensus document (Klepac et al., 2012) of the Inter-Organizational Task Force on Cognitive and Behavioral Psychology Doctoral Education, in part, because that document shows how the field at large is developing greater sophistication about what is needed to reorient the field in a post-DSM era.

When theory and processes of change became more central, the task force correctly argued that more training is needed in philosophy of science, scientific strategy, ethics, and the broad range of domains from which principles can arise. More training is needed in linking procedures to principles, and in fitting procedures to the particular needs of the particular case in an ethical and evidence-sensitive manner. We agree with the task force's conclusions, and the chapters in this volume are in part an effort to respond to that challenge. This book is not a comprehensive response—that will take a whole series of volumes, of which this is the first we plan to publish.

At this point in the volume it is worth considering what the future may hold if the field develops a greater empirical linkage between procedures and processes that alleviate problems and promote prosperity in people. Stated another way: What will unfold in an era of process-based empirical therapy? We cannot say for sure, but the broad outlines seem clear enough. In several areas, the chapters in the present volume anticipate some of the changes that appear to lie ahead.

# Likely Future Developments

**The decline of named therapies.** As packages and protocols are broken down into procedures linked to processes, named therapies will become much less dominant. Indeed, the term "cognitive behavioral therapy" has become too narrow because the therapeutic change that occurs is by no means restricted to cognitive and behavioral processes; there are also social, motivational, emotional, epigenetic, neurobiological, evolutionary, and many other evidence-based processes involved. Many of these have been outlined in the chapters of this book.

One could further argue that CBT is not a singular term, but that there are many CBTs, some more evidence based, theory grounded, and process oriented than others. But allowing evidence-based treatment to continue to develop under a mountain of specifically named treatments (e.g., eye movement desensitization and reprocessing, cognitive processing therapy, dialectical behavior therapy, and so on) will keep the field stuck in an era of packages and protocols. Those names that are linked to well-developed and specific theoretical models can be accommodated as names for theoretical models, but in a process-based era there is just no need to name every technological combination and sequence, any more than there is a need to name every architectural design or layout of city roads.

Very few of the chapters in section 3 present methods that would need to be linked to a named therapy in order to be effective. Chapter 3 emphasizes that clinicians often need to move beyond protocols by using case formulation that specifies how evidence-based treatment targets will be linked to robust processes of change. Named protocols will continue to have a role for some time, but as procedures and processes take center stage, most of them will begin to move to the sidelines.

**The decline of general theories and the rise of testable models.** Amorphous systems and general theoretical claims will either fold into more specific and testable models and theories or be recognized as broad philosophical claims. Distinct sets of philosophical assumptions will remain distinct, precisely because assumptions establish the grounds for empirical testing and thus are not fully subject to empirical testing (this issue is covered extensively in chapter 2 on the philosophy of science). This reality does not mean that philosophically distinct approaches cannot coexist and even cooperate. In this volume we argue that cooperation is more likely if differences in assumptions are appreciated. In some ways this very volume is a test of that idea by bringing together methods from the different wings and traditions in CBT.

Testable models and specific theories are highly useful in science, especially if more of an eye is given to their utility. In the era of syndromal protocols, theory was often given short shrift as it bore on intervention. That seems sure to change going forward. Pragmatically useful models and theories will be subjected to great scrutiny on several key dimensions, however, including the next four we are about to mention.

**The rise of mediation and moderation.** Even now, with the handwriting on the wall, agencies and associations that certify evidence-based intervention methods, such as Division 12 (clinical psychology) of the American Psychological Association, have failed to require evidence of processes of change linked to the underlying theoretical model and procedures deployed (Tolin, McKay, Forman, Klonsky, & Thombs, 2015). That cannot continue in a process-based era. Theoretical models that underlay an intervention procedure need to specify the processes of change linked to that procedure for a particular problem. Even if the procedure works well, if the specified process of change cannot be shown to be consistently applicable, the underlying model is wrong. The field can tolerate short delays while measurement issues are worked out, but the task of developing adequate assessment falls on those proposing models and theories, not on those properly demanding evidence for processes of change.

The distinction between a model failure and a procedural failure is important in the other direction as well. For example, if a procedure fails to alter putatively critical processes of change that may have been shown to be important in longitudinal studies of developmental psychopathology, then the model remains untested even if the procedure fails. In this case, the field can tolerate short delays while procedural details are worked out to produce better impact on processes of change in specific areas.

The most important point is that a procedure should be thought of as evidence based only when science supports that procedure, its underlying model, and their linkage. If a procedure reliably produces gains *and* manipulates a process that mediates these gains, *then* it is ready to be admitted into the armamentarium of process-based empirical therapy.

Even then, there is more to do on practical grounds. If moderation is not specified, it still needs to be investigated vigorously because the history of evidence-based methods shows that few processes are always positive regardless of context (e.g., Brockman, Ciarrochi, Parker, & Kashdan, 2016). Thus, in a mature, process-oriented field, evidence of theoretically coherent mediators and moderators will be as important as evidence of procedural benefits. We look forward to the day when meta-analyses of procedural mediation are as common and as important as meta-analyses of procedural impact.

**New forms of diagnosis and functional analysis.** As process-based approaches evolve, core processes that are used in new forms of functional analysis, and person-based applications, will become more central. The rise of statistical models that can delve into individual growth curves and personal cognitive and behavioral networks holds out the hope for a reemergence of the individual in evidence-based approaches. For example, the complex network approach can offer an alternative to the latent disease model. This approach holds that psychological problems are not expressions of underlying disease entities but rather are interrelated elements of a complex network. This approach, which is an extension of functional analysis, not only provides a framework for psychopathology, but it might be used to predict therapeutic change, relapse, and recovery at some point in time (Hofmann, Curtiss, & McNally, 2016).

We need an approach for targeting interventions that is not so much trans-diagnostic (a term with feet placed uncomfortably across a divide that seems likely to widen) as it is an alternative approach to diagnosis. For process-based CBT and EBT to prosper, well-developed alternatives to the DSM that can guide research and practice are needed.

**From nomothetic to idiographic approaches.** Contemporary psychiatric nosology, which views psychiatric problems as expressions of latent disease entities, forces a nomothetic system onto human suffering. Consistent with this approach, in the protocol for syndrome-era CBT, protocol X was developed to treat psychiatric disease X, whereas CBT protocol Y was developed to treat disease Y, while all but ignoring any differences among individuals.

However, in order to answer Paul's (1969) clinical question, a purely top-down, nomothetic approach will not be useful. This question requires a bottom-up idiographic approach in order to understand why in a particular case a psychological problem is maintained and how the change process can be initiated. Nomothetic principles are key, but their basis and their application need to include the intense analysis of the individual. Often qualitative research will inform these developments. Psychologists are already well equipped with many of the methodological tools to deal with these issues, ranging from single-case experimental designs (Hayes, Barlow, & Nelson-Gray, 1999) to ecological momentary assessments, and the use of these methodological tools will likely increase, especially as they are linked to modern statistical methods, as we noted with the immediately preceding trend.

**Processes need to specify modifiable elements.** The practical needs of practitioners present the field with a natural analytic agenda. This is one reason that different philosophies of science (see chapter 2) can more readily coexist within CBT than in many other areas of science: contextualists may view pragmatic outcomes as truth criteria in and of themselves, whereas elemental realists may view them as the natural outgrowth of ontological knowledge, but both can agree on the practical importance of the outcomes for intervention work. One implication is that processes that are clearly modifiable, and theories and models that specify contextual elements that can be used to modify processes of change, are inherently advantaged in a process-based approach to empirical therapy. Cognitions, emotions, and behavior are all the dependent variables of intervention science. Awareness of that simple fact adds the next key feature.

**The importance of context.** If a dependent variable is going to change in psychology, ultimately it needs to be done by changing history or situational circumstance. Said in another way, context needs to change. That is exactly what a therapeutic technique does.

Intervention scientists are far better at measuring the emotional, cognitive, or behavioral responses of people than they are at measuring the historical, social, and situational context. That is understandable, but the latter needs continuing attention in a process-based approach.

This truism about measuring suggests that theories and models that specify the relationship of processes of change to methods of manipulating these processes should be advantaged over theories and models that leave off this key step. Identifying this relationship is a demanding criterion that few current models and theories meet. It is easier to develop models of change that are not specifically tied to intervention components.

To some degree process-based therapy can solve this problem empirically: trial and error can determine which components move which change processes. In the long run, however, we need to know *why* certain methods move certain processes, not just that they do. Theories that explain the link between evidence-based processes and evidence-based procedures and components will thus become more important as a process-based empirical approach matures.

**Component analyses and the reemergence of laboratory-based studies.** The considerations we have touched on are part of why carefully crafted component studies have had a reemergence in CBT. It is possible to drill down in a very fine-grained way to specific process-based questions with clinical populations in the laboratory, but doing so in randomized controlled trials of packages and protocols would be harder to do (e.g., Campbell-Sills, Barlow, Brown, & Hofmann, 2006). It is unwise to allow packages to exist for many years before they are dismantled, but in a more process-based era, information about component processes can be built from the bottom up, allowing even a meta-analysis of scores of component studies to inform clinical work (Levin, Hildebrandt, Lillis, & Hayes, 2012).

**Integration of behavioral and psychological science with the other life sciences.** Behavioral and psychological science does not and cannot live in a world unto itself: behavior is part of the life sciences more generally. The enormous increase in attention to the neurosciences in modern intervention science reflects this more holistic and biologically friendly zeitgeist—in the modern era we want to know how psychological events change us as organisms and vice versa. There are other shoes still to fall, however, that are part of this same zeitgeist. We know, for example, that epigenetic processes impact the organization of the brain (Mitchell, Jiang, Peter, Goosens, & Akbarian, 2013), but they are themselves affected by experiences that are protective in mental health areas (e.g., Dusek et al., 2008; Uddin & Sipahi, 2013). Some of this is covered in chapter 10, on evolution science.

An interest in biology does not need to be reductionistic. History and context are as important to an evolutionary biologist as they are to a psychotherapist; this is one reason why we included a chapter on evolution science in this volume. Every level of analysis has its own place in a unified fabric of science. In the modern era, however, it's likely that intervention scientists will be increasingly called upon to be broadly trained in the life sciences and to be knowledgeable about developments in them.

**New forms of delivery of care.** As chapter 4 on the changing role of practice shows, the world of apps, websites, telemedicine, and phone-based intervention is upon us. For decades psychotherapy trainers have worried that there will never be enough psychotherapists to go around given the enormous human need for psychological care. That sense of overwhelming need only increases when we think of global mental health needs, or when we realize that therapy methods are relevant to social problems (e.g., prejudice) or to human prosperity (e.g., positive psychology and quality of life).

Fortunately, there is no reason to think of psychotherapy as being limited to a fifty-minute, one-on-one, face-to-face intervention. Human beings can change because they read a book (Jeffcoat & Hayes, 2012), use an app on their smartphone (Bricker et al., 2014), or receive a short follow-up call from a nurse (Hawkes et al., 2013). A process-based approach is able to encompass these methods because of the relatively controlled research strategies that can document and study process changes as these methods are used, and because of the branching, interactive, and dynamic possibilities that many forms of technological intervention permit.

**A science of the therapeutic relationship.** As discussed in chapter 3, the therapeutic relationship and other common core processes themselves require an analysis. It is not enough to know that general therapy features predict outcome; common core processes need to be manipulated and shown to matter *experimentally*. As we mentioned in the book's introduction, evidence-based intervention methods are having an impact on our understanding of the therapeutic relationship itself (Hofmann & Barlow, 2014). For example, it has been shown empirically that psychological flexibility can account for the impact of acceptance and commitment therapy, but it can also help account for the impact of the therapeutic alliance (e.g., Gifford et al., 2011).

**Using the clinic as a source of data.** CBT research began in the clinic. A process-based empirical approach seems likely to empower practitioners to stay involved in knowledge generation, especially as more individually focused analytic methods continue to emerge. Diversity matters in a process-focused approach, and front-line practitioners see a more diverse group of clients than do academic medical centers in large urban areas.

**Using the world community as a source of data.** Only a few countries on the planet can afford the kind of grant infrastructure that funds large, well-controlled outcome studies. All are in the West, and all are dominantly white. Yet at the same time, the world is awakening to the enormous health needs around the globe, including mental and behavioral health needs.

It is important to examine whether processes of change in EBT are culture bound—in the main, the answer so far appears to be reassuring (e.g., Monestès et al., 2016). Process-based empirical therapy holds out hope that it can better fit itself to the needs of and draw additional information from the world community. For example, if a process mediates outcome and it's culturally valid, clinical creativity can be put to use figuring out how to best move that process in culturally sound and contextually appropriate procedures that are adjusted to fit specific needs.

**The change of CBT as we know it.** Ironically, over time a process-based approach seems likely to shorten the life of CBT as a clearly distinct approach compared with EBT more generally. This will not occur because all evidence-based methods will be shown to emerge from CBT. Rather, as CBT reorients toward issues that were previously the focus only of other therapy traditions, there will be fewer and fewer reasons to distinguish CBT from analytic, existential, humanistic, or systemic work.

There will always be a need for clarity about philosophical assumptions, but many theoretical systems already exist within CBT, and better training in philosophy of science should empower CBT researchers to walk into the lion's den of more diverse theoretical systems without losing balance and bearing. We are not (yet) calling for an end to the use of the term "cognitive behavioral therapy." If the approach contained within this volume is pursued, however, we can see a day when the term will add little to our description of the current field. It is possible that if all the trends discussed in this volume unfold, it will mean the end of CBT as we know it—but this will only be the case if considerable progress is made toward a new and empowering future of a broader and deeper form of EBT.

We are not sure if all these trends will unfold, nor if they will do so anytime soon. Many of them are already under way, however, so there can be no doubt that the world of psychological intervention is going to change. In the main, we believe that these trends are positive, and a more process-focused approach will help today's students push out the boundaries of tomorrow's consensus. The goal is not upheaval; the goal is progress. People are in need and are seeking answers from our field. It is up to us to provide for them. We hope this volume offers not just a snapshot of where we are today but also shines a beacon toward a place where we can go.

# References

Bricker, J. B., Mull, K. E., Kientz, J. A., Vilardaga, R. M., Mercer, L. D., Akioka, K. J., et al. (2014). Randomized, controlled pilot trial of a smartphone app for smoking cessation using acceptance and commitment therapy. *Drug and Alcohol Dependence, 143*, 87–94.

Brockman, R., Ciarrochi, J., Parker, P., & Kashdan, T. (2016). Emotion regulation strategies in daily life: Mindfulness, cognitive reappraisal and emotion suppression. *Cognitive Behaviour Therapy, 46*(2), 91–113.

Campbell-Sills, L., Barlow, D. H., Brown, T.A., & Hofmann, S. G. (2006). Effects of suppression and acceptance on emotional responses of individuals with anxiety and mood disorders. *Behaviour Research and Therapy, 44*(9), 1251–1263.

Dusek, J. A., Otu, H. H., Wohlhueter, A. L., Bhasin, M., Zerbini, L. F., Joseph, M. G., et al. (2008). Genomic counter-stress changes induced by the relaxation response. *PLoS One, 3*(7), e2576.

Eysenck, H. J. (1952). The effects of psychotherapy: An evaluation. *Journal of Consulting Psychology, 16*(5), 319–324.

Gifford, E. V., Kohlenberg, B. S., Hayes, S. C., Pierson, H. M., Piasecki, M. P., Antonuccio, D. O., et al. (2011). Does acceptance and relationship focused behavior therapy contribute to bupropion outcomes? A randomized controlled trial of functional analytic psychotherapy and acceptance and commitment therapy for smoking cessation. *Behavior Therapy, 42*(4), 700–715.

Hawkes, A. L., Chambers, S. K., Pakenham, K. I., Patrao, T. A., Baade, P. D., Lynch, B. M., et al. (2013). Effects of a telephone-delivered multiple health behavior change intervention (CanChange) on health and behavioral outcomes in survivors of colorectal cancer: A randomized controlled trial. *Journal of Clinical Oncology, 31*(18), 2313–2321.

Hayes, S. C. (2004). Acceptance and commitment therapy, relational frame theory, and the third wave of behavioral and cognitive therapies. *Behavior Therapy, 35*(4), 639–665.

Hayes, S. C., Barlow, D. H., & Nelson-Gray, R. O. (1999). *The scientist practitioner: Research and accountability in the age of managed care* (2nd ed.). New York: Allyn and Bacon.

Hofmann, S. G., & Barlow, D. H. (2014). Evidence-based psychological interventions and the common factors approach: The beginnings of a rapprochement? *Psychotherapy, 51*(4), 510–513.

Hofmann, S. G., Curtiss, J., & McNally, R. J. (2016). A complex network perspective on clinical science. *Perspectives on Psychological Science, 11*(5), 597–605.

Insel, T., Cuthbert, B., Garvey, M., Heinssen, R., Pine, D. S., Quinn, K., et al. (2010). Research Domain Criteria (RDoC): Toward a new classification framework for research on mental disorders. *American Journal of Psychiatry, 167*(7), 748–751.

Jeffcoat, T., & Hayes, S. C. (2012). A randomized trial of ACT bibliotherapy on the mental health of K-12 teachers and staff. *Behaviour Research and Therapy, 50*(9), 571–579.

Klepac, R. K., Ronan, G. F., Andrasik, F., Arnold, K. D., Belar, C. D., Berry, S. L., et al. (2012). Guidelines for cognitive behavioral training within doctoral psychology programs in the

United States: Report of the Inter-Organizational Task Force on Cognitive and Behavioral Psychology Doctoral Education. *Behavior Therapy, 43*(4), 687–697.

Levin, M. E., Hildebrandt, M. J., Lillis, J., & Hayes, S. C. (2012). The impact of treatment components suggested by the psychological flexibility model: A meta-analysis of laboratory-based component studies. *Behavior Therapy, 43*(4), 741–756.

Mitchell, A. C., Jiang, Y., Peter, C. J., Goosens, K., & Akbarian, S. (2013). The brain and its epigenome. In D. S. Charney, P. Sklar, J. D. Buxbaum, & E. J. Nestler (Eds.), *Neurobiology of mental illness* (4th ed., pp. 172–182). Oxford: Oxford University Press.

Monestès, J.-L., Karekla, M., Jacobs, N., Michaelides, M., Hooper, N., Kleen, M., et al. (2016). Experiential avoidance as a common psychological process in European cultures. *European Journal of Psychological Assessment.* DOI: 10.1027/1015-5759/a000327.

Paul, G. L. (1967). Strategy of outcome research in psychotherapy. *Journal of Consulting Psychology, 31*(2), 109–118.

Paul, G. L. (1969). Behavior modification research: Design and tactics. In C. M. Franks (Ed.), *Behavior therapy: Appraisal and status* (pp. 29–62). New York: McGraw-Hill.

Tolin, D. F., McKay, D., Forman, E. M., Klonsky, E. D., & Thombs, B. D. (2015). Empirically supported treatment: Recommendations for a new model. *Clinical Psychology: Science and Practice, 22*(4), 317–338.

Uddin, M., & Sipahi, L. (2013). Epigenetic influence on mental illnesses over the life course. In K. C. Koenen, S. Rudenstine, E. S. Susser, & S. Galea (Eds.), *A life course approach to mental disorders* (pp. 240–248). Oxford: Oxford University Press.

**Steven C. Hayes, PhD**, is Foundation Professor in the department of psychology at the University of Nevada, Reno. An author of forty-four books and over 600 scientific articles, his career has focused on an analysis of the nature of human language and cognition, and the application of this to the understanding and alleviation of human suffering and the promotion of human prosperity. Among other associations, Hayes has been president of the Association for Behavioral and Cognitive Therapies (ABCT), and the Association for Contextual Behavioral Science. He has received several awards, including the Impact of Science on Application Award from the Society for the Advancement of Behavior Analysis, and the Lifetime Achievement Award from the ABCT.

**Stefan G. Hofmann, PhD**, is a professor in Boston University's department of psychological and brain sciences clinical program, where he directs the Psychotherapy and Emotion Research Laboratory (PERL). His research focuses on the mechanism of treatment change, translating discoveries from neuroscience into clinical applications, emotions, and cultural expressions of psychopathology. He is past president of the Association for Behavioral and Cognitive Therapies (ABCT), and the International Association for Cognitive Psychotherapy. He is also editor in chief of *Cognitive Therapy and Research*, and is associate editor of *Clinical Psychological Science*. He is author of many books, including *An Introduction to Modern CBT* and *Emotion in Therapy*.

# Index

# B

# C

# MORE BOOKS *from*
# NEW HARBINGER PUBLICATIONS

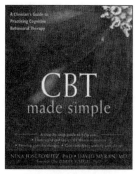
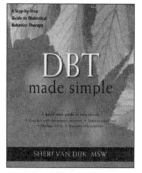
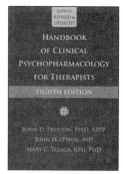
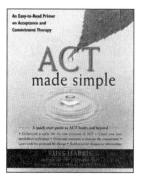
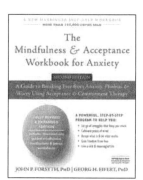
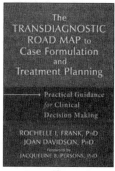

Register your **new harbinger** titles for additional benefits!

When you register your **new harbinger** title—purchased in any format, from any source—you get access to benefits like the following:

- Downloadable accessories like printable worksheets and extra content

- Instructional videos and audio files

- Information about updates, corrections, and new editions

Not every title has accessories, but we're adding new material all the time.

Access free accessories in 3 easy steps:

**1.** Sign in at NewHarbinger.com (or **register** to create an account).

**2.** Click on **register a book**. Search for your title and click the **register** button when it appears.

**3.** Click on the **book cover or title** to go to its details page. Click on **accessories** to view and access files.

That's all there is to it!

If you need help, visit:

NewHarbinger.com/accessories

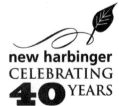

new harbinger
CELEBRATING
**40** YEARS